AIIMS Protocols in
Neonatology

AIIMS Protocols in
Neonatology

Ramesh Agarwal

MD DM (Neonatology)
Additional Professor
Department of Pediatrics
Newborn Health Knowledge Centre
All India Institute of Medical Sciences
New Delhi, India

Ashok Deorari

MD FAMS
Professor
Department of Pediatrics
WHO Collaborating Centre for Education
and Research in Newborn Care
All India Institute of Medical Sciences
New Delhi, India

Vinod K Paul

MD PhD DNB FAMS FIAP FNNF
Professor and Head
Department of Pediatrics
All India Institute of Medical Sciences
New Delhi, India

CBS Publishers & Distributors Pvt Ltd

New Delhi • Bengaluru • Chennai • Kochi • Kolkata • Mumbai
Bhopal • Bhubaneswar • Hyderabad • Jharkhand • Nagpur • Patna • Pune
• Uttarakhand • Dhaka (Bangladesh)

AIIMS Protocols in
Neonatology

ISBN: 978-81-239-2335-2

First Edition: 2015
   Reprint: 2016, 2017, 2019

Published by Satish Kumar Jain and produced by Varun Jain for
CBS Publishers & Distributors Pvt Ltd
4819/XI Prahlad Street, 24 Ansari Road, Daryaganj, New Delhi 110 002, India.
Ph: 23289259, 23266861, 23266867   Website: www.cbspd.com
Fax: 011-23243014   e-mail: delhi@cbspd.com;
                                   cbspubs@airtelmail.in.

Corporate Office: 204 FIE, Industrial Area, Patparganj, Delhi 110 092
Ph: 4934 4934   Fax: 4934 4935   e-mail: publishing@cbspd.com;
                                     publicity@cbspd.com
*   **Bengaluru:** Seema House 2975, 17th Cross, K.R. Road, Banasankari 2nd Stage, Bengaluru 560 070, Karnataka
    Ph: +91-80-26771678/79   Fax: +91-80-26771680   e-mail: bangalore@cbspd.com
*   **Chennai:** 7, Subbaraya Street, Shenoy Nagar, Chennai 600 030, Tamil Nadu
    Ph: +91-44-26680620/26681266   Fax: +91-44-42032115   e-mail: chennai@cbspd.com
*   **Kochi:** 42/1325, 1326, Power House Road, Opp KSEB, Power House, Ernakulam 682 018, Kochi, Kerala
    Ph: +91-484-4059061-65   Fax: +91-484-4059065   e-mail: kochi@cbspd.com
*   **Kolkata:** 6/B, Ground Floor, Rameswar Shaw Road, Kolkata-700 014, West Bengal
    Ph: +91-33-22891126, 22891127, 22891128   e-mail: kolkata@cbspd.com
*   **Mumbai:** 83-C, Dr E Moses Road, Worli, Mumbai-400018, Maharashtra
    Ph: +91-22-24902340/41   Fax: +91-22-24902342   e-mail: mumbai@cbspd.com

Representatives

• **Bhubaneswar**	0-9911037372	• **Hyderabad**	0-9885175004	• **Jharkhand**	0-9811541605
• **Nagpur**	0-9421945513	• **Patna**	0-9334159340	• **Pune**	0-9623451994
• **Uttarakhand**	0-9716462459	• **Dhaka (Bangladesh)**	01912-003485		

Printed at: HT Media Ltd., Greater Noida, UP, India

to
The Newborn Babies

Contributors

Ramesh Agarwal MD, DM
Additional Professor
Department of Pediatrics
AIIMS, New Delhi

Rajiv Aggarwal MD
Consultant Neonatologist
Sakra World Hospitals and
Daffodils Clinic
Bengaluru

Kamal Arora MD, DM
Assistant Professor
Dayanand Medical College and
Hospital
Ludhiana

Arvind Bagga MD
Professor
Division of Pediatric Nephrology
Department of Pediatrics
AIIMS, New Delhi

Madhumati Bose MSc
Special Educator
National Child Trust
New Delhi

Aparna Chandrasekaran MD, DM
Jr Consultant, Neonatology
Kanchi Kamakoti Child Trust
Hospital
Chennai

Suman Chaurasia MD
PhD Scholar
Department of Pediatrics
AIIMS, New Delhi

Deepak Chawla MD, DM
Associate Professor
Department of Pediatrics
Government Medical College
Chandigarh

Poonam Coshic
BTO
Main Blood Bank
AIIMS, New Delhi

Ashok Deorari MD, FAMS
Professor
Department of Pediatrics
WHO Collaborating Centre for
Education and Research in
Newborn Care
AIIMS, New Delhi

Sheffali Gulati MD
Professor
Division of Neurology and
Child Development
Department of Pediatrics
AIIMS, New Delhi

Shuchita Gupta MD
PhD Scholar
Department of Pediatrics
AIIMS, New Delhi

Girish Gururaj MD, DM
Consultant Neonatologist
Apollo Hospital
Mysore

Ashish Jain DNB, DM
Assistant Professor
Department of Neonatology
Maulana Azad Medical College
New Delhi

Vandana Jain MD
Additional Professor
Division of Pediatric
Endocrinology
Department of Pediatrics
AIIMS, New Delhi

Madhulika Kabra MD
Professor
Division of Genetics and
Metabolism
Department of Pediatrics
AIIMS, New Delhi

Sushil Kabra MD
Professor
Division of Pulmonology
Department of Pediatrics
AIIMS, New Delhi

Chandra Kumar DNB, DM
Consultant Neonatologist
Cloudnine Hospital
T Nagar, Chennai

Ranjith Kumar M MD
DM (Pediatric Neurology)
Resident
Department of Pediatrics
AIIMS, New Delhi

V Kannan DNB, DM
Senior Advisor
Pediatrics and Neonatologist
Head, Department of Pediatrics
Command Hospital
Pune

Rakesh Lodha MD
Additional Professor
Department of Pediatrics
AIIMS, New Delhi

Manisha Mehta MD
Research Officer
Division of Neonatology
Department of Pediatrics
AIIMS, New Delhi

Satish Mishra DM
Neonatologist and Pediatrician
Lifeline Advanced Neonatal
Centre
Jalandhar

Deeksha Mittal
Research Officer
Division of Neonatology
Department of Pediatrics
AIIMS, New Delhi

Tejopratap Oleti DM
Consultant Neonatologist
Fernandez Hospital
Hyderabad

Vinod K Paul MD, PhD, DNB, FAMS,
FIAP, FNNF
Professor and Head
Department of Pediatrics
AIIMS, New Delhi

Aathira Ravindranath MD
Resident
Department of Pediatrics
AIIMS, New Delhi

Sunil Saharan MD
Pediatric Cardiology Fellow
Doernbecher Children's Hospital
Oregon Health and Science
University
Portland, USA

M Jeeva Sankar DM
Assistant Professor
Division of Neonatology
Department of Pediatrics
AIIMS, New Delhi

Savita Sapra PhD
Clinical Psychologist
Department of Pediatrics
AIIMS, New Delhi

Arun Sasi DM
Clinical Fellow
Monash Medical Center
Melbourne

Manju Saxena PhD
Physician Scientist
Division of Neonatology
Department of Pediatrics
AIIMS, New Delhi

Amanpreet Sethi MD
DM (Neonatology) Resident
Department of Pediatrics
AIIMS, New Delhi

Aditi Sinha MD
Assistant Professor
Division of Neonatology
Department of Pediatrics
AIIMS, New Delhi

Suvasini Sharma DM
Assistant Professor
Department of Pediatrics
Lady Hardinge Medical College
New Delhi

Subhash C Shaw MD, DNB, DM
Lt Col
Command Hospital, Kolkata

Pradeep Kumar Sharma DM
Consultant
SPS Apollo Hospital
Ludhiana

Sindhu Sivanandan MD
DM Resident
Division of Neonatology
Department of Pediatrics
AIIMS, New Delhi

S Sreeram DM
Department of Neonatology
Fernandez Hospital
Hyderabad

Anu Thukral DM, DNB
Assistant Professor
Department of Pediatrics
Lady Hardinge Medical College
New Delhi

Amit Upadhyay DNB, DM
Associate Professor and Head
Department of Pediatrics
LLRM Medical College
Meerut

Manas Upadhyay MD, DM
Neonatologist
Cuttack, Orissa

V Prakash MD
DM (Neonatology) Resident
Department of Pediatrics
AIIMS, New Delhi

Preface

Protocols are instrumental for adoption of evidence-based practices and elimination of unnecessary or potentially harmful practices. Protocol based approach makes sure that there is a uniform clinical practice irrespective of disparate players and their views. Unit protocols also facilitate learning of the trainee doctors and nurses.

Protocols have been an integral part of NICU life at AIIMS right since its inception. As part of its philosophy of unrestricted sharing of the knowledge and resources, the neonatology faculty at AIIMS decided way back to publish the protocols in Indian Journal of Pediatrics. There was an overwhelming response from the neonatal fraternity to the extent that AIIMS protocols practically became part of majority of the neonatal units in India as well as other countries in South East Asia. For postgraduate students, it served as first hand resource for learning neonatology. The AIIMS protocols have been cited for over 400 times across the globe including in many major publications of recent times.

Initially, we published the protocols in Indian Journal of Pediatrics, which were periodically updated. Subsequently, the journal published them in form of a manual that enhanced their usability and outreach. The full texts of the protocols were made available on our website (www.newbornwhocc.org), which was one of the reasons of its popularity receiving nearly 200,000 hits over the last few years.

This publication is a manifestation of our desire to bring out a physician manual that contains relevant protocols based on context specific and updated evidence as well as other necessary resources and tools for day-to-day neonatology practice in level 2 and 3 neonatal units in South East Asia.

The current manual has 33 protocols. These are focused on the operational aspects of a condition rather than discussing the theory. There are summaries of relevant evidence and management algorithms at appropriate places. There is a substantial amount of additional resource material such as resuscitation algorithm, hand hygiene poster, BP charts, drugs to be avoided in G6PD deficiency, online resources for self learning and drugs use in pregnancy and lactation. There is a section that deals with main findings on chest X-ray of common conditions. A section on drug dosages has also been included.

India produces over 1200 postgraduate theses in pediatrics every year; however, the quality of research is too low to teach research methods to the students and generate a good piece of evidence. We have included a section that provides a number of research questions and optimum design to be used and relevant outcomes to be studied.

AIIMS protocols have been an outcome of intense efforts of the faculty, scientists and many past and present residents and fellows over a long time. All of them have shown an extraordinary commitment for this cause. We wish to acknowledge the immense contribution of Drs M Jeeva Sankar, Anu Thukral, Deepak Chawla, Kamal Arora and Aparna Chandrasekaran who not only contributed substantially in terms of contents but also in process of editing. We wish to thank Mr YN Arjuna of CBS Publishers who patiently accommodated our changing philosophy and style.

No book is flawless and we are unlikely to be exception. We would really appreciate your constructive criticism (ra.aiims@gmail.com).

Ramesh Agarwal
Ashok Deorari
Vinod K Paul

Contents

Section V

Gastrointestinal Disorders

Section VI

Infections

Section VII

Metabolic and Hematological Disorders

Section VIII

Miscellaneous

Section IX

Therapies and Diagnostic Modalities

Section X

Annexures

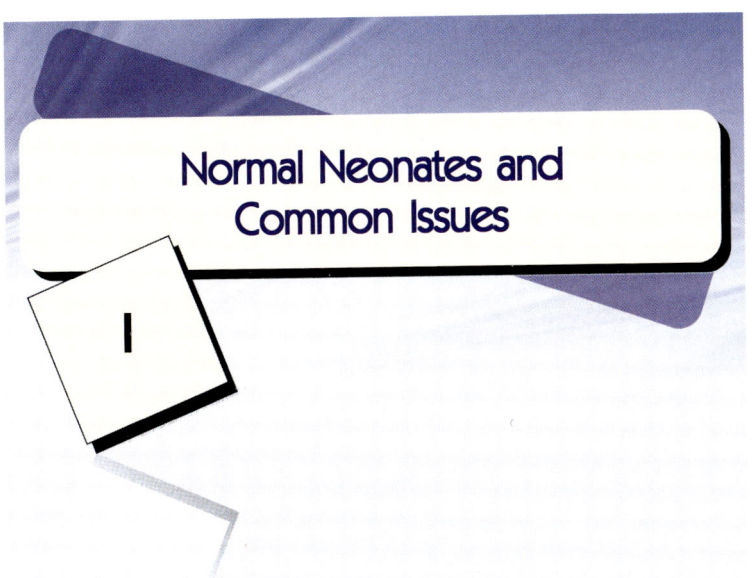

Normal Neonates and Common Issues

I

1. Care of Normal Neonates
2. Thermal Management
3. Management of Fluids and Electrolytes

1   Care of Normal Neonates

Normal neonate for the purpose of this protocol has been defined as:

- Birth weight greater than 2500 g and gestation of 37 weeks or more
- Birth weight between 10th and 90th percentiles as per intra-uterine growth charts
- Absence of maternal illness or intra-partum event that may put the neonate at risk of illness (e.g. gestational diabetes and antepartum hemorrhage)
- Normal Apgar scores, no need for resuscitation at birth
- No postnatal illness such as respiratory distress, sepsis, dyselectrolemia, hypoglycemia or polycythemia.

CARE AT BIRTH

Personnel and equipment:[1, 2] One health provider (physician or nurse) trained in neonatal resuscitation must be physically available at time of birth of all infants irrespective of their risk status (high or low). *It is not good enough to have someone on call.*

If the delivery is anticipated to be high risk because of presence of risk factors identified before birth, more advanced neonatal resuscitation may be required. In these cases, two persons should be present solely to manage the baby. There should be a 'resuscitation team', with specified leader and an identified role of each member. For multiple births, there should be separate teams.

The resuscitation corner must be physically located in the delivery room itself. The health professional designated to care for the baby at birth should check for the *"Resuscitation preparedness"* well in time before the baby is delivered

(Table 1.1). One may refer the 'Neonatal Resuscitation Programme' for details of resuscitation.[3]

Table 1.1: Checklist for "Resuscitation preparedness"	
For providing warmth	Preheat the warmer by turning on manual mode for at least 20 minutes. Make available at least 3 towels and a blanket
Thermoregulation	Plastic bag or plastic wrap for small babies
For positioning	The shoulder rolls should be prepared and kept ready
For clearing airway	10 to 12F suction catheter attached to wall suction set at 80–100 mmHg, meconium aspirator
For ventilation	Check for availability and the functioning of self-inflating bags. Check for availability of all sizes of the masks (00, 0) and 8F feeding tube and 20 mL syringe
For oxygen delivery	Oxygen tubing or T piece resuscitator that can deliver the free flow oxygen, pulse oximeter, option for providing varying concentration of oxygen (blender, air, oxygen)

What is Evidence?

The Neonatal Resuscitation Programme guidelines are based on the American Academy of Pediatrics (AAP) and American Heart Association (AHA) guidelines for cardiopulmonary resuscitation and emergency cardiovascular care of the neonate.[3] The evidence-based guidelines originally published in October 2010 are based on the International Liaison Committee on Resuscitation (ILCOR) consensus on science statement. The evidence-based worksheets can be viewed at www.aap.org/nrp.

Time of birth: The attending physician/nurse should note the time of birth. It is important to call out the time of birth loudly; this helps in accurate recording of the time and alerts other personnel in case any help is needed.

Standard precautions and asepsis at birth: The personnel attending the delivery must exercise all the universal/standard precautions in *all cases*.[4] All fluid products from the baby/mother should be treated as potentially infectious. Gloves, masks and gowns should be worn when resuscitating the newborn. The protective eyewear or face shields should be worn during procedures that are likely to generate droplets of blood or other bodily fluids.

It is important to prevent infection at birth by observing five cleans:[5]
1. Clean hands: Appropriate hand-hygiene and wearing sterile gloves.
2. Clean surface: Use clean and sterile towel to dry and cover the baby.
3. Clean cord: The umbilical cord should be cut with a clean and sterile blade/scissors.
4. Clean thread: The cord should be clamped with a clean and sterile clamp or tie.
5. Do not apply anything to the cord.

PREVENTION AND MANAGEMENT OF HYPOTHERMIA

Immediately after birth, the newborn is at maximum risk of hypothermia. This early hypothermia may have a detrimental effect on the health of the infant. Special care should be taken to prevent and manage hypothermia. It should be ensured that the temperature of delivery room is 25°C and free from draft of air. The pediatrician should receive the baby directly (no middle person should be allowed) in a pre-warmed sterile linen sheet.

The infant should be dried thoroughly including the head and face areas.[6] Any wet linen should not be allowed to remain in contact with the infant. The infant may be placed on the mother's abdomen immediately after the birth to ensure early skin-to-skin (STS) contact with the mother.[7] This will not only maintain the newborn's temperature but also promote early breastfeeding and decreases the pain and bleeding in the mother. The baby should be observed for the transition period and made wear the caps and socks.

What is Evidence?

A review by Puieg J et al (2007)[8] found that skin-to-skin contact between the mother and her baby immediately after birth reduces crying, improves mother–infant interaction, keeps the baby warm and helps the mother to breastfeed successfully. No important negative effects were identified.

Delayed clamping of umbilical cord: Umbilical cord clamping must be delayed for nearly 2 minutes in order to allow transfer of additional amount of blood from placenta to the infant. This delayed cord clamping in term babies is associated with improved hematologic status, iron status and clinical anemia at 2 to 6 months. Even though, there was an increase in polycythemia among infants in whom late clamping was done, this appeared to be benign.

What is Evidence?

A meta-analysis including 15 trials (1912 neonates)[9] showed that delayed cord clamping in term neonates was associated with benefits at 2 to 6 months:
• Improved hematocrit (WMD: 3.7 g/dL, 95% C.I. 2.00–5.40)
• Iron status measured by ferritin concentration
• Clinical anemia (RR; 0.53; 95% C.I. 0.40–0.70).

Cleaning of baby: The baby should be dried and cleaned at birth with a clean and sterile cloth. The cleaning should be gentle and should only wipe out the blood and the meconium and not to remove the vernix caseosa (white greasy material on the skin). The vernix protects skin of the infant and helps maintain temperature.[10] This gets absorbed on its own after sometime.

Clamping of the cord: The umbilical cord should be clamped at 2–3 cm away from the abdomen using a commercially available clamp, a clean and autoclaved thread or a sterile rubber band. The stump should be away from the genitals to avoid contamination. When the commercial clamps are not available, the rubber band could be a better option than a thread as once cord starts shriveling, the rubber band would still maintain its grip while the thread might loosen up.[11] Inspect the cord every 15–30 minutes for initial few hours after birth for early detection of any oozing from the cord.[12]

Routine stomach wash: Performing routine stomach wash in the babies to prevent gastritis (amniotic fluid or meconium) should not be done. There are no studies that report the advantage of this ritual.

Care of the eye: At birth, both the eyes of the neonates should be cleaned with separate swabs. The sterile water or the normal saline may be used for this purpose. The swipe to clean the eyes should be gentle and from the inner canthus area to the outer canthus. Currently, there is insufficient evidence to recommend the routine antibiotic prophylaxis for prevention of ophthalmia neonatorum in Indian settings.[13–15] The cleaning on a daily basis is not recommended as a routine.

Placement of identity band: The birthing places with high birth rates should take utmost care to ensure the identity of the mother-baby dyad by an appropriate method as per the hospital policy. Each infant must have an identity band containing name of the mother, hospital registration number, gender and birth weight of the infant.[16] Reliability of the foot prints for identification has not been investigated.

Recording of Apgar scores: The apgar scores should be recorded at 1 minute and 5 minutes of birth.[17] This score has a limited value in guiding resuscitation. The prediction of the subsequent outcomes by Apgar scores is also poor.[18] However, Apgar scores may help deciding the need for nursery admission.

CARE OF BABY DURING THE INITIAL FEW HOURS AFTER BIRTH

Weight record of the baby: The baby should be weighed after stabilization. A sterile preheated sheet (or a single use paper towel) should be placed on a 5 to 10 g sensitivity weighing machine. Zeroing of the machine should be performed. The baby is then gently placed on the weighing machine and the weight is recorded.[19] Weighing of the baby is a complex skill and it requires adequate training of health providers.

Initiation of breastfeeds: The breastfeeding should be initiated at the earliest possible time. The health provider should actively assist the mother to initiate breastfeeding irrespective of the mode of delivery. Breastfeeding counseling alone without any proactive support is unlikely to result in high rates of successful breastfeeding.[20] Time of initiation of the breastfeeding should be documented.

Vitamin K administration: Vitamin K should be administered to all the babies (0.5 mg for babies less than 1000 g and 1 mg for babies more than 1000 g).[21] It is preferable to administer the K1 preparation, however, if it is not available, the K3 preparation may be administered.[22] This should be administered as an IM injection using the 26 G (½ inch) needle and a 1 mL syringe on the anterolateral aspect of the thigh.

First examination: The baby should be thoroughly examined by the attending person from head to toe and the findings should be recorded in neonatal record sheet. Examine midline structures for malformations (e.g. cleft lip, neck masses, chest

abnormality, omphalocele, meningocele and cloacal abnormality). Special attention should be given to identify and document the anal opening. There is no need for routine passage of
catheter in the stomach, nostrils and the rectum for detection
of esophageal atresia, choanal atresia and ano-rectal malformation, respectively. The baby should be examined for presence
of birth injuries in cases with difficult extraction. The axillary
temperature of the baby should be recorded before the baby is
shifted out from the birthing place.

Communication with the family: Before leaving the birthing
place, the health professional should communicate with the
mother and the family members. The following facts should
be clearly told to the family: (1) gender of the baby, (2) birth
weight, (3) well being of the baby. Ensure that the family
members and the mother get to witness the gender and the
identity number of the baby.

Rooming in: Under no circumstances, a normal newborn
should be separated from the mother. In the initial few hours
of life, the baby is very active, and the closeness of the baby to
the mother will facilitate the early breastfeeding and bonding.
The studies have shown that any separation during initial
hours may have a significant adverse impact on successful
breastfeeding.

CARE OF BABY BEYOND FEW HOURS AFTER BIRTH

Care of the cord: The umbilical stump should be kept dry and
devoid of any application. The nappy of the baby should be
folded well below the stump to avoid any contamination.[23,24]
Renal evidence supports application of 4%. Colorhexidine is
community settings with high NMR and unhygienic cord
practices.[15, 26, 27]

Oil massage: The benefits of the oil application have been
described for the low birth weight babies in both the developed
and the developing countries.[28–30] However, a paucity of data
still exists for the oil application and/or massage in the term
babies.[31] Oil massage is a low cost traditional practice that is
well ingrained into the Indian culture, with no reported adverse
outcome. The same may be allowed in a gentle way and with
clean hands. Care should be taken not to use oils with additives
or the irritant oils (such as mustard oil) for this purpose.

Exclusive breastfeeding: A proactive and a systematic approach should be followed to initiate, support and maintain breast-feeding. The advantages of the breastfeeding should be discussed with the mother to motivate her. Availability of a dedicated lactation nurse or councilor would significantly increase the chances of successful breastfeeding.

Bath: The routine dip baths should be avoided till the baby is in the hospital as this increases the risk of hypothermia.[32] The sponging of the baby should be done once a day with clean water as per the requirement. The dip bath may be undertaken once the cord has fallen and the baby is discharged from the hospital.

Powder application: Currently, there is no evidence to suggest the regular use of any powder and the same should be avoided.

Position of sleep: There is substantial evidence in the literature from the developed countries of an independent association of prone position and occurrence of SIDS.[33,34] Healthy term newborns should be preferably made to sleep on their backs.

Traditional practices that should be discouraged: The application of kajal/surma in the eyes, putting oil in the ear or applying the cow-dung on cord must be strongly discouraged.[35]

Timing of discharge in a normal newborn: Whenever possible, the baby should undergo an observation period of 48 to 72 hrs in the health facility (for establishment of breastfeeding and observation for any morbidity including jaundice). However, an early discharge within 24 to 48 hrs may be considered for the non-primigravida mothers who have a history of successful breastfeeding.

The following criteria should be met in all the babies prior to discharge planning:
- The routine formal examination of the newborn has been performed and documented.
- The newborn has received the immunization as per schedule.
- The mother is confident and trained to take care of the neonate.

- The newborn is not having a significant jaundice or any other illness requiring close observation by a health provider.
- The newborn is breastfeeding adequately.
  The adequacy of feeds can be determined by:
  – Passage of urine 6 to 8 times every 24 hrs
  – Baby sleeping well for 2–3 hrs after feeds
  – There is no excessive weight loss (normally babies do not lose more than 8 to 10% in initial 3 to 4 days)
- The mother has been counseled regarding routine newborn care and her queries are answered.
- Follow-up advice should be communicated to the mother of the baby. Babies, particularly born to primigravida mothers should be called for follow-up visit at 48 hrs of discharge if discharged before 48 hours. The breastfeeding and the jaundice in these babies should be evaluated.[38]

ADVICE ON DISCHARGE: NORMAL NEWBORN

1. Exclusive breastfeeding: All mothers should be advised to exclusively breastfeed the babies till 6 months of age. The advantages of the breast milk should be discussed with the mother.
2. Immunization: The mother should be explained the schedule of the immunization and the date of the next immunization should be mentioned on the discharge card.
3. The follow-up date for the babies discharged early (within 48 hrs) for assessment of jaundice should be communicated to the parents.
4. The danger signs should be documented and mother should be educated to recognize the same and report early when they are recognized:[36–39]
   a. Difficulty in feeding
   b. Convulsions
   c. Lethargy (movement only when stimulated)
   d. Fast breathing (RR >60/min)
   e. Severe chest in drawing
   f. Temperature of more than 37.5°C or below 35.5°C.

What is Evidence?

- **The Young Infant Study** published in Lancet 2008;371;S135–147; evaluated 3177 children aged 0–6 days and 5712 infants aged 7–59 days for clinical signs and symptoms, and determined the specificity and sensitivity of each one in predicting a severe illness. The study reported that (a) history of feeding difficulty; (b) history of convulsions; (c) movement only when stimulated; (d) respiratory rate of 60 breaths per minute or more; (e) severe chest in drawing, temperature of 37.5°C or more or below 35.5°C, had the highest sensitivity (85%) and specificity (75%) for severe illness.

- *Cochrane review by* Brown S et al[40] looked at 7 studies (n = 3435) at the early postnatal discharge from hospital for healthy mothers and term infants and the re-admission within 8 weeks. They found that the failure of breastfeeding was an important cause for the re-admission. Hence, a review of cases discharged early at 2–3 days after discharge, may have a role in preventing re-admission.

REFERENCES

1. Martines J, Paul VK, Bhutta ZA, Koblinsky M, Soucat A, Walker N, Bahl R, Fogstad H, Costello A. Neonatal survival: a call for action. Lancet 2005;365:1189–97.

2. Sibley L and Ann Sipe T. What can a meta-analysis tell us about traditional birth attendant training and pregnancy outcomes? Midwifery 2004;20:51–60.

3. Kattwinkel, (Ed.) Textbook of Neonatal Resuscitation, 6th edn. American Academy of Pediatrics and American Heart Association, 2011.

4. Sridhar MR, Bopathi S, Lodha R, Kabra SK. Standard precautions and post exposure prophylaxis for preventing infections. Indian J Pediatr 2004;71:617–26.

5. Government of India, 1993. Child survival and safe motherhood programme—India. New Delhi: Ministry of Health and Family Welfare.

6. Dahm LS, James LS. Newborn temperature and calculated heat loss in the delivery room. Pediatrics 1972;49:504–13.

7. Moore ER, Anderson GC, Bergman N. Early skin-to-skin contact for mothers and their healthy newborn infants. Cochrane Database of Systematic Reviews 2007, Issue 3. Art. No.: CD003519. DOI: 10.1002/14651858.CD003519.pub2.

8. Puig G, Sguassero Y. Early skin-to-skin contact for mothers and their healthy newborn infants: RHL commentary (last revised: 9 November 2007). The WHO Reproductive Health Library; Geneva: World Health Organization.

9. Hutton EK, Hassan ES. Late *versus* Early clamping of the umbilical cord in full-term neonates: A systematic review and meta-analyses of controlled trials. JAMA 2007;297:1241–52.

10. Moraille R, Pickens WL, Visscher SB et al. A novel role for vernix caseosa as a skin cleanser. Biol Neonate 2005;87:8–14.

11. Anderson JM, Phillip AGS. Management of the umbilical cord: Care regimens, colonization, infection and separation. Neoreviews 2004;5:e155–63.

12. Neligan GA, Smith MC. Prevention of hemorrhage from the umbilical cord. Arch Dis Child 1963;38:471–75.

13. Ali Z, Khadije D, Elahe A, Mohammad M, Fateme Z, Narges Z. Prophylaxis of ophthalmia neonatorum comparison of betadine, erythromycin and no prophylaxis. J Trop Pediatr. 2007 Dec; 53(6):388–92.

14. Ramirez-Ortiz MA, Rodriguez-Almaraz M, Ochoa-Diazlopez H, Diaz-Prieto P, Rodriguez-Suárez RS. Randomised equivalency trial comparing 2.5% povidone-iodine eye drops and ophthalmic chloramphenicol for preventing neonatal conjunctivitis in a trachoma endemic area in southern Mexico. Br J Ophthalmol 2007 Nov;91(11):1430–4.

15. Matinzadeh ZK, Beiragdar F, Kavemanesh Z, Abolgasemi H, Amirsalari S. Efficacy of topical ophthalmic prophylaxis in prevention of ophthalmia neonatorum. Trop Doct 2007 Jan; 37(1):47–9. Original Text.

16. Robus JB et al. Guidelines on preventing abduction of infants from Hospital. National center for missing and exploited children. J Healthe Prot Manage 1992;4:36–49.

17. Behnke M, Eyler FD, Carter RL, et al. Predictive value of Apgar score for developmental outcome in premature infants. Am J Perinatol 1989;6:18–21.

18. Pinheiro JMB. The Apgar cycle: a new view of a familiar scoring system. Arch. Dis. Child. Fetal Neonatal Ed 2009;94:F70–2.

19. WHO Collaborating Center for Training and Research in Newborn Care. Teaching Aids on Newborn Care. URL: http//www. newbornwhocc.org. Accessed on 10th October 2009.

20. Moore ER, Anderson GC. Randomized controlled trial of very early mother-infant skin-to-skin contact and breastfeeding status. Journal of Midwifery & Women's Health 2007;52:116–125.

21. Puckett RM, Offringa M. Prophylactic vitamin K for vitamin K deficiency bleeding in neonates. Cochrane Database of Systematic Reviews 2000, Issue 4. Art. No.: CD002776. DOI: 10.1002/14651858.CD002776.

22. Chawla D, Deorari AK, Saxena R, Paul VK, Agarwal R, Biswas A et al. Vitamin K1 *versus* Vitamin K3 for prevention of subclinical vitamin deficiency: A Randomized Controlled Trial. Indian Pediatr 2007;22:817–22.

23. Zupan J, Gamer P, Omari AA. Topical umbilical cord care at birth. Cochrane Database Syst Rev 2004(3):CD001057.

24. Lawn J, Cousens S, Bhutta ZA, Darmstadt GL, Martines J, Paul VK, Knippenberg R, Fogstadt H, Shetty P, Horton R. Why are 4 million newborn babies dying each year? Lancet 2005;364: 399–401.

25. LC Mullany L, Darmstadt G, Khatry S et al. Topical applications of chlorhexidine to the umbilical cord for prevention of omphalitis and neonatal mortality in southern Nepal: a community-based, cluster-randomised trial. Lancet 2006;367:910–18.

26. Arifeen El, Mullany LC, Shah R, Rahman M, Radwanur M et al. The effect of cord cleansing with chlorhexidine on neonatal mortality in rural Bangladesh: A community-based, cluster-randomised trial. Lancet 2012;379:1022–28.

27. Sajid Soofi, Simon Cousens, Aamer Imdad, Naveed Bhutto, Nabeela Ali, Zulfiqar A Bhutta. Topical application of chlorhexidine to neonatal umbilical cords for prevention of omphalitis and neonatal mortality in a rural district of Pakistan: a community-based, cluster-randomised trial. Lancet 2012;379:1029–39.

28. Solanki K, Matnani M, Kale M, Joshi K, Bavdekar A, Bhave S, Pandit A. Transcutaneous absorption of topically massaged oil in neonates. Indian Pediatr 2005;42:998–1005.

29. Sankaranarayanan K, Mondkar JA, Chauhan MM, Mascarenhas BM, Mainkar AR, Salvi RY. Oil massage in neonates: an open randomized controlled study of coconut *versus* mineral oil. Indian Pediatr 2005;42:877–84.

30. Agarwal KN, Gupta A, Pushkarna R, Bhargava SK, Faridi MM, Prabhu MK. Effects of massage and use of oil on growth, blood flow and sleep pattern in infants. Indian J Med Res 2000;112: 212–17.

31. Bhutta ZA, Darmstadt GL, Hasan BS, Haws RA. Outcomes in developing countries: A review of the evidence community-based interventions for improving perinatal and neonatal health. Pediatrics 2005;115:519–617.

32. Bergström A, Byaruhanga R, Okong P. The impact of newborn bathing on the prevalence of neonatal hypothermia in Uganda: a randomized, controlled trial. Acta Paediatr. 2005;94:1462–7.

33. Kattwinkel J, Brooks J, Myerberg D; American Academy of Pediatrics, Task Force on Infant Positioning and SIDS. Positioning and SIDS. Pediatrics 1992;89:1120–6.

34. American Academy of Pediatrics, Task Force on Infant Sleep Position and Sudden Infant Death Syndrome. Changing concepts of sudden infant death syndrome: implications for infant sleeping environment and sleep position. Pediatrics 2000;105:650–6.

35. Mehrotra SK, Maheshwari BB. Prevalence of ocular lesions in a rural community. Indian J Ophthalmol 1975;23:17–20.

36. Young Infants Clinical Signs Study Group. Clinical signs that predict severe illness in children under age 2 months: a multicentre study. Lancet. 2008;371:135-42.

37. Bang AT, Bang RA, Reddy MH, Baitule SB, Deshmukh MD, Paul VK, de C Marshal TF. Simple clinical criteria to identify sepsis or pneumonia in neonates in the community needing treatment or referral. Pediatr Infect Dis J. 2005;24:335-41.

38. Deorari AK, Chellani H, Carlin JB, Greenwood P, Prasad MS, Satyavani A, Singh J, John R, Taneja DK, Paul P, Meenakshi M, Kapil A, Paul VK, Weber M. Clinicoepidemiological profile and predictors of severe illness in young infants (<60 days) reporting to a hospital in North India. Indian Pediatr. 2007;44:739–48.

39. Narang A, Kumar P, Narang R, Ray P, Carlin JB, Greenwood P, Muley P, Misra S, Weber M. Clinico-epidemiological profile and validation of symptoms and signs of severe illness in young infants (<60 days) reporting to a district hospital. Indian Pediatr. 2007; 44:751–9.

40. Brown S, Small R, Argus B, Davis PG, Krastev A. Early postnatal discharge from hospital for healthy mothers and term infants. Cochrane Database of Systematic Reviews 2008, Issue 3. Art. No: CD002958.

2

Thermal Management

A newborn baby is homeothermic, but his ability to maintain his body temperature can be easily overwhelmed by environmental temperatures. Thermal protection of the newborn is a set of continuing measures, which starts at birth to ensure that he maintains a body temperature of 36.5 to 37.5°C (Table 2.1).[1] According to NNPD 2002–2003, incidence of hypothermia among extramural babies was 18.4%.[2]

Table 2.1: Temperature ranges

Normal axillary temperature	36.5–37.5°C
Mild hypothermia or cold stress	36–36.4°C
Moderate hypothermia	32–35.9°C
Severe hypothermia	<32°C
Hyperthermia	>37.5°C

THERMONEUTRAL ENVIRONMENT (TNE)

TNE refers to a narrow range of environmental temperature at which the basal metabolic rate (BMR) of the baby is at a minimum, oxygen consumption is least and the baby maintains its normal body temperature.[2] Range of TNE varies accordingly to the gestation and postnatal age (Table 2.2).

As opposed to TNE, thermoregulatory environment refers to environmental temperature beyond TNE range, at which baby would be able to maintain its body temperature but by increasing its BMR.

The infants therefore should be kept in TNE so that their energy is utilized for growth and other vital functions.

Table 2.2: Thermoneutral zone

Weight of the baby	Recommended ambient temperature			
	35°C	34°C	33°C	32°C
Less than 1500 gm	1 to 10 days old	11 days to 3 wks old	3 to 5 wks old	More than 5 wks old
1500 to 1999 gm		1 to 10 days old	11 days to 4 wks old	More than 4 wks old
2000 to 2499 gm		1 to 2 days old	3 days to 3 wks old	More than 3 wks old
2500 g or more		1 to 2 days old	3 days to 3 wks old	More than 3 wks old

RECORDING TEMPERATURE

It is not necessary to measure the temperature of healthy newborn babies routinely, particularly when the warm chain is followed.

Temperature should be monitored every 1–2 hour for a baby with serious illness, twice daily for babies weighing between 1500 to 2499 g, four times daily for babies below 1500 g and once a day for other babies who are doing well.

METHODS OF RECORDING TEMPERATURE

Touch Method

Abdomen skin temperature is assessed by touch with dorsum of hand. Abdominal temperature is representative of the core temperature. Baby's temperature can be assessed with reliable accuracy by human touch, which can be easily taught to parents and can be practiced at home as well. The interpretation is as follows:

- Baby's feet and hands are warm   : Normal body temperature
- Peripheries are cold, the trunk is warm   : Cold stress
- Peripheries and the trunk both are cold   : Hypothermia

Thermometers

WHO recommends the use of low reading thermometer which can record up to 30°C. American Academy of Pediatrics (AAP) recommends against using mercury thermometers because the glass can break and mercury is poisonous.[3] The best is to use a digital thermometer.

Thermister Probe

Skin temperature can be recorded by a thermister. The probe is attached to skin over upper abdomen. The thermister will sense the skin temperature and display on the panel.

THE CONCEPT OF WARM CHAIN

The warm chain is a set of ten interlinked steps carried out at birth and later which will reduce the chances of hypothermia in all newborns.

Thermal Care in Delivery Room

After birth, newborn's temperature can drop at a rate of 0.1°C and 0.3°C per minute for core and skin temperature, respectively. Delivery room should be clean, warm (at least 25–28°C) and free from draughts from open windows and doors or from fans.

If the temperature of the room is less than optimal, a heater should be available to warm the room. All the towels, blankets, caps, baby's clothes should be pre-warmed. The radiant warmer should be switched on at least 20 to 30 minutes in advance and put in the manual mode with 100% heater output.

Warm Resuscitation

All the equipment, supplies and linen coming in contact should be warmed up to prevent hypothermia.

Immediate Drying

After birth, the baby should be immediately dried with a dry towel, starting with the head. After drying thoroughly, the baby should then be covered with a second, dry towel and a cap put on its head.

Skin-to-Skin Contact

Baby can be kept on mother's chest in skin contact while mother is being attended, and later in postnatal ward for initial few hours. If a baby is in cold stress, the baby should be immediately put in skin-to-skin contact with mother.

Breastfeeding

Breastfeeding should begin as soon as possible after birth preferably within an hour. This ensures adequate supply of calories for heat generation.

Postpone Bathing/Weighing

Bathing should be postponed in a term baby at least till next day. Weighing should be done only after covering the baby adequately and making zero correction for clothing.

Clothing and Bedding

Newborns should be covered with one or two layers of clothes and cap, socks and hand gloves.

Rooming in

Babies and mother should be kept together for 24 hrs in the same bed.

Warm Transportation

In case of transport: Whether to home or to another hospital/ ward, thermal protection should be ensured. Stable babies including preterm and LBW babies should be transported well wrapped and in skin-to-skin contact with mother.

Small, sick and unstable babies should be transported using an incubator. Temperature should be checked before and after transport. All peripheral hospitals caring for high risk mothers should go for in utero transfer as early as possible.

Training and Awareness

All the health care personnel involved in the newborn care should be adequately trained and informed about the principles of warm chain.

THERMAL MANAGEMENT IN PRETERM BABIES

Apart from the routine procedures and adhering to warm chain, extra care is required for preterm babies.

Polythene Occlusive Wraps

NRP 2010 recommends the use of polythene wraps for all babies <28 weeks. This technique involves placing the premature infant in a food grade polyethylene bag. The baby should be placed under a radiant warmer. Wrapping reduces evaporative heat loss, while allowing radiant heat delivery to the baby.[4]

Polythene Occlusive Wraps: What is Evidence?

A Cochrane review has confirmed the efficacy of plastic bags in addition to radiant warming in improving the NICU admission temperature of premature babies <28 weeks gestation.[5]

All preterm babies <34 weeks should be admitted and nursed either under a radiant warmer or in an incubator. Kangaroo mother care should be started as soon as the baby is stable.

Incubators

Incubators are preferred over radiant warmer for the care of preterm babies less than 28–30 wks of gestation.[6] Incubators decrease the insensible water loss (IWL).

What is Evidence?

Double wall incubators have an additional inner wall. These incubators have advantages of having lesser radiative heat loss.[7]

a. Mechanisms

The incubators reduce the exposure of babies to air currents minimizing convective heat loss. Evaporative heat loss is limited by maintaining humidity within the incubator. Radiative heat losses are minimized by double walled incubators.

The incubators have a transparent canopy and a heating element installed under the bassinet. A fan pushes the air over the heating element. The heated air maintains the desired temperature inside the canopy. The heater output is servo-controlled by baby's temperature.

Practical Tips

- In air mode, desired temperature of the environment is set and the heater output adjusts itself to maintain this. The appropriate set temperature is decided by using the thermo neutral temperature charts.
- In skin mode, the desired skin temperature is set to 36.5°C. The feedback system modifies heater output to keep the baby's temperature constant.
- For sick babies, skin mode is preferred because it helps to assess the temperature requirement for the baby. Set the temperature at 36.5°C. The probe should be properly positioned, if it gets dislodged, there is a danger of overheating.
- Air mode is preferred for procedures. When switching over to air mode, set the air temperature similar to the average incubator air temperature in skin mode.

b. Humidification

Since humidity is a potent source of infection (especially psuedomonas), its use should be restricted to babies < 28 weeks gestation during initial few days.

c. Weaning from Incubator

There is no clear cut recommendation with respect to when to wean the baby from incubator.[8]

The baby can be weaned, when the baby starts consistently gaining weight, maintain normal body temperature at the ambient temperature of < 30°C.

Radiant Warmers (RW)

Radiant warmer is an 'open care system'. It is easy to maintain and allows easy access during procedures, but has the disadvantage of having high insensible water loss.

a. Principle

The radiant warmers employ a heating rod usually made of quartz crystal to generate heat. The heat gets uniformly reflected to the baby by reflectors. RW also reduce conductive heat loss by heating up the microenvironment.

b. Modes

There are two modes—servo and manual. Servo mode of control is preferred over manual mode. Servo mode controls the heater output based on the skin temperature. In servo, skin temperature is set at 36.5°C. Covering the infant's head, arms and legs improves the efficacy of RW. Room temperature should be at least 25°C for optimal functioning of RW.

Operator determines the heater output in manual mode. It is not routinely used because of risk of overheating or under heating. Manual mode is used for prewarming the linen, rapid rewarming of hypothermic baby and if the baby has fever.

Practical Tips

- If on manual mode, baby's temperature should be checked every 15 minutes.
- There should not be more than one baby under a warmer as this results in cross infection and unequal heat distribution.
- In small babies, cling wraps (polythene sheets) can be used for covering the tops of side walls, which helps in reducing the insensible water loss.

Heated Water Filled Mattress

It is an economical device for keeping LBW/sick babies. Generally, the mattress has a capacity to hold 5 L of water. An electric heating plate and control units are fitted into the bottom of the mattress that keep the temperature of water at 35–38°C. This is not routinely used because of practical difficulties and safety.

Phase Changing Material (PCM)

It consists of a sealed pouch containing PCM. It maintains a temperature of 37°C for 4–6 hours without electricity. The pouch can be reheated repeatedly.

Small studies have proven the efficacy of phase changing materials for maintaining the temperature of the LBW baby over a defined time period. Trials are needed to assess the efficacy of PCM as a modality for effective thermal management in newborns.

Kangaroo Mother Care

For LBW babies, who are stable, KMC is the effective way of keeping babies warm. KMC is a no cost, easy, applicable at home, which has multiple added advantages. Prolonged KMC is recommended for all LBW babies (<2 kg).

CLINICAL FEATURES OF HYPOTHERMIA

Clinical features of hypothermia can be discussed under the four different situations:

a. Initial signs of hypothermia are generally related to peripheral vasoconstriction like pallor, acrocyanosis, cool extremities and decreased peripheral perfusion. There can be signs of CNS manifestations like irritability.

b. Late signs include those related to CNS depression like lethargy, bradycardia, apnea, poor feeding, hypotonia and weak suck or cry. As there is increase in pulmonary artery pressure, fast breathing and chest retractions can be present. Abdominal signs like increased gastric residuals and abdominal distention can also be present.

c. Prolonged hypothermia increases the metabolic rate resulting in hypoglycemia, hypoxia, metabolic acidosis and coagulation abnormalities.

d. Chronic cold stress results in poor weight gain.

MANAGEMENT OF HYPOTHERMIA

Cold Stress

- Remove cold/wet clothes and cover the baby adequately with warm clothes.
- Warm the room.
- Ensure skin-to-skin contact with mother.
- Breastfeed the baby.
- Monitor axillary temperature every ½ hr till it reaches 36.5°C, then hourly for next 4 hours, 2 hourly for 12 hours thereafter.

Moderate Hypothermia

- Maintain skin-to-skin contact.
- Take measures to reduce heat loss.
- Provide extra heat by room heater, radiant warmer, incubator or apply warm towel.

Severe Hypothermia

- Admit the baby.
- Rapid rewarming is done up to 34°C, then slow rewarming to 36.5°C.
- Take measures to reduce heat loss.
- Start IVF at 60–80 mL/kg of 10% dextrose.
- Start supplemental oxygen if needed.
- Give Inj. vitamin K.
- If not improving, consider sepsis.

CAUSES, SYMPTOMS AND MANAGEMENT OF HYPERTHERMIA

Hyperthermia is also a common problem with neonates. Temperature of more than 37.5°C is defined as hyperthermia in newborns.

Causes

- Too hot environment—high room temperature
- The baby has many layers of covers/clothes

- Dehydration fever—the baby may be in a dehydration state
- Sepsis (especially in term babies)

Dehydration Fever

Dehydration results in excess weight loss for the baby. Fever generally subsides with correction of breastfeeding issues or when extra feeds given properly.

Symptoms

Early: Irritable, tachycardia, tachypnea, flushed face, hot and dry skin

Late: Apathy, lethargic and then comatose

Severe forms of hyperthermia can lead to shock, convulsions, even death.

Management

Place the baby in a normal environment (25–28°C) away from heat source.

- Undress the baby partial/fully.
- Give frequent breastfeeds/give breast milk.
- If temperature is >39°C, sponging can be done with tap water.

Practical Tips

- Don't use cold/ice water for sponging. Tap water is good enough.
- Measure the temperature hourly until it becomes normal.
- Examine the baby for any infection.

REFERENCES

1. Thermal Protection of Newborns: A Practical Guide, WHO–1997.

2. NNPD report 2002–2003, www.newbornwhocc.org.

3. Caring for Your Baby and Young Child: Birth to age 5: American Academy of Pediatrics.

4. International Consensus on Cardiopulmonary Resuscitation and Emergency Cardiovascular Care Science with Treatment Recommendations, Circulation 2010;122;S516–38.

5. McCall EM, Alderdice F, Halliday HL, Jenkins JG, Vohra S. Interventions to prevent hypothermia at birth in preterm and/or low birth weight infants. Cochrane Database of Systematic Reviews 2010, Issue 3. Art. No.:CD004210.

6. Flenady V, Woodgate PG. Radiant warmers *versus* incubators for regulating body temperature in newborn infants. Cochrane Database of Systematic Reviews 2003, Issue 4. Art. No.: CD000435. DOI:10.1002/14651858.CD000435.

7. Laroia N, Phelps D, Roy J. Double wall *versus* single wall incubator for reducing heat loss in very low birth weight infants in incubators. Cochrane Database of Systematic Reviews 2007, Issue 2. Art. No.:CD004215. DOI:10.1002/14651858.CD004215.

8. Gray PH, Flenady V. Cot-nursing *versus* incubator care for preterm infants. Cochrane Database of Systematic Reviews 2001, Issue 2. Art. No.:CD003062. DOI: 10.1002/14651858.CD003062.

3

Management of Fluids and Electrolytes

Adaptation to extrauterine life consists of three phases of fluid balance. After birth, there is efflux of fluid from the intracellular to the extracellular compartment.[1] This results in salt and water diuresis by 48–72 hours of age. Loss of this excess extracellular fluid (ECF) and evaporative water loss from immature skin result in physiological weight loss during first week of life. Since the ECF compartment is larger in preterm neonates, the weight loss is greater in them. Term infants are expected to lose up to 7–10% of their birth weight as compared to 10–15% weight loss in premature neonates. First phase of transition ends with maximum weight loss. Second intermediate phase is characterized by diminished insensible water loss along with increasing maturation of skin barrier, a fall in urine volume to less than 1–2 mL/kg per hour, and a low sodium excretion. Third phase consists of stable growth and is characterized by continuous weight gain with a positive net balance for water and sodium.

RENAL FUNCTION

Kidneys in the neonate have limited capacity to excrete either concentrated (due to immaturity of the distal nephron with an anatomically shortened loop of Henle) or diluted urine (due to physiologically low glomerular filtration rate). Physiological range for urine osmolality in neonates varies from a lower limit of 50 mmol/L to upper limits of 600 mmol/L in preterm neonates and 800 mmol/L in term neonates.[2,3] An acceptable osmolality range of 300–400 mmol/L corresponds to a daily urine output of 2–3 ml/kg/hr.

Neonatal kidneys have limited capacity to excrete or conserve sodium. Normally, there is salt and water diuresis in the first 48–72 hours of life. Therefore, sodium supplementation should be started after ensuring initial diuresis or at least 5–6% weight loss.[3–6] Preterm neonates have a limited tubular capacity to reabsorb sodium and hence have increased urinary losses. Failure to supplement sodium after the first week of life can result in low body stores of sodium and poor weight gain.[3,6–8] Sodium requirements range from 3 to 5 mEq/kg/day in preterm neonates after the first week of life.[8,9]

FLUID LOSSES

In addition to mandatory water loss by the kidneys and gastro-intestinal system (termed as sensible loss), additional water losses occur due to evaporation from the skin and respiratory tract. This water loss is termed as insensible water loss (IWL). Insensible water losses tend to be higher in preterm infants (Table 3.1).

Table 3.1: Insensible water loss by birth weight on day 1

Birth weight	Insensible water loss (mL/kg/day)
<1000 g	60–80
1000–1500 g	40–60
>1500 g	20

Evaporation loss through the skin usually contributes to 70% of IWL.[1] The remaining 30% is contributed by losses from the respiratory tract. The emphasis in fluid and electrolyte therapy should be on prevention of excessive IWL rather than replacement of increased IWL. Hence, incubators, plastic barriers and heat shields should be used liberally in the management of extremely premature neonates.

GUIDELINES FOR FLUID AND ELECTROLYTE THERAPY

First Week of Postnatal Life

The goals for fluid and electrolyte administration during first week after birth are to allow contraction of ECF (without compromising intravascular fluid volume and cardiovascular function) with negative water balance of not more than 10%, to allow a negative net balance for sodium of 2–5 mmol/kg per day, to maintain normal serum electrolyte concentrations, to avoid oliguria (0.5–1.0 ml/kg per hour) for longer than twelve hours and to ensure avoiding excessive transepidermal water loss. Once period of transition is over, goals are to replace actual water and electrolytes losses and requirements.

What is Evidence?

Restricted fluids in preterm neonates

A review of four randomized clinical studies with different levels of fluid intake during the first week of life concluded that fluid restriction reduces the risk of patent ductus arteriosus, necrotizing enterocolitis and death with trend towards reduction in risk of bronchopulmonary dysplasia.[10]

Amount of actual fluid intake to be prescribed from recommended range for each day (Table 3.2) is selected with careful monitoring to achieve physiological weight loss, normal tissue perfusion and normal serum electrolytes.

Table 3.2: Parenteral fluid and electrolyte requirements during first week after birth

	Parenteral fluid in mL/kg/d *Day after birth*					
	1	2	3	4	5	6
Term neonate	60–120	80–120	100–130	120–150	140–160	140–180
Preterm neonate ≥1500 g	60–80	80–100	100–120	120–150	140–160	140–160
Preterm neonate <1500 g	80–90	100–110	120–130	130–150	140–160	160–180

Electrolyte requirement (mEq/kg)*	
Sodium	0–3 (carefully adjust for neonates <1000 g)
Potassium	0–2 (start after onset of diuresis)
Chloride	0–5

*No electrolyte supplementation is required during initial 48 hrs of life

After First Postnatal Week

Table 3.3: Parenteral fluid and electrolyte requirements after first postnatal week

	Fluid (ml/kg/d)	*Sodium (mmol/kg/d)*	*Potassium (mmol/kg/d)*
Term neonate	140–160	2.0–3.0	1.5–3.0
Preterm neonate	140–160	3.0–5.0 (to 7.0)	2.0–5.0

Sodium and potassium should be started in the IV fluids after 48 hours, each in a dose of 2–3 mEq/kg/day. Dextrose infusion should be maintained at 4–6 mg/kg/min. Dextrose 10% may be used in babies with birth weight more than 1250 grams and 5% dextrose in babies with birth weight less than 1250 grams.

EXAMPLES

Babies 1500 grams or more (mostly term and preterm babies)

Day 1

A full term infant on intravenous fluids would need to excrete a solute load of about 15 mOsm/kg/day through kidneys. To excrete this solute load at a urine osmolarity of 300 mOsm/L, the infant would need a minimum of 50 mL/kg free water. Allowing for an additional IWL of 20 mL/kg, the initial fluids should be 60–70 mL/kg/day. The initial fluids should be 10% dextrose with no electrolytes in order to maintain a glucose infusion rate of 4–6 mg/kg/min.

Day 2–Day 7

As the infant grows and receives enteral milk feeds, the solute load presented to the kidneys increases and the infant requires more fluid to excrete the solute load. Water is also required for fecal losses and for growth purposes. The fluid requirements increase by 15–20 mL/kg/day till a maximum of 150 mL/kg/day. Sodium and potassium should be added after 48 hrs of age and glucose infusion should be maintained at 4–6 mg/kg/min.

Babies <1500 grams (mostly preterm babies <32 wks)

Day 1

The urine output in a preterm baby would be similar to a term baby. However, the fluid requirement will be higher due to increased IWL and increased weight loss (extracellular fluid loss). It is recommended that caps, socks and plastic barriers to be used to reduce the IWL under the radiant warmer. Using this method, it is possible to manage VLBW infants with fluids of 80 mL/kg/day on day 1 of life.

Day 2–Day 7

As the skin matures in a preterm baby, the IWL progressively decreases and becomes similar to a term baby by the end of the first week. Hence, the fluid requirement in a preterm baby would become similar to a term baby by the end of the first week. Plastic barriers, caps and socks are used throughout the first week in order to reduce IWL from the immature skin. Fluids need to be increased at 10–15 mL/kg/day till a maximum of 150 mL/kg/day. Sodium and potassium should be added after 48 hours and glucose infusion should be maintained at 4–6 mg/kg/min.

STRATEGIES TO REDUCE INSENSIBLE WATER LOSS

Double wall incubators reduce insensible water loss in VLBW neonates by about 30%. The use of radiant warmers for VLBW care may increase water loss and impair thermoregulation. Thin, transparent plastic barriers (e.g. cling-wrap) may be used to increase the local humidity and limit air movement.[11] These transparent plastic films may be fixed to the supporting walls of the radiant warmer in order to create a micro-environment around the baby. These plastic barriers are effective in reducing IWL without interfering with the thermal regulation of the warmer. The use of emollient ointments or coconut oil decreases insensible water loss of up to 50% in open care conditions.[12–14] Endotracheal intubation and mechanical ventilation using warmed and humidified air significantly reduce insensible respiratory water loss.

Monitoring of Fluid and Electrolyte Status

Body weight: Term neonates lose 1–2% of their birth weight daily with a cumulative loss of 7–10% in the first week of life. Preterm neonates lose 2–3% of their birth weight daily with a cumulative loss of 10–15% in the first week of life. Failure to lose weight in the first week of life should be an indication for fluid restriction. However, excessive weight loss in the first 7 days or later would be non-physiological and would merit correction with fluid therapy.

Clinical examination: The usual physical signs of dehydration are unreliable in neonates. Infants with 10% (100 mL/kg) dehydration may have sunken eyes and fontanel, cold and clammy skin, poor skin turgor and oliguria. Infants with 15% (150 mL/kg) or more dehydration would have signs of shock (hypotension, tachycardia and weak pulses) in addition to the above features. Dehydration would merit correction of fluid and electrolyte status gradually over the next 24 hours.

Serum biochemistry: Hyponatremia with weight loss suggests sodium depletion and would merit sodium replacement. Hyponatremia with weight gain suggests water excess and necessitates fluid restriction. Hypernatremia with weight loss suggests dehydration and would require fluid correction over 48 hours. Hypernatremia with weight gain suggests salt and water load and would be an indication of fluid and sodium restriction.

Urine output, specific gravity (SG) and osmolarity: The acceptable range for urine output is 1–3 mL/kg/hr, for specific gravity between 1.005 and 1.012. Specific gravity can be checked by dipstick or by a hand-held refractometer.

Laboratory Guidelines for Fluid and Electrolyte Therapy

Intravenous fluids should be increased in the presence of: (a) Increased weight loss (>3%/day or a cumulative loss >15%); (b) Increased serum sodium (Na >145 mEq/L); (c) Increased urine specific gravity (>1.020); (d) Decreased urine output (<1 mL/kg/hr). Similarly, fluids should be restricted in the presence of: (a) Decreased weight loss (<1%/day or a cumulative loss <5%); (b) Decreased serum sodium in the presence of weight gain (Na <130 mEq/L); (c) Decreased urine specific gravity (<1.005); (d) Increased urine output (>3 mL/kg/hr).

SPECIFIC CLINICAL CONDITIONS

Extreme prematurity (gestation <28 weeks, birth weight <1000 grams): These babies have large insensible water losses due to thin, immature skin barrier. The stratum corneum matures rapidly in 1–2 weeks and therefore fluid requirements become comparable to larger infants by the end of the second week. Fluid requirement in the first week may be decreased substantially by reducing the IWL with the use of plastic transparent barriers, coconut oil application on the skin or using double walled incubators.[2,11,12] The initial fluids on day 1 and 2 should be electrolyte free and should be made using 5% dextrose solutions to prevent risks of hyperglycemia. Sodium and potassium should be added after 48 hrs of life.

Respiratory distress syndrome (RDS): The renal function in preterm babies may be further compromised in the presence of hypoxia and acidosis due to RDS. Positive pressure ventilation may lead to increased secretion of aldosterone and ADH, leading to water retention. Symptomatic patent ductus arteriosus (PDA) is more likely to occur in the presence of RDS. Results from various studies have shown that restricted water intake has a beneficial effect on the incidence of PDA, CLD, NEC and death.[4] Hence, fluid therapy in sick preterm infants should be monitored strictly using the above mentioned clinical and laboratory criteria.

Perinatal asphyxia and brain injury: Perinatal asphyxia may be associated with syndrome of inappropriate ADH (SIADH) secretion. However, routine restriction of fluid is not recommended in these infants. Fluid restriction in this condition should be done only in the presence of hyponatremia. The intake should be restricted to two-thirds maintenance fluids till serum sodium values return to normal. Once urine production increases by the third postnatal day, fluids may be gradually restored to normal levels. Renal parenchyma injury from perinatal asphyxia may result in acute tubular necrosis (ATN), which is commonly accompanied by oliguria or anuria. In case of oliguric renal failure, fluid intake should be restricted to replenishment of IWL and metabolic water requirement (400 mL/m^2 or 40 mL/kg) and any other losses (urine output, gastric secretions, etc.). During the recovery phase of ATN, there can be large urinary sodium and potassium losses, which should be calculated and replaced.

Diarrhea: The correction of fluid deficit is done over 24 hours. Ongoing losses need to be assessed and corrected 6–8 hourly.

REFERENCES

1. Bell EF, Oh W. Fluid and electrolyte management. In: Avery GB, Fletcher MA, MacDonald MG, eds. Neonatology: Pathophysiology of the Newborn. 5th ed. Philadelphia: Lippincott Williams & Wilkins, 1999;345–61.
2. Chevalier RL. Developmental renal physiology of the low birth weight pre-term newborn. J Urol 1996;156:714–9.

3. Modi N. Renal function, fluid and electrolyte balance and neonatal renal disease. In: Rennie JM, Roberton NRC, eds. Textbook of Neonatology. 3rd edn. Edinburgh: Churchill Livingstone, 1999; 1009–36.

4. Hartnoll G, Betremieux P, Modi N. Randomised controlled trial of postnatal sodium supplementation in infants of 25–30 weeks gestational age: effects on cardiopulmonary adaptation. Arch Dis Child Fetal Neonatal Ed 2001;85:F29–32.

5. Hartnoll G, Betremieux P, Modi N. Randomised controlled trial of postnatal sodium supplementation on oxygen dependency and body weight in 25–30 week gestational age infants. Arch Dis Child Fetal Neonatal Ed 2000;82:F19–23.

6. Al-Dahhan J, Haycock GB, Nichol B, Chantler C, Stimmler L. Sodium homeostasis in term and preterm neonates. III. Effect of salt supplementation. Arch Dis Child 1984;59:945–50.

7. Mbiti MJ, Ayisi RK, Orinda DA. Sodium supplementation in very low birth weight infants fed on their own mother's milk: II. Effects on protein and bone metabolism. East Afr Med J 1992;69:627–30.

8. Ayisi RK, Mbiti MJ, Musoke RN, Orinda DA. Sodium supplementation in very low birth weight infants fed on their own mother's milk I: Effects on sodium homeostasis. East Afr Med J 1992;69:591–5.

9. Higgins ST, Baumgart S. Fluid and electrolyte disorders. In: Spitzer AR, ed. Intensive care of the fetus and neonate. St. Louis Mosby-Year book, 1996;1034–49.

10. Bell EF, Acarregui MJ. Restricted *versus* liberal water intake for preventing morbidity and mortality in preterm infants. Cochrane Database Syst Rev 2008:CD000503.

11. Kaushal M, Agarwal R, Aggarwal R, et al. Cling wrap, an innovative intervention for temperature maintenance and reduction of insensible water loss in very low-birth weight babies nursed under radiant warmers: a randomized, controlled trial. Ann Trop Paediatr 2005;25:111–8.

12. Nangia S, Paul VK, Chawla D, Agarwal R, Deorari AK, Sreenivas V. Topical coconut oil application reduces trans-epidermal water loss (TEWL) in very low birth weight (VLBW) neonates: A randomized clinical trial. In: Pediatric Academic Society. Toronto, 2007;7933.21.

13. Nopper AJ, Horii KA, Sookdeo-Drost S, Wang TH, Mancini AJ, Lane AT. Topical ointment therapy benefits premature infants. J Pediatr 1996;128:660–9.

14. Lane AT, Drost SS. Effects of repeated application of emollient cream to premature neonates' skin. Pediatrics 1993;92:415–9.

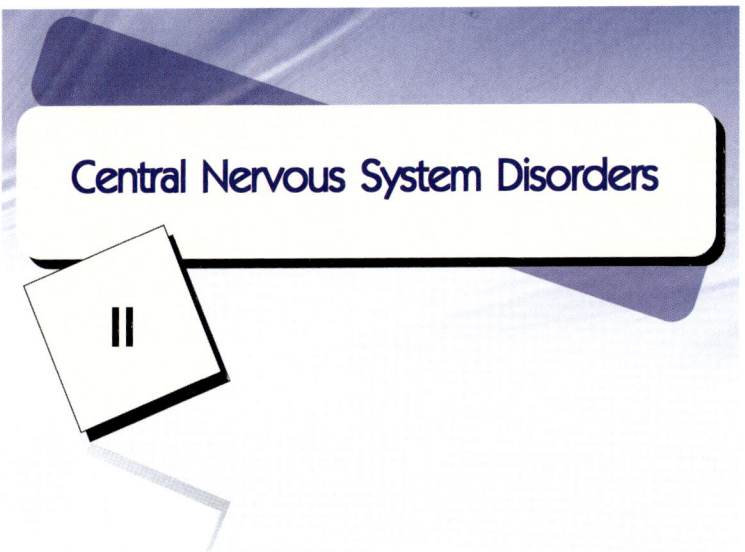

Central Nervous System Disorders

II

4

Post Resuscitation Management of Asphyxiated Neonates

Perinatal asphyxia (PA) is a major public health problem. As per the latest estimates, PA accounts for 9% (i.e. 0·8 million) of total Under-5 mortality (i.e. 8.8 millions) worldwide, being one of the three most common causes of neonatal deaths along with prematurity and bacterial infections.[1] Of a total of 2.7 million stillbirths globally, approximately 1.2 million occur during intrapartum period, largely owing to asphyxia.[2,3] NNPD (2002–2003) reported PA to be the commonest cause of still-births, accounting for 45.1% of all such cases.[4]

As reported in NNPD (2002–2003), Apgar scores of <7 was found at 1 minute in 8.4% while 2.4% had scores of <7 at 5 minutes of life of all intramural births at 18 neonatal units in India.[4] Oxygen was the most commonly used resuscitative measure in 9.5%, bag and mask ventilation in 6.3% and chest compressions in 0.8% while use of other medications in 0.5%. PA was responsible for 28.8% of all neonatal deaths. Manifestations of hypoxic ischemic encephalopathy (HIE) were seen in approximately 1.4% of all babies. Apart from neonatal deaths, asphyxia is responsible for lifelong neuromotor disability in a large number of children.

DEFINITIONS

There is no one definition of PA (Table 4.1). The definition of PA is context specific and can be sensitive, e.g. those given by WHO and NNPD for the purpose of deciding immediate care of newborn or a specific definition such as the one given by AAP for the purpose of giving a label or predicting the long-term outcome.

Table 4.1: Different definitions of perinatal asphyxia	
World Health Organization[3]	Failure to initiate and sustain breathing
NNPD Network[4]	• Moderate PA: Slow/gasping breathing or an Apgar score of 4 to 6 at 1 minute· Severe PA: No breathing or an Apgar score of 0–3 at 1 minute of age
American Academy of Pediatrics and American College of Obstetrics and Gynecology[5]	**Presence of all of the following criteria:** • Profound metabolic or mixed acidemia (pH <7.00) in umbilical cord blood • Persistence of low Apgar scores less than 3 for more than 5 minutes • Signs of neonatal neurologic dysfunction (e.g. seizures, encephalopathy, tone abnormalities) • Evidence of multiple organ involvement (such as that of kidneys, lungs, liver, heart and intestine).

CONSEQUENCES OF ASPHYXIA

PA is a multi-organ system disorder affecting virtually every organ system in the body including brain, heart, lungs, kidneys and intestine. Care of asphyxiated infant therefore should be oriented towards determining the severity of dysfunction of critical organ systems and provide appropriate support to allow recovery to happen. Many of these complications are potentially fatal. In term infants with asphyxia, renal, CNS, cardiac and lung dysfunction occur in 50%, 28%, 25% and 25% cases, respectively.[6] The extent of organ system dysfunction determines the early and late outcomes of an asphyxiated neonate (Table 4.2).

Table 4.2: Organ system dysfunction in perinatal asphyxia	
CNS	Hypoxic ischemic encephalopathy, intracranial hemorrhage, seizures, long-term neurological sequelae
Cardiac	Myocardial dysfunction, valvular dysfunction, rhythm abnormalities, congestive cardiac failure
Renal	Hematuria, acute tubular necrosis, renal vein thrombosis
Pulmonary	Delayed adaptation, respiratory failure, meconium aspiration, surfactant depletion, primary pulmonary hypertension
GI tract	Necrotizing enterocolitis, hepatic dysfunction
Hematological	Thrombocytopenia, coagulation abnormalities
Metabolic	Acidosis, hypoglycemia, hypocalcemia, hyponatremia

Hypoxic ischemic encephalopathy (HIE) refers to the CNS dysfunction associated with PA, and is often the prime concern while managing asphyxiated neonate as it can kill the neonate, and carries a potential to cause serious long-term neuromotor sequelae among survivors.

A detailed classification of HIE in terms of neonates was proposed by Sarnat and Sarnat.[7] A simpler and practical classification of HIE by severity of manifestations provided by Levene et al is recommended for routine use (Table 4.3).[8] Thomson score is based on features of HIE and it can have a maximum (worst) score of 22. A score of 15 or more has shown a positive predictive value of 92%, negative predictive value of 82%, sensitivity of 71% and specificity of 96% for abnormal outcome at 12 months of age.[21]

Table 4.3: Classification of HIE

Levene[8]

Feature	Mild	Moderate	Severe
Consciousness	Irritable	Lethargy	Comatose
Tone	Hypotonia	Marked hypotonia	Severe hypotonia
Seizures	No	Yes	Prolonged
Sucking/ respiration	Poor suck	Unable to suck	Unable to sustain spontaneous respiration

Thompson score[21]

Sign	0	1	2	3
Tone	Normal	Hypertonia	Hypotonia	Flaccid
Level of consciousness	Normal	Hyperalert/Stare	Lethargic	Comatose
Fits	Normal	<3 per day	>2 per day	
Posture	Normal	Fisting, cycling	Strong distal flexion	Decerebrate
Moro	Normal	Partial	Absent	
Grasp	Normal	Poor	Absent	
Suck	Normal	Poor	Absent	
Respiration	Normal	Hyperventilation	Brief apnea	IPPV (apnea)
Fontanel	Normal	Full, not tense	Tense	

Evolution of HIE Changes

HIE evolves gradually beginning from the time of insult to hours and days later (Table 4.4). The initial hypoxic-ischemic

Table 4.4: Clinical features of severe HIE in time frame	
Birth to 12 hours	• Decreased alertness and tone
	• Convulsions
	• Periodic breathing or respiratory failure
	• Intact pupillary and occulomotor responses
12 to 24 hours	• Change in alertness level
	• Apneic spells
	• Increase in convulsions
	• Jitteriness
	• Weakness in proximal limbs
	• In term babies, upper limbs more involved than lower limbs and hemiparesis
	• In preterms, lower limbs more involved
24 to 72 hours	• Further decrease in alertness
	• Pupillary and occulomotor disturbances
	• Respiratory arrest
	• In premature babies, intraventricular hemorrhage and periventricular hemorrhagic infarction
After 72 hours	• Persistent and diminishing stupor
	• Abnormal sucking, swallowing, gag and tongue movements
	• Hypotonia more common than hypertonia, weakness in proximal limbs
	• In term babies, upper limbs more involved than lower limbs and hemiparesis
	• In preterms, lower limbs more involved, hemiparesis

event results in infarction of the brain tissue (primary energy failure). The subsequent injury (secondary injury) is mediated by reperfusion and free radicals in an-area surrounding the necrotic area (penumbra). The penumbra undergoes a programmed neuronal death (apoptosis) even after the hypoxic insult is over. The time gap between these two phases could be 6 to 24 hrs, and provides a window to institute specific therapeutic intervention.

MANAGEMENT OF A NEONATE WITH PERINATAL ASPHYXIA

The management of asphyxiated babies is mainly supportive and involves maintaining optimum oxygenation, ventilation, perfusion, metabolic milieu and control of seizures.

Delivery Room Care

- Obtain arterial cord blood for analysis: After cutting the cord, apply additional clamp on umbilical cord on placental side keeping a cord segment of 10 to 15 cm between two clamps.
- Take a heparinized syringe and puncture the cord (from clamped segment, once placenta is out and resuscitation is over) to take blood sample from umbilical artery.

Presence of metabolic acidosis (pH <7.00 and base deficit greater than 16 mmol/L) indicates relatively long standing asphyxia (many minutes to hours), while presence of respiratory acidosis in absence of metabolic acidosis indicates presence of acute asphyxia (minutes) as in cord prolapse, acute abruption of placenta, etc.

Cord Blood Gas in Asphyxia: What is Evidence?

A recent meta-analysis has shown a good correlation of cord ABG abnormalities (pH <7.00 and base deficit e"16 mmol/l) with short term (mortality, HIE, IVH or PVL) and long term prognosis (cerebral palsy).

Low arterial cord pH was significantly associated with neonatal mortality (odds ratio 16.9, 95% CI 9.7 to 29.5), HIE (OR: 13.8, 95% CI-6.6 to 28.9), IVH or PVL (OR: 2.9, 95% CI-2.1 to 4.1), and cerebral palsy (OR: 2.3, 95% CI: 1.3 to 4.2).[17]

Transfer the infant to NICU if
- Apgar score 0–3 at 1 minute
- Prolonged bag and mask ventilation (60 seconds or more)
- Chest compression

Even babies transferred to mother should be monitored frequently in the first 48–72 hours for development of any features suggestive of HIE.

NICU Care

1. Maintain normal temperature
   - After drying, place the baby under the radiant warmer.
   - Maintain normal body temperature of the baby.
   - Avoid hyperthermia.[9]
2. Maintain normal oxygenation and ventilation
   - Assess the infant for adequacy of oxygenation and ventilation and provide support as needed.
   - Keep under oxygen hood in case of adequate spontaneous breathing.

- Assisted ventilation is required if there is apnea or spontaneous respiration is inadequate or there is continuing hypoxia or hypercarbia.
- Maintain saturations between 90% and 95% and avoid any hypoxia or hyperoxia.
- Measure arterial blood gas if any respiratory or perfusion abnormalities are present (maintain pO_2 between 60 torr and 90 torr and pCO_2 at 40 to 45 torr). Avoid hypocarbia, as this would reduce the cerebral perfusion, and hypercarbia, which can increase intracranial pressure and predispose the baby to intracranial bleed.

3. Maintain normal tissue perfusion
   - Ensure normal perfusion, i.e. normal blood pressure, capillary refill time of less than 3 seconds, normal urine output, and absence of metabolic acidosis.
   - Start intravenous fluid in all infants with Apgar scores <4 at 1 minute or <7 at 5 minutes of age or a baby that is having respiratory problems, encephalopathy or abnormal tone.
   - In sick babies, place arterial line for guiding management of blood pressure. BP should be tightly maintained in normal range according to gestation and postnatal age specific BP charts avoiding wider fluctuation.[11]
   - If the tissue perfusion is inadequate, infuse normal saline (or Ringer's lactate) 10 mL/kg over 5–10 min.
   - Administer dobutamine (preferred) or dopamine to maintain adequate cardiac output as required.
   - Do not restrict fluid routinely as this practice may predispose the babies to hypoperfusion. Restrict fluid only if there is hyponatremia (serum sodium <120 mg/dL) secondary to syndrome of inappropriate secretion of ADH (SIADH) or if there is renal failure. Do echocardiography in infants needing ionotropic support and to assess contractibility. It helps in appropriate management of perfusion.[20]

4. Maintain normal hematocrit and metabolic milieu
   - Check blood glucose levels and maintain it between 75 mg/dL and 100 mg/dl.
   - Check hematocrit. Correct Anemia and maintain hematocrit between 45% and 55%. If the venous hematocrit in a baby is above 65%, bring it down to 55% by partial exchange transfusion using normal saline.

- Check blood gases to detect metabolic acidosis as needed and maintain pH above 7.30.
- In case of severe asphyxia, provide calcium in a maintenance dose of 4 mL/kg/day (of 10% calcium gluconate) for 1–2 days as a continuous infusion or as 1:1 diluted boluses, slowly under cardiac monitoring and maintain serum calcium concentration in the normal range.

5. Treat seizures
   - Refer to seizure protocol.
6. Nutrition
   - Start oral feeding once baby is hemodynamically stable, does not require vasopressors and has a normal abdominal examination (no distension, passing stool and normal bowel sounds).
7. Miscellaneous
   - Administer Vitamin K (1 mg IM) to all infants with perinatal asphyxia.

ROLE OF SPECIAL INVESTIGATIONS

Electroencephalography (EEG)

EEG is not indicated routinely in all asphyxiated babies but it helps in the diagnosis and management of seizures and prognosticating the babies for long-term outcomes.

The prognosis is likely to be poor if the EEG shows:
1. Long periods of inactivity (more than 10 seconds)
2. Brief period of bursts (less than 6 seconds) with small amplitude bursts
3. Interhemispheric asymmetry and asynchrony
4. Isoelectric and low voltage (less than 5 microvolts)[25]

Amplitude-integrated electroencephalography (aEEG) is simplified form and can be performed on continuous basis in NICU. Following abnormalities would indicate poor prognosis:
- Wide fluctuations in the amplitude with the baseline voltages dropping to near zero
- Peak amplitudes under 5 mV
- Seizure spikes

While a normal aEEG may not necessarily mean that the brain is normal, a severe or moderately severe aEEG abnormality may indicate brain injury and a poorer outcome.

The time of onset of sleep wake cycling (SWC) has a prognostic value. If SWC returns before 36 hours then outcome is good.[22]

Cranial Ultrasound (US)

Cranial US is not a good modality for detecting changes of HIE in the term babies. However, hypoechoic areas can be seen in very severe cases (having large areas of infection).

In preterm babies, US can pick up periventricular leuko-malacia and intraventricular-periventricular hemorrhage by serial cranial US during the first week of life.

Computed Tomography (CT)

CT has a role in initial evaluation of a baby with HIE if MRI is not readily accessible. In acute stage of HIE, CT in term babies show generalized low attenuation of brain parenchyma. However, several weeks after asphyxial insult, CT readily picks up diffuse cortical neuronal injury, injury to basal ganglia and thalamus, focal and multifocal ischemic brain injury as well as periventricular leucomalacia. CT has a limited role in identification of parasagittal cerebral injury.

Magnetic Resonance Imaging (MRI)

MRI is the best imaging modality for determining prognosis mostly in the term infants. Diffusion weighted MRI can pick up abnormalities within 24 to 48 hours after birth (though optimal time is 2 to 3 days), whereas conventional MRI shows abnormalities in the first 3 to 4 days. An altered signal at the level of the posterior limb of the internal capsule and abnormalities of thalami and basal ganglia in term infants and that of white and grey matter at term equivalent age in preterm infants are strong predictors of subsequent risk of poor neurodevelopmental outcome.[13,14,24] Another common pattern of injury is injury to the watershed regions.

NEWER MODES OF THERAPY

Therapeutic Hypothermia

Institution of moderate therapeutic hypothermia (TH; 33–34°C) in infants of at least 36 wks gestation (not preterm) with moderate to severe encephalopathy (not mild) in intensive care unit settings initiated within 4–6 hrs and continued for

72 hrs of age has shown to reduce mortality and neuro-morbidity by 18 months of age.[10,12] TH can be instituted by selectively cooling the head or the whole body. It is a safe modality in settings where intensive care facilities to manage sickest neonates are available.

TH has become standard of care in developed countries. However, in low to middle income countries where the patient profile is different (concomitant IUGR, infection and nutritional deficiencies), and there is a paucity of intensive care, and many births occur out of hospital, small studies have shown that there may be increase in mortality with TH. The true value of TH in low to middle income countries is yet to be tested.[18]

Therapeutic Hypothermia: What is Evidence?
A Cochrane review (8 RCTs; 638 term infants with moderate/severe encephalopathy and evidence of intrapartum asphyxia) showed that TH reduced combined outcome of mortality or major neurodevelopmental disability by 24% to 18 months of age.

Prophylactic Phenobarbitone

Some interest has been generated in the protective role of prophylactic phenobarbitone in newborns with perinatal asphyxia. A dose of 40 mg/kg administered prophylactically was associated with a better neurodevelopmental outcome at 3 years of age.[15] However, the Cochrane review database systematic review by Evans' et al (2007) that included the 5 RCTs derived no difference in the risk of death, neuro-disability.[16] Another study using 40 mg/kg within 1st hour showed a significant reduction in HIE with no difference in complications.[19] Recommendation for use of prophylactic phenobarbitone still awaits further studies.

Drugs under Investigation

A large number of drugs is under investigation for neuro-protection in HIE. These need to be used in the early period of hypoxic ischemic injury. They act by causing blockade of free radical generation (allopurinol, oxypurinol), scavenging of oxidants (superoxide dismutase, glutathione, N-acetyl cysteine and alpha tocopherol), calcium channel blockade (flunarizine, nimodipine), blockage of NMDA receptors (magnesium, MK801, dextromethorphan) and blockage of inflammatory mediators (phospholipase A_2, indomethacin). Corticosteroids have no role on the treatment of HIE. Likewise, the current evidence does not support the use of mannitol in the management of HIE.

FOLLOW-UP

Follow all the neonates with the moderate and severe asphyxia, especially those with stage II and III HIE staging. They should have a complete neurological assessment and intervention if needed during the follow-up. A formal psychometric assessment at 18 months should be performed in all these babies.

LONG-TERM OUTCOME

Among the infants who survive severe HIE, the sequelae include mental retardation, epilepsy and cerebral palsy of varying degrees. The latter can be in the form of hemiplegia, paraplegia or quadriplegia. Such infants need careful evaluation and support. They may need to be referred to specialized clinics capable of providing coordinated comprehensive follow-up care.

Predictors of mortality and neurological morbidity after perinatal hypoxic ischemic insult

- Extended very low Apgar scores (at 20 minutes)
- Time to establish spontaneous respiration (for 30 or more minutes)
- Abnormal neurological examination (severe HIE)
- Brain imaging (USG, MRI)
- Other investigations (EEG, amplitude integrated EEG, evoked potentials like BERA)

The incidence of long-term complications depends on the severity of HIE. Up to 80% of babies with severe HIE die whereas rest 20% have neurological sequelae. Up to 80% of surviving infants with severe HIE develop serious complications, 10–20% develop moderately serious disabilities. The incidence of death is up to 5% and that of neurological sequelae is up to 24% after moderate birth asphyxia. Infants with mild HIE tend to be free from death or any neurological sequelae.[26,27]

A recently published follow-up study on long-term outcomes of whole body hypothermia for neonatal hypoxic ischemic encephalopathy revealed the rate of combined end point of death or an IQ score of less than 70 at 6 to 7 years of age to be lower (though not a significant difference) among children undergoing whole body hypothermia (47%) than among those undergoing usual care (62%) (P=0.06). Death occurred in 28% and 44% (P=0.04), respectively and death or severe disability occurred in 41% and 60% (P=0.03), respectively.[28]

REFERENCES

1. Black RE, Cousens S, Johnson HL, Lawn JE, Rudan I, Bassani DG, Jha P, Campbell H, Walker CF, Cibulskis R, Eisele T, Liu L, Mathers C. Child Health Epidemiology Reference Group of WHO and UNICEF. Global, regional and national causes of child mortality in 2008: a systematic analysis. Lancet 2010 Jun 5;375(9730):1969–87. Epub 2010 May 11.

2. Lawn JE, Blencowe H, Pattinson R, Cousens S, Kumar R, Ibiebele I, Gardosi J, Day LT, Stanton C. Lancet's Stillbirths Series Steering Committee. Stillbirths: Where? When? Why? How to make the data count? Lancet 2011 Apr 23;377(9775):1448–63. Epub 2011 Apr 13.

3. World Health Organizaton. Perinatal mortality: A Listing of Available Information. FRH/MSM.96.7. Geneva:WHO,1996.

4. Report of the National Neonatal Perinatal Database (National Neonatology Forum, India) 2003.

5. Committee on fetus and newborn, American Academy of Pediatrics and Committee on Obstetric Practice, American College of Obstetrics and Gynecology. Use and abuse of the APGAR score. Pediatr 1996;98:141–2.

6. Perlman JM, Tack ED, Martin T, Shackelford G, Amon E. Acute systemic organ injury in term infants after asphyxia. Am J Dis Child 1989;143:617–20.

7. Sarnat HB, Sarnat MS. Neonatal encephalopathy following fetal distress: A clinical and electroencephalographic study. Arch Neurol 1976;33:695–706.

8. Levene MI. The asphyxiated newborn infant. In: Levene MI, Lilford RJ. Fetal and neonatal neurology and neuro-surgery. Edinburgh: Churchil Livingstone 1995;405–26.

9. Laptook A, Tyson J, Shankaran S, McDonald S, Ehrenkranz R, Fanaroff A, Donovan E, Goldberg R, O'Shea TM, Higgins RD, Poole WK. National Institute of Child Health and Human Development Neonatal Research Network. Elevated temperature after hypoxic-ischemic encephalopathy: risk factor for adverse outcomes. Pediatrics 2008;122:491–9.

10. Edwards AD, Brocklehurst P, Gunn AJ, Halliday H, Juszczak E, Levene M, Strohm B, Thoresen M, Whitelaw A, Azzopardi D. Neurological outcomes at 18 months of age after moderate hypothermia for perinatal hypoxic ischaemic encephalopathy: synthesis and meta-analysis of trial data. BMJ. 2010 Feb 9;340:c363. doi:10.1136/bmj.c363.

11. Zubrow AB, Hulman S, Kushner H, Falkner B. Determinants of blood pressure in infants admitted to neonatal intensive care units: a prospective multicentre study. Journal of Perinatology 1995;15:472–9.

12. John S. Wyatt, Peter D. Gluckman, Ping Y. Liu, Denis Azzopardi, Roberta Ballard, A. David Edwards, Donna M. Ferriero, Richard A. Polin, Charlene M. Robertson, Marianne Thoresen, Andrew Whitelaw, Alistair J. Gunn for the CoolCap Study Group Determinants of Outcomes after Head Cooling for Neonatal Encephalopathy. Pediatrics 2007;119:912–21.

13. Lianne J, Woodward, Peter J Anderson, Nicole C Austin, Kelly Howard, Terrie E Inder. Neonatal MRI to predict neuro-developmental outcomes in preterm infants. NEJM 2006; 355: 685–94.

14. Thayyil S, Chandrasekaran M, Taylor A, Bainbridge A, Cady EB, Chong WK, Murad S, Omar RZ, Robertson NJ. Cerebral magnetic resonance biomarkers in neonatal encephalopathy: a meta-analysis. Pediatrics 2010 Feb;125:e382–95. Epub 2010, Jan 18.

15. Hall RT, Hall FK, Daily DK. High-dose phenobarbital therapy in term newborn infants with severe perinatal asphyxia: a randomized, prospective study with three-year follow-up. J Pediatr. 1998;132:345–8.

16. Evans DJ, Levene MI, Tsakmakis M. Anticonvulsants for preventing mortality and morbidity in full term newborns with perinatal asphyxia. Cochrane Database Syst Rev 2007;18:CD001240.

17. Malin GL, Morris RK, Khan KS. Strength of association between umbilical cord pH and perinatal and long term outcomes: systematic review and meta-analysis. BMJ. 2010;340:c1471.

18. Thayyil S. Brain Cooling in Babies: Are We Ready for Clinical Trials in Developing Countries? Indian Pediatr 2011;48:441–2.

19. Vargas-Origel A, Espinosa- Garcia JO, Muniz-Quezada E, Vargas-Nieto MA, Aguilar Garcia G, Prevention of hypoxic-ischemic encephalopathy with high dose, early phenobarbitol therapy. Gac Med Mex, 2004;140:147–53.
20. Ranjit MS. Cardiac abnormalities in birth asphyxia Indian J Paediatr 2000;67:529–32.
21. Thompson CM, et al. The value of a scoring system for hypoxic encephalopathy in predicting neurodevelopmental outcome, Acta Paediatr 1997;86:757.
22. Osredkar D, et al. Sleep wave cycling on amplitude integrated electroencephalography in term newborns with hypoxic ischaemic encephalopathy, Paediatrics 2005;115:327.
23. Ilves P, et al. Changes in Doppler ultrasonography in asphyxiated term infants with hypoxic ischemic encephalopathy, Acta Paediatr 1998;87:680.
24. Rutherford MA, et al. Abnormal magnetic resonance signal in the internal capsule predicts poor neurodevelopmental outcome in infants with hypoxic ischaemic encephalopathy, Paediatrics 1998; 102:323.
25. Menache CC, et al. Prognostic value of neonatal discontinuous EEG, Paediatr Neurol 2002;27:93.
26. Robertson C, Finer N. Term infants with hypoxic ischaemic encephalopathy: outcome at 3.5 years, Dev Med Child Neurol 1985;27:473–84.
27. Thornberg E, Thringer K, Odeback A, Milsom I. Birth Asphyxia: Incidence, clinical course and outcome in a Swedish population, Acta Paediatr 1995;84:927–32.
28. Shankaran S et al. Childhood outcomes after hypothermia for neonatal encephalopathy, N Engl J Med 2012;366:2985–92.

5

Seizures

Neonatal seizures (NS) are the most frequent and distinctive clinical manifestation of neurological dysfunction in the newborn infant. Infants with NS are at a high risk of neonatal death or neurological impairment/epilepsy disorders in later life. Though mortality due to NS has decreased from 40% to about 20% over the years, the prevalence of long-term neuro-development sequelae has largely remained unchanged at around 30%.[1] Improper and inadequate management of seizures could be one of the major reasons behind this phenomenon.

DEFINITION

A seizure is defined clinically as a paroxysmal alteration in neurologic function, i.e. motor, behavior and/or autonomic function. This definition includes:[2]

1. Epileptic seizures: Phenomena associated with corres-ponding EEG seizure activity, e.g. clonic seizures
2. Non-epileptic seizures: Clinical seizures without corres-ponding EEG correlate, e.g. subtle and generalized tonic seizures
3. EEG seizures: Abnormal EEG activity with no clinical correlation.

EPIDEMIOLOGY

The National Neonatal Perinatal Database (NNPD; 2002–03), which collected data from 18 tertiary care units across the country, has reported an incidence of 10.3 per 1000 live-births.[3] The incidence was found to increase with decreasing gestation and birth weight—for example, preterm infants had almost twice the incidence when compared to term neonates

(20.8 *versus* 8.4 per 1000 live-births) while very low birth weight infants had more than 4-fold higher incidence (36.1 per 1000 live-births).[4]

CLASSIFICATION

Four major types of NS have been identified[3] (Table 5.1).

Table 5.1: Investigations required in a neonate with seizures

Essential investigations (required in all with few exceptions*)	Additional investigations
• Blood sugar • Serum sodium and calcium • Cerebrospinal fluid (CSF) examination • Cranial ultrasound (US), and • Electroencephalography (EEG) and/or amplitude integrated EEG	• Hematocrit (if plethoric and/or at-risk for polycythemia) • Serum bilirubin (if icteric) • Serum magnesium • Arterial blood gas and anion gap (lethargy, vomiting, family history, etc.) • Imaging: CT and/or MRI (if no etiology found after essential investigations) • TORCH screen for congenital infections • Work-up for inborn errors of metabolism

*Given in the text

Subtle seizures: They are called subtle because the clinical manifestations are mild and are often missed. They are the commonest type, constituting about 50% of all seizures. Common examples of subtle seizures include:

1. *Ocular:* Tonic horizontal deviation of eyes or sustained eye opening with ocular fixation or cycled fluttering
2. *Oral–facial–lingual movements:* Chewing, tongue-thrusting, lip-smacking, etc.
3. *Limb movements:* Cycling, paddling, boxing-jabs, etc.
4. *Autonomic phenomena:* Tachycardia or bradycardia
5. *Apnea* may be a rare manifestation of seizures, particularly in term infants. Apnea due to seizure activity has an accelerated or a normal heart rate when evaluated 20 seconds after onset. Bradycardia is thus not an early manifestation in convulsive apnea but may occur later due to prolonged hypoxemia.

Clonic seizures: They are rhythmic movements of muscle groups. They have both fast and slow components, occur with a frequency of 1–3 jerks per second, and are commonly associated with EEG changes.

Tonic seizures: This type refers to a sustained flexion or extension of axial or appendicular muscle groups. These seizures may be focal or generalized and may resemble decerebrate (tonic extension of all limbs) or decorticate posturing (flexion of upper limbs and extension of lower limbs). Usually there are no EEG changes in generalized tonic seizures.

Myoclonic seizures: These manifest as single or multiple lightning fast jerks of the upper or lower limbs and are usually distinguished from clonic movements because of more rapid speed of myoclonic jerks, absence of slow return and predilection for flexor muscle groups. Common changes seen on the EEG include burst suppression pattern, focal sharp waves and hypsarrhythmia.

Myoclonic seizures carry the worst prognosis in terms of neurodevelopmental outcome and seizure recurrence. Focal clonic seizures have the best prognosis.

COMMON CAUSES OF NEONATAL SEIZURES[3, 5–9]

The most common causes of seizures as per the recently published studies from the country are hypoxic ischemic encephalopathy, metabolic disturbances (hypoglycemia and hypocalcemia) and meningitis.[8,9] Etiology could, however, vary between different centres depending upon the patient population (term *versus* preterm), level of monitoring (only clinical *versus* electrical and clinical seizures), etc.

Hypoxic-ischemic encephalopathy (HIE): HIE secondary to perinatal asphyxia is the commonest cause of NS. Most seizures due to HIE (about 50–65%) start within the first 12 hrs of life while the rest manifest by 24–48 hours of age. Additional problems like hypoglycemia, hypocalcemia and intracranial hemorrhage may co-exist in neonates with perinatal asphyxia and these should always be excluded. Subtle seizures are the most common type of seizures following HIE.

Metabolic causes: Common metabolic causes of seizures include hypoglycemia, hypocalcemia and hypomagnesemia. Rare causes include pyridoxine dependency and inborn errors of metabolism (IEM).

Infections: Meningitis should be excluded in all neonates with seizures. Meningoencephalitis secondary to intrauterine infections (TORCH group, syphilis) may also present as seizures in the neonatal period.

Intracranial hemorrhage: Seizures due to subarachnoid, intraparenchymal or subdural hemorrhage occur more often in term neonates, while seizures secondary to intraventricular hemorrhage (IVH) occur in preterm infants. Most seizures due to intracranial hemorrhage occur between 2 and 7 days of age. Seizures occurring in a term 'well baby' on day 2–3 of life is often due to subarachnoid hemorrhage.

Developmental defects: Cerebral dysgenesis and neuronal migration disorders are rare causes of seizures in the neonatal period.

Miscellaneous: They include polycythemia, maternal narcotic withdrawal, drug toxicity (e.g. theophylline, doxapram), local anesthetic injection into scalp and phacomatosis (e.g. tuberous sclerosis, incontinentia pigmenti). Accidental injection of local anesthetic into scalp may be suspected in the presence of fixed and dilated pupil and absence of doll's eye reflex. Multifocal clonic seizures on the 5th day of life may be related to low zinc levels in the CSF fluid (benign idiopathic neonatal convulsions).

Seizures due to SAH and late onset hypocalcemia carry a good prognosis for long-term neurodevelopmental outcome while seizures related to hypoglycemia, cerebral malformations and meningitis have a high risk for adverse outcome.

APPROACH TO AN INFANT WITH NEONATAL SEIZURES
(Fig. 5.1)[3, 6-7]

History

Seizure history: A complete description of the seizure should be obtained from the parents/attendant. History of associated eye movements, restraint of episode by passive flexion of the affected limb, change in color of skin (mottling or cyanosis), autonomic phenomena and whether the infant was conscious or sleeping at the time of seizure should be elicited. The day of life on which the seizures occurred may provide an important clue to its diagnosis. While seizures occurring on day 0–3 might be related to perinatal asphyxia, intracranial hemorrhage and metabolic causes, those occurring on day 4–7 may be due to sepsis, meningitis, metabolic causes and developmental defects.

Antenatal history: History suggestive of intrauterine infection, maternal diabetes and narcotic addiction should be elicited in the antenatal history. A history of sudden increase in fetal movements may be suggestive of intrauterine convulsions.

Perinatal history: Perinatal asphyxia is the commonest cause of neonatal seizures and a detailed history including history of fetal distress, decreased fetal movements, instrumental delivery, need for resuscitation in the labor room, Apgar scores and abnormal cord pH (< 7) and base deficit (>10 mEq/L) should be obtained. Use of a pudendal block for mid-cavity forceps may be associated with accidental injection of the local anesthetic into the fetal scalp.

Feeding history: Appearance of clinical features including lethargy, poor activity, drowsiness and vomiting after initiation of breastfeeding may be suggestive of inborn errors of metabolism. Late onset hypocalcemia should be considered in the presence of top feeding with cow's milk.

Family history: History of consanguinity in parents, family history of seizures or mental retardation and early fetal/ neonatal deaths would be suggestive of inborn errors of metabolism. History of seizures in either parent or sib(s) in the neonatal period may suggest benign familial neonatal convulsions (BFNC).

Examination

Vital signs: Heart rate, respiration, blood pressure, capillary refill time and temperature should be recorded in all infants.

General examination: Gestation, birth weight and weight for age should be recorded as they may provide important clues to the etiology—for example, seizures in a term 'well baby' may be due to subarachnoid hemorrhage while seizures in a large for date baby may be secondary to hypoglycemia. The neonate should also be examined for the presence of any obvious malformations or dysmorphic features.

CNS examination: Presence of a bulging anterior fontanel may be suggestive of meningitis or intracranial hemorrhage. A detailed neurological examination should include assessment of consciousness (alert/drowsy/comatose), tone (hypotonia or hypertonia) and fundus examination for chorioretinitis.

Systemic examination: Presence of hepatosplenomegaly or an abnormal urine odor may be suggestive of IEM. The skin should be examined for the presence of any neuro-cutaneous markers. Presence of hypopigmented macules or ash-leaf spot would be suggestive of tuberous sclerosis.

Investigations

Essential investigations: Investigations that should be considered in all neonates with seizures include blood sugar, serum sodium and calcium, cerebrospinal fluid (CSF) examination, cranial ultrasound (US), and electroencephalo-graphy (EEG). CSF examination should be done in all cases as seizure may be the first sign of meningitis. It should not be omitted even if another etiology such as hypoglycemia is present. CSF study may be withheld temporarily if severe cardio-respiratory compromise is present or even omitted in infants with severe birth asphyxia (documented abnormal cord pH/base excess and onset of seizures within 12–24 hrs of life).

One should carry out all these investigations even if one or more investigations are positive as multiple etiologies may coexist, e.g. sepsis, meningitis and hypoglycemia.

Additional investigations: These may be considered in neonates who do not respond to a combination of pheno-barbitone and phenytoin or earlier in neonates with specific features. These include neuroimaging (CT, MRI) screen for congenital infections (TORCH) and for inborn errors of metabolism (IEM). An arterial blood gas may have to be performed if IEM is strongly suspected.

Imaging: Neurosonography is an excellent tool for detection of intraventricular and parenchymal hemorrhage but is unable to detect SAH and subdural hemorrhage. It should be done in all infants with seizures. CT scan should be done in all infants where an etiology is not available after the first line of investigations. It can be diagnostic in subarachnoid hemorrhage and developmental malformations. Magnetic resonance imaging (MRI) is indicated only if investigations do not reveal any etiology and seizures are resistant to usual anti-epileptic therapy. It can be diagnostic in cerebral dysgenesis, lissencephaly and other neuronal migration disorders.

Electroencephalogram (EEG): EEG has both diagnostic and prognostic role in seizures. It should be done in all neonates who need anti-convulsant therapy. Ictal EEG may be useful for the diagnosis of suspected seizures and also for diagnosis of seizures in muscle-relaxed infants. It should be done as soon as the neonate is stable enough to be transported for EEG, preferably within first week. EEG should be performed for at least one hour.[10] Inter-ictal EEG is useful for long-term prognosis of neonates with seizures. A background abnormality in both term and preterm neonates indicates a high risk for neurological sequelae. These changes include burst-suppression pattern, low voltage invariant pattern and electro-cerebral inactivity.

Amplitude integrated EEG (aEEG): This new method provides continuous monitoring of cerebral electrical activity at the bedside in critically sick newborns. aEEG is helpful in evaluating the background as well in identification of seizure activity in NS. As with conventional EEG, background abnormalities like burst-suppression or continuous low voltage pattern in aEEG also help in prognosticating the infant with seizures particularly in the setting of HIE. Seizure activity on aEEG is characterized by a rapid rise in both the lower and upper margins of the trace. Some seizures that are focal or relatively brief are, however, missed by this technique.[3]

Screen for congenital infections: TORCH screen and VDRL should be considered in the presence of hepatosplenomegaly, thrombocytopenia, intrauterine growth restriction, small for gestational age and presence of chorioretinitis.

Metabolic screen: This includes blood and urine ketones, urine reducing substances, blood ammonia, anion gap, urine and plasma aminoacidogram, serum and CSF lactate/pyruvate ratio.

MANAGEMENT OF SEIZURES

Initial Medical Management

The first step in successful management of seizures is to nurse the baby in thermoneutral environment and to ensure airway, breathing and circulation (TABC). Oxygen should be started, IV access should be secured and blood should be collected for glucose and other investigations. A brief relevant history should be obtained and quick clinical examination should be performed. All this should not require more than 2–5 minutes.

Correction of Hypoglycemia and Hypocalcemia

If glucostix shows hypoglycemia or if there is no facility to test blood sugar immediately, 2 mL/kg of 10% dextrose should be given as a bolus injection followed by a continuous infusion of 6–8 mg/kg/min.

If hypoglycemia has been treated or excluded as a cause of convulsions, the neonate should receive 2 mL/kg of 10% calcium gluconate IV over 10 minutes under strict cardiac monitoring. If serum calcium levels are suggestive of hypocalcemia, the newborn should receive calcium gluconate at 8 mL/kg/d for 3 days. If seizures continue despite correction of hypocalcemia, 0.25 mL/kg of 50% magnesium sulfate should be given intramuscularly.

Anti-epileptic Drug Therapy[3]

Anti-epileptic drugs (AED) should be considered in the presence of even a single clinical seizure since clinical observations tend to grossly under-estimate electrical seizures and facilities for continuous EEG monitoring are not universally available. If aEEG is being used, eliminating all electrical seizure activity should be the goal of AED therapy.[3] AED should be given if seizures persist even after correction of hypoglycemia/hypocalcemia (Fig. 5.1).

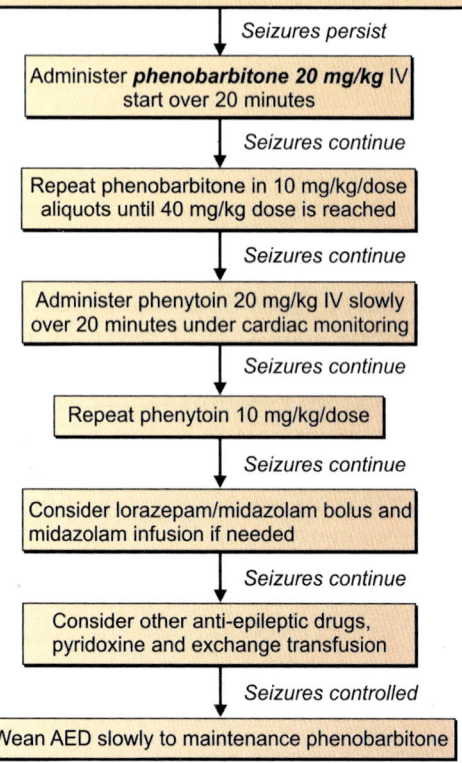

Fig. 5.1: Acute management of neonatal seizures

Phenobarbitone (Pb)

It is the drug of choice in neonatal seizures. The dose is 20 mg/kg/IV slowly over 20 minutes (not faster than 1 mg/kg/min). If seizures persist after completion of this loading dose, additional doses of phenobarbitone 10 mg/kg may be used every 20–30 minutes until a total dose of 40 mg/kg has been given. The maintenance dose of Pb is 3–5 mg/kg/day in 1–2 divided doses, started 12 hours after the loading dose.

Phenytoin

Phenytoin is indicated if the maximal dose of phenobarbitone (40 mg/kg) fails to resolve seizures or earlier, if adverse effects like respiratory depression, hypotension or bradycardia ensue with phenobarbitone. The dose is 20 mg/kg IV at a rate of not more than 1 mg/kg/min under cardiac monitoring. Phenytoin should be diluted in normal saline as it is incompatible with dextrose solution. A repeat dose of 10 mg/kg may be tried in refractory seizures. The maintenance dose is 3–5 mg/kg/d (maximum of 8 mg/kg/d) in 2–4 divided doses. Oral suspension has erratic absorption from gut and should be avoided in neonates.

Fosphenytoin, the prodrug of phenytoin, does not cause the same degree of hypotension or cardiac abnormalities, has high water solubility (can be given IM), and is less likely to lead to soft-tissue injury when compared with phenytoin. It is dosed in phenytoin equivalents—1.5 mg/kg of fosphenytoin is equivalent to 1 mg/kg of phenytoin.

Benzodiazepines

This group of drugs may be required in up to 15–20% of neonatal seizures. The commonly used benzodiazepines are lorazepam and midazolam. Diazepam is generally avoided in neonates because of its short duration of anti-epileptic effect but very prolonged sedative effect, narrow therapeutic index and the presence of sodium benzoate as a preservative. Lorazepam is preferred over diazepam as it has a longer duration of action and results in less adverse effects (sedation and cardiovascular effects). Midazolam is faster acting than lorazepam and may be administered as an infusion. It causes less respiratory depression and sedation than lorazepam. However, when used as continuous infusion, the infant has to be monitored for respiratory depression, apnea and brady-cardia *(equipment for resuscitation and assisted ventilation should be available at the bedside of all neonates given multiple doses of AED).*

Second-line AED: Evidence and Recommendations

The Cochrane review[11] found one study that randomized infants who failed to respond to phenobarbital to receive either lidocaine or midazolam as second-line agents. There was a trend for lidocaine to be more effective in reducing seizure burden (RR 0.40 95% CI 0.14 to 1.17) but both groups had similarly poor long-term outcomes assessed at one year.

Based on the available evidence, the WHO guidelines on neonatal seizures recommend either midazolam or lidocaine as the second-line AED in neonatal seizures.[12]

However, given the lack of robust evidence and constraints involved in providing respiratory support and/or monitoring in most neonatal units in India, it seems appropriate to use phenytoin as the second-line agent in neonates with seizures.

The doses of these drugs are given below:
- Lorazepam: 0.05 mg/kg IV bolus over 2–5 minutes; may be repeated
- Midazolam: 0.15 mg/kg IV bolus followed by infusion of 0.1 to 0.4 mg/kg/hour.
- According to Volpe, the expected control rate of neonatal clinical seizures to anti-convulsants is 40% to the initial 20 mg/kg loading dose of phenobarbitone, 70% to a total of 40 mg/kg of Pb, 85% to a 20 mg/kg of phenytoin and 95% to 100% to 0.05 to 0.1 mg/kg lorazepam.[1]

Anti-epileptic Drugs for Seizures Refractory to Above Treatment

In exceptional circumstances, when the seizures are refractory to phenobarbitone, phenytoin and midazolam, the following drugs might be tried:
- *Lidocaine:* It is usually administered as a bolus dose of 4 mg/kg IV followed by an infusion rate of 2 mg/kg/hr. It

is tapered over several days. Adverse effects include arrhythmias, hypotension and seizures. It should not be administered with phenytoin.
- *Paraldehyde:* A dose of 0.1–0.2 mL/kg/dose may be given IM or 0.3 mL/kg/dose mixed with coconut oil in 3:1 may be used by per rectal route. Additional doses may be used after 30 minutes and every 4–6 hourly. Adverse effects include pulmonary hemorrhage, pulmonary edema, hypotension and liver injury.
- *Sodium valproate:* Per rectal or IV route may be used in acute condition. The dose is 20–25 mg/kg/d followed by 5–10 mg/kg every 12 hours. It should, however, be used with caution in newborns given the uncertain risk of hepatotoxicity following its use.
- *Vigabatrin:* It has been used in neonates with infantile spasms. The dose is 50 mg/kg/day.
- *Topiramate:* It shows promise in neonatal seizures because of its potential neuroprotective effect against injury caused by seizures. It has been used for refractory infantile spasms in infants. The higher volume of distribution when compared with other drugs requires higher initial and maintenance doses of approximately 3 mg/kg.

Other Therapies

Pyridoxine: A therapeutic trial of pyridoxine is reserved as a last resort in refractory seizures. Intravenous route is the preferred method; however, suitable IV preparations are not universally available. Hence, intramuscular (IM) route may have to be used (1 mL of injection neurobion has 50 mg pyridoxine and 1 mL each may be administered both the sides in either the gluteal region or anterolateral aspect of thigh). It should ideally be done in the NICU as hypotension and apnea can occur.

Exchange transfusion: This is indicated in life-threatening metabolic disorders, accidental injection of local anesthetic, trans-placental transfer of maternal drugs (e.g. chlorpropamide) and bilirubin encephalopathy.

Maintenance of Anti-epileptic Therapy

Principles of AED used in older children and adults are applicable to neonates also. Monotherapy is the most appropriate strategy to control seizures. Attempts should be made to stop all anti-epileptic drugs and wean the baby to only phenobarbitone at 3–5 mg/kg/day. If seizures are uncontrolled or if clinical toxicity appears, a second AED may be added. The choice may vary from phenytoin, carbamazepine and valproic acid.

When to Discontinue AED

This is highly individualized and no specific guidelines are available. The goal is to discontinue phenobarbitone as early as possible. We usually try to discontinue all medications at

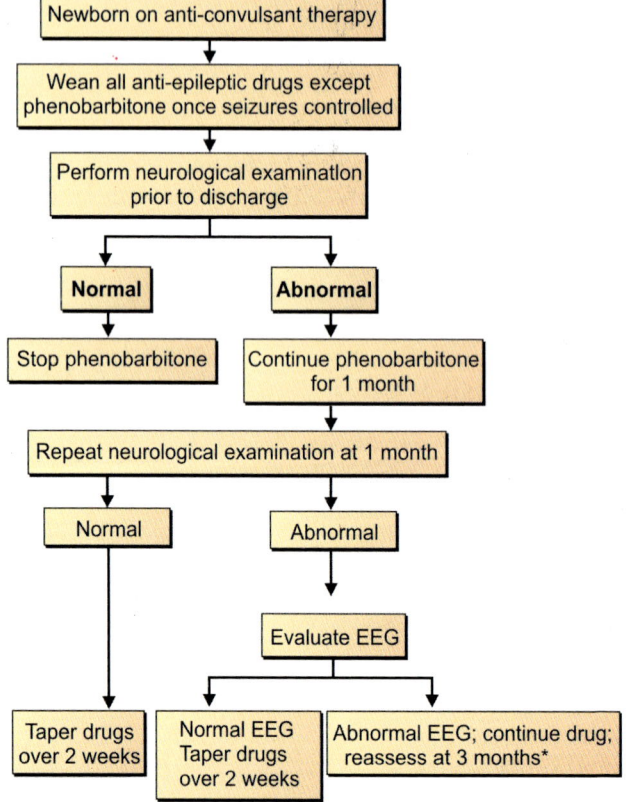

* Intractable seizures may need lifelong therapy; consider switching over to other (phenytoin or carbamazepine)

Fig. 5.2: Weaning of anti-convulsant therapy

discharge if clinical examination is normal, irrespective of etiology and EEG. If neurological examination is persistently abnormal at discharge, AED is continued and the baby is reassessed at one month. If the baby is normal on examination and seizure free at 1 month, phenobarbitone is discontinued over 2 weeks. If neurological assessment is not normal, an EEG is obtained. If EEG is not overtly paroxysmal, phenobarbitone is tapered and stopped. If EEG is overtly abnormal, the infant is reassessed in the same manner at 3 months and then 3 monthly till 1 year of age (Fig. 5.2*).*

REFERENCES

1. Tekgul H, Gauvreau K, Soul J, Murphy L, Robertson R, Stewart J, et al. The current etiologic profile and neurodevelopmental outcome of seizures in term newborn infants. Pediatrics 2006;117:1270–80.

2. Volpe JJ, editor. Neurology of the newborn. 5th edn. Philadelphia: Saunders Elsevier, 2008; p. 203–44.

3. Mizrahi EM, Kellaway P, eds. Diagnosis and management of neonatal seizures. Lippincott-Raven, 1998; p. 15–35.

4. National Neonatal Perinatal Database. Report for the year 2002–03. http://www.newbornwhocc.org/pdf/nnpd_report_2002–03.PDF (accessed Jan 8, 2012).

5. Painter MJ, Scher MS, Stein MD, Armatti S, Wang Z, Gardner JC, et al. Phenobarbitone compared with phenytoin for treatment of neonatal seizures. N Engl J Med 1999;341:485–9.

6. Rennie JM. Neonatal seizures. Eur J Pediatr 1997;156:83–7.

7. Laroia N. Controversies in diagnosis and management of neonatal seizures. Indian Pediatr 2000;37:367–72.

8. Iype M, Prasad M, Nair PM, Geetha S, Kailas L. The newborn with seizures—a follow-up study. Indian Pediatr 2008;45:749–52.

9. Kumar A, Gupta A, Talukdar B. Clinico-etiological and EEG profile of neonatal seizures. Indian J Pediatr 2007;74:33–7.

10. Wical BS. Neonatal seizures and electrographic analysis: evaluation and outcomes. Pediatr Neurol 1994;10:271–5.

11. Booth D, Evans DJ. Anticonvulsants for neonates with seizures. Cochrane Database Syst Rev. 2004 Oct. 18;(4):CD004218.

12. WHO. Guidelines on Neonatal Seizures. Geneva: World Health Organization, 2012.

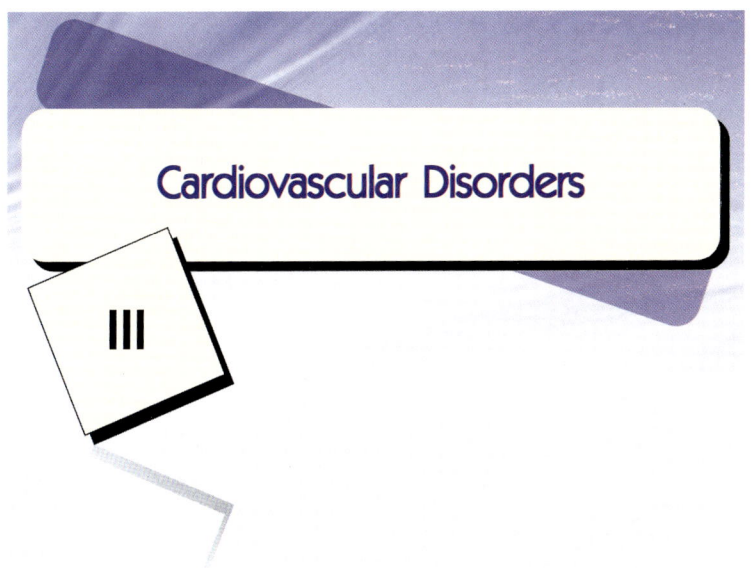

Cardiovascular Disorders

III

6. Patent Ductus Arteriosus in Preterm Neonates

Patent Ductus Arteriosus
in Preterm Neonates

INTRODUCTION

Patent ductus arteriosus (PDA) is a major morbidity seen in premature infants, with its incidence being inversely related to gestational age. Studies report incidence of 15–40% in very low birth weight infants (<1500 g) whereas in premature extremely low birth weight infants (<28 weeks; <1000 g), it is as high as 50–65%.[1,2]

The ductus arteriosus functionally close in term infants by 12–24 hrs, whereas the closure may be delayed by 3–5 days in preterm neonates.[3]

HEMODYNAMIC CONSEQUENCES OF PDA

The presence of PDA has significant effects on myocardial functions as well as systemic and pulmonary blood flow. Preterm newborns adapts by increasing the left ventricular contractility and thereby maintaining the effective systemic blood flow even when the left to right shunts equals 50% of the left ventricular output.[4] This is mainly accomplished by increase in stroke volume (SV) rather than heart rate.

Despite the increased left ventricular output, there is significant redistribution of blood flow to major organ systems. Usually there is shunting from systemic to pulmonary circulation called *ductal steal*, the maximum of which occurs at the beginning of the cardiac systole when the pressure gradient is maximum. Contrary to the belief that ductal run off occurs only in diastole, it is present all throughout the cardiac cycle. However, its effect on systemic circulation is best demonstrated on echocardiogram during diastole, as a retrograde flow in the descending aorta or other systemic vessels. This steal phenomenon may lead to systemic hypoperfusion, despite increased cardiac output. Hence, hemodynamically significant PDA has negative effect on cerebral circulation and oxygenation, which may lead to injury to the immature brain.

DIAGNOSIS OF PDA

Clinical Diagnosis of PDA and its Pitfalls

The clinical features of a PDA are mainly because of the hyperdynamic circulation caused by the shunt, resulting in bounding peripheral pulses (diagnosed clinically by easily palpable dorsalis pedis artery pulsation), wide pulse pressure (>25 mm of Hg), hyperactive precordium (visible precordial pulsations in more than 2 rib spaces), systolic murmur (usually ejection systolic; rarely pansystolic or continuous), persistent tachycardia, etc.

In a ventilated infant, fluctuating FiO_2, increasing pressure requirements, unexplained CO_2 retention or metabolic acidosis, recurrent apnea, etc. suggests a symptomatic ductus. However, diagnosis of PDA based on clinical features alone has mainly two pitfalls, i.e. low sensitivity and delay in detection. In studies, comparing clinical examination *versus* echocardiography, there was a delay of 1–4 days in diagnosis of PDA based on clinical findings alone.[5] Moreover, these signs were insensitive (sensitivity of 30–40%) and had low predictive value (60%).

Role of Echocardiography

Echocardiography is the gold standard for diagnosis as well as for assessing the severity of PDA.[6] The features suggestive of PDA include:

a. 2-D and color Doppler-short axis view: Direct visualization of the ductus is classically described as 'three-legged stool' appearance. In color Doppler, there is continuous flare in the main pulmonary artery (MPA).
b. Short axis view, pulsed Doppler: Turbulence in MPA due to left to right shunt jet flowing into MPA.
c. Four chamber view: Bowing of interatrial septum to right with enlarged left atrium and left ventricle.
d. Long axis view: LA/Ao ratio >1.5:1.
e. Raised left ventricular stroke volume.

However, these signs only establish the presence of a patent ductus and do not reflect the hemodynamic significance of the ductus. The echocardiographic markers indicating the hemodynamic significance and degree of shunting have been well described in a recent review (Table 6.1).[7]

Echocardiography also helps in ruling out other structural heart diseases and facility for in-house echocardiography enables serial monitoring as well as determines treatment responses.

Table 6.1: Echocardiographic markers of hemodynamically significant PDA

Echocardiography parameter*	No PDA	Mild	Moderate	Large
Features of ductus arteriosus				
Transductal diameter (mm)	0	<1.5	1.5–3.0	>3.0
Ductal velocity V_{max} (cm/sec)	0	>2	1.5–2.0	<1.5
Antegrade PA diastolic flow (cm/sec)	0	>30	30–50	>50
Pulmonary overcirculation				
Left atrial/aortic root width ratio	1.1 ± 0.2	<1.4:1	1.4–1.6	>1.6:1
Left ventricular/aortic root width ratio	1.9 ± 0.3	–	2.2 ± 0.4	2.27± 0.27
E wave/A wave ratio	<1	<1	1–1.5	>1.5
IVRT (ms)	<55	46–54	36–45	<35
LVSTI Systemic hypoperfusion	0.34 ± 0.09	–	0.26 ± 0.03	0.24 ± 0.07
Retrograde diastolic flow (as % of forward flow)	10	<30	30–50	>50
Aortic stroke volume (mL/kg)	≤ 2.25	–	–	≤ 2.34
Left ventricular output (mL/kg/min)	190–310	–	–	>314
LVO/SVC flow ratio	2.4 ± 0.3	–	–	4.5 ± 0.6

Empty boxes imply data not available. Reproduced with permission.[7]
*LVO: left ventricular output, SVC: superior vena cava, LVSTI: left ventricular stroke volume index, IVRT: isovolumic relaxation time, PWD: pulse wave Doppler, CWD: continuous wave Doppler, PA: pulmonary artery.

LIMITATIONS OF ECHOCARDIOGRAPHY

Even though echocardiography is the gold standard for diagnosis of PDA, it has its own limitations especially with regard to decisions on treatment.[8]

a. There is limited data to prove that functional echocardiography alters the neonatal outcomes.

b. Though the criteria for assessment of degree of shunting are established, there is lack of universal consensus regarding the best criteria for initiating treatment of PDA. No data till date supports decision to treat PDA based on echocardiography criteria alone.

c. Many neonatal units lack easy access to echocardiography and it is still a consultative tool, making serial assessments practically difficult.

d. Last but not the least, echocardiography is highly operator dependent and hence, it always needs to be used in conjunction with clinical findings.

Recommendations on Use of Echocardiography in PDA
1. In all infants in whom treatment of PDA is considered, echocardiography before treatment is essential to establish the diagnosis as well as to rule out other structural heart disease (e.g. duct dependent condition in which closure of PDA is contraindicated).
2. Post treatment echocardiography is required to document the response to treatment and assess the ductus.
3. Early targeted treatment based on echocardiographic criteria alone cannot be recommended at this point of time even though some large RCT (DETECT Trial, Australia) is currently evaluating the same.

Other Diagnostic Tests

The other diagnostic tests have very limited role, especially in preterm babies with PDA. Chest radiograph findings are non-specific and features like cardiomegaly and pulmonary plethora occurs late when significant PDA leads to congestive heart failure.

Biomarkers like brain natriuretic peptide (BNP) and N-terminal-pro-BNP which has shown good sensitivity and specificity. Though these markers are promising, their routine clinical use is yet to be proven.[9]

MANAGEMENT OF PDA

The management of PDA could be broadly divided into three aspects: pharmacological closure of ductus, general supportive measures and surgical ligation of the PDA.

To Treat or not to Treat a PDA

Despite three decades of intense research enrolling thousands of preterm infants, yet evidence for the long-term benefits of pharmacological closure of PDA is inconclusive and debatable.[9] The decision to treat PDA depends on the three factors—the spontaneous closure rate, adverse effect of ductal patency and risk-benefit of treatment.

In a recent systematic review, Benitz et al evaluated the effect of medical and surgical treatment either prophylactic or therapeutic on various outcomes.[10] Although all modes of interventions effectively closed the ductus, there was little beneficial effect on the outcomes. Hence, the therapeutic decision to treat ductus arteriosus is complex and there is a hot debate for conservative approach, especially in preterm infants more than 1000 g in whom the spontaneous closure rate is high.

PHARMACOLOGICAL CLOSURE OF PDA

Indications for Treatment*

Treatment should be considered in preterm infants with echocardiographically proven *hemodynamically significant* ductus arteriosus with one of the following conditions:

1. Features of congestive heart failure
2. Requiring prolonged respiratory support (invasive or non-invasive) unlikely to be due to other reasons

---

* These indications are based on pragmatic clinical decision and not based on high quality evidence.
* Treatment of all infants otherwise clinically asymptomatic based on echocardiography findings of hs-PDA alone is not warranted.
* Definition of hs-PDA: Presence of PDA > 1.5 mm with one of the following: LA/Ao ratio >1.5:1, LV/Ao ratio > 2.2:1, retrograde flow diastolic flow in descending aorta, celiac or cerebral arteries > 30% of antegrade flow; Left ventricular output > 320 mL/kg/min.

3. Unexplained oxygen requirement ($FiO_2 \geq 30\%$) or rising O_2 requirement on respiratory support
4. Recurrent apnea requiring respiratory support (CPAP/Nasal IMV/invasive ventilation) attributed to PDA

Mechanism and Agents of Pharmacological Closure

The pharmacological basis for medical therapy is the use of non-selective cyclo-oxygenase (COX) inhibitors, which inhibits prostaglandin synthesis and causes ductal constriction.[11] The two most widely studied and used non-selective COX inhibitors are
- Indomethacin
- Ibuprofen

Indomethacin Versus Ibuprofen

In the Cochrane meta-analysis, comparing ibuprofen with indomethacin in preterm <37 weeks gestation or low birth weight (<2500 gm), involving 20 trials enrolling 1092 infants, there was no difference in the failure of duct closure (RR = 0.94; 95% CI 0.76, 1.17).[12] Oral ibuprofen was used in 3 trials, while intravenous preparation was used in the rest. The ibuprofen group had significantly lower serum creatinine levels and decreased incidence of oliguria. There was 32% reduction in NEC in ibuprofen group (RR = 0.68; 95% CI 0.47, 0.99). There was no difference in other outcomes like mortality, reopening rate of PDA, need for surgical ligation of PDA, duration of ventilator support, chronic lung disease (CLD), IVH or ROP. Studies have shown a closure rate of 70–80% with either indomethacin or ibuprofen in preterm babies ≤ 32 weeks.

Oral Ibuprofen

Considering the fact that intravenous ibuprofen is not available in Indian market and the high cost for imported indomethacin injections, oral ibuprofen is a promising alternative. In randomized controlled trial of oral *versus* intravenous ibuprofen for VLBW infants with PDA, the rate of ductal closure was higher (oral = 84.3% *versus* IV = 62.5%; P = 0.04) and renal side effects were lesser in the oral ibuprofen group. Hence, oral ibuprofen may be a safe and easily available cheap option for treatment of PDA.[13]

There is very limited data on use of oral indomethacin and it is not generally recommended especially with oral iboprufen being easily available.

There is some evidence that oral paracetamol therapy has equal efficacy and lesser side effects, however, it requires confirmation in randomized trials.

Recommendations
1. Both indomethacin and ibuprofen are equally effective in closing PDA with closure rate of 70–80%.
2. Ibuprofen currently appears to be the superior option with its better safety profile, especially reduced NEC rates.
3. Infants
a. On significant amount of enteral feeds (at least 120 mL/kg/day)—oral ibuprofen
b. On parenteral fluids, partial feeds—IV indomethacin*
4. The question of which drug confers better long-term intact survival is yet unanswered.
*IV ibuprofen is not available in Indian market.

DOSAGE AND DURATION OF TREATMENT

Indomethacin (Short versus Long Course)

The two most commonly followed dosing schedules for indomethacin are the short course (3 intravenous doses at 12 hourly intervals with starting dose of 0.2 mg/kg followed by 0.1 mg/kg for babies less than 2 days of age, 0.2 mg/kg for 2–7 days and 0.25 mg/kg for >7 days old infants) and the long course (0.1 mg/kg per day for 6 doses) therapy (Table 6.2).

Table 6.2: Dosage of indomethacin and ibuprofen for pharmacological treatment of a PDA[16]

Indomethacin	IV Infusion over 30 min	• Loading dose: 0.2 mg/kg/dose
		• Subsequent doses (adjusted as per postnatal age)
		  – <2 days: 0.1 mg/kg/dose 12 hourly × 2 doses
		  – 2–7 days: 0.2 mg/kg/dose 12 hourly × 2 doses
		  – >7 days: 0.25 mg/kg/dose 12 hourly × 2 doses

Ibuprofen	IV or oral	• Loading dose: 10 mg/kg/dose • Subsequent dose: 5 mg/kg/dose 24 hourly × 2 doses

• *Following the first course, a second course with same dosage could be used in case of persistent PDA needing treatment or re-opening of the ductus with symptoms.*

• *Failure of medical treatment: Persistence of hemodynamically significant ductus or reopening despite two courses of treatment defines failure of medical treatment.*

The basis for the long course therapy is that, indomethacin induced prostaglandin inhibition is a transient phenomenon and the prostaglandin levels normalizes within 6–7 days after the short course therapy, which increases the chance for reopening of the duct.

A Cochrane meta-analysis compared short course (0.3 to 0.6 mg/kg, 3 doses) with the long course (0.6 to 1.6 mg/kg, 6 to 8 doses). Indomethacin therapy for PDA included 431 preterm infants from 5 randomized controlled trials, failed to reveal significant difference between the two groups as regards to PDA closure rate, need for surgical ligation or re-opening rates. The prolonged course group had nearly two times more risk of necrotizing enterocolitis (NEC) as compared to the conventional dose group (RR = 1.87, 95% CI 1.07, 3.27). Hence, prolonged long course treatment cannot be recommended for routine treatment of PDA.[14,15]

RECOMMENDATION ON DOSAGE

Side Effects and Monitoring

Adverse effects of treatment with NSAIDS include
- Renal compromise due to its effect on COX 1,
- Bleeding tendency due to its effect on platelet function, and
- Increased risk of necrotizing enterocolitis.

Monitoring during Therapy

- Baseline   Urine output, RFT, platelet count
- Daily   Urine output
- Alternate day   RFT, platelet counts (daily if baseline counts are < 150,000/mm^3

Contraindications

- Renal: Urine output < 0.6 mL/kg/h, blood urea > 40 mg/dL, creatinine > 1.8 mg/dL
- Bleeding: Bleeding from IV sites, skin bleeds, gastrointestinal bleeding, enlarging or evolving intraventricular hemorrhage (IVH), platelet count < 60,000/mm^3
- Gastrointestinal: Necrotizing enterocolitis; blood in stool

GENERAL SUPPORTIVE MEASURES

Fluid Restriction

In Cochrane meta-analysis, restriction of mean fluid intake to 120 mL/kg/day as compared to 160 mL/kg/day in the initial few weeks of life is found to be beneficial with lower incidence of PDA, BPD and mortality.[17]

Role of Furosemide and Dopamine in Medical Management of PDA

Routine use of furosemide in indomethacin treated symptomatic PDA is not recommended and is contraindicated in presence of dehydration.[19,20]

Low dose dopamine is considered to be beneficial in reversing indomethacin induced oliguria in preterm babies with PDA. However, there is no evidence to support this notion. In the Cochrane meta-analysis by Barrington et al[21] use of dopamine in indomethacin treated symptomatic PDA showed improvement in urine output but there was no effect on serum creatinine or incidence of oliguria. The use of dopamine had no effect on the rate of failure for ductal closure. The evidence for effect of dopamine on cerebral circulation, IVH or death before discharge is insufficient. Hence, use of dopamine for prevention of renal dysfunction induced by COX inhibitors cannot be recommended.

Mechanical Ventilation Strategy

In infants on ventilator support with hs-PDA, using slightly higher PEEP and lower Ti might be helpful, though data is very limited.[18]

Recommendations

1. In clinically symptomatic or echocardiographically diagnosed PDA, it is recommended to restrict parenteral fluid intake to 120 mL/kg/day, provided other parameters like urine output, serum Na, urine specific gravity, etc. are within normal limits.
2. Infants on full enteral feeds with hs-PDA, a fluid intake of up to 150 ml/kg/day may be used and calorie density may be increased in case of inadequate weight gain.
3. No role for routine use of dopamine in treating NSAID induced oliguria.
4. No role for routine use of furosemide in treatment of PDA except in case of established congestive heart failure.

SURGICAL LIGATION OF PDA

It is reserved for infants with symptomatic hs-PDA with
1. Failure of medical therapy
2. Contraindications to medical therapy

Studies have also shown in preterm <28 weeks gestation that need for surgical ligation of PDA is an independent risk factor for increased rates of BPD, ROP and adverse neuro-developmental outcome.[22]

PDA and Neonatal Outcomes

The presence of PDA has been associated with adverse neonatal outcomes like BPD and NEC.[23,24] However, none of the studies have shown any cause-effect relationship and studies have failed to consistently show association between symptomatic PDA and adverse outcomes like cerebral palsy, cognitive delay, ROP, NEC or BPD once adjusted for prematurity and perinatal factors.[22]

REFERENCES

1. Van Overmeire B, Van de Broek H, Van Laer P, Weyler J, Vanhaesebrouck P. Early *versus* late indomethacin treatment for patent ductus arteriosus in premature infants with respiratory distress syndrome. J Pediatr 2001;138:205–11.
2. Fanaroff AA, Stoll BJ, Wright LL, et al. Trends in neonatal morbidity and mortality for very low birth weight infants. Am J Obstet Gynecol. 2007;196:147e1–8.
3. Clyman R I. Mechanisms regulating the ductus arteriosus. Biol Neonate 2006;89:330–35.
4. Shimada S, Kasai T, Konishi M, Fujiwara T. Effects of patent ductus arteriosus on left ventricular output and organ blood flows in preterm infants with respiratory distress syndrome treated with surfactant. J Pediatr 1994;125:270–77.
5. Skelton R, Evans N, Smythe J. A blinded comparison of clinical and echocardiographic evaluation of the preterm infant for patent ductus arteriosus. J Paediatr Child Health 1994;30:406–11.
6. Evans N, Malcolm G, Osborn D, Kluckow M. Diagnosis of patent ductus arteriosus in preterm infants. NeoReviews 2004;5:86–97.

7. Sehgal A, McNamara PJ. Does echocardiography facilitate determination of hemodynamic significance attributable to the ductus arteriosus? Eur J Pediatr 2009;168:907–14.

8. Kluckow M, Seri I, Evans N· Functional Echocardiography: an emerging clinical tool for the Neonatologist. J Pediatr. 2007 Feb;150(2):125–30.

9. Sasi A, Deorari AK. Patent ductus arteriosus in preterm infants. Indian Pediatr 2011;48:301–8.

10. Benitz WE. Treatment of persistent patent ductus arteriosus in preterm infants: time to accept the null hypothesis. Journal of Perinatology 2010;30:241–52.

11. Narayanan-Sankar M, Clyman RI. Pharmacologic closure of patent ductus arteriosus in the neonate. NeoReviews 2003;4:215–21.

12. Ohlsson A, Walia R, Shah SS. Ibuprofen for the treatment of patent ductus arteriosus in preterm and/or low birth weight infants. Cochrane Database Syst Revs. 2010;4:CD003481.

13. Cherif A, Khrouf N, Jabnoun S, Mokrani C, Amara MB, Guellouze N, et al. Randomized pilot study comparing oral ibuprofen with intravenous ibuprofen in very low birth weight infants with patent ductus arteriosus. Pediatrics 2008;122: e1256–61.

14. Herrera C, Holberton J, Davis PG. Prolonged *versus* short course of indomethacin for the treatment of patent ductus arteriosus in preterm infants. Cochrane Database Syst Rev. 2007;2:CD003480.

15. Gork AS, Ehrenkranz RA, Bracken MB. Continuous *versus* intermittent bolus doses of indomethacin for patent ductus arteriosus closure in symptomatic preterm infants. Cochrane Database Syst Rev. 2008;1:CD006071.

16. Clyman RI. Patent ductus arteriosus in preterm neonates. In Avery's diseases of the newborn. Eds: Taeush HW, Ballard RA. 7th edn. WB Saunders, p.699–710.

17. Bell EF, Acarregui MJ. Restricted *versus* liberal water intake for preventing morbidity and mortality in preterm infants. Cochrane Database Syst Rev 2000;(2):CD000503.

18. Vanhaesebrouck S, Zonnenberg I, Vandervoort P, Bruneel E, Van Hoestenberghe M, Theyskens C. Conservative treatment for patent ductus arteriosus in the preterm Arch. Dis. Child Fetal Neonatal Ed 2007;92:F244–7.

19. Green TP, Thompson TR, Johnson De, Lock JE. Furosemide promotes patent ductus arteriosus in premature infants with respiratory distress syndrome. N Engl J Med 1983;308:743–8.

20. Brion LP, Campbell DE. Furosemide for prevention of morbidity in indomethacin treated infants with patent ductus arteriosus. Cochrane Database Syst Rev. 2001;3:CD001148.

21. Barrington KJ, Brion LP. Dopamine *versus* no treatment to prevent renal dysfunction in indomethacin treated preterm newborn infants. Cochrane Database Syst Rev. 2002;3:CD003213.

22. Chrone N, Leonard C, Piecuch R, Clyman R I. Patent ductus arteriosus and its treatment as risk factors for neonatal and neurodevelopmental morbidity. Pediatrics 2007;119:1165–74.

23. Rojas MA, Gonzalez A, Bancalari E, Claure N, Poole C, Silva-Neto G: Changing trends in the epidemiology and pathogenesis of neonatal chronic lung disease. J Pediatr 1995;126:605–10.

24. Dollberg S, Lusky A, Reichman B. Patent ductus arteriosus, indomethacin and necrotizing enterocolitis in very low birth weight infants: a population-based study. J Pediatr Gastroenterol Nutr 2005;40:184–8.

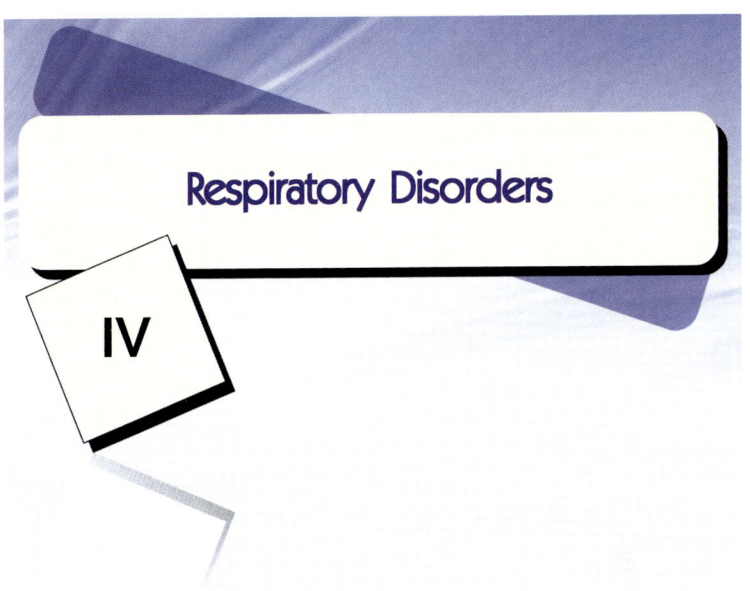

Respiratory Disorders

IV

7 Respiratory Distress

Respiratory distress in newborn is one of the commonest conditions contributing to 30–40% of admissions in NICU.[1] Respiratory distress occurs in 2.2% of all newborns and in almost 60% of the infants below 1000 g (ELBW infants).[2]

DEFINITION

Respiratory distress is defined as presence of any two of the following features[3]:
1. Respiratory rate >60/minute
2. Subcostal/intercostal recessions
3. Expiratory grunt/groaning

In addition, presence of nasal flaring, suprasternal retractions, decreased air entry on auscultation of the chest also will indicate the presence of respiratory distress. An infant who has an advanced degree of respiratory distress may exhibit additional signs, such as cyanosis, gasping, choking, apnea and stridor.[4]

INCIDENCE

Respiratory distress occurs in almost 2.2–3.3% of the live born infants.[2,5] According to the NNPD data (2002–03), 5.8% of the live born infants had respiratory morbidities.[3] The incidence is inversely proportional to the gestational age and birth weight.

CAUSES OF RESPIRATORY DISTRESS

Respiratory distress in a newborn can be due to a wide variety of conditions, majority of which are uncommon and should be considered in cases with unusual presentations (Table 7.1). The frequency of a particular condition as the cause of respiratory distress in an infant depends on various factors with gestation being the most important one. In preterm infants, respiratory distress syndrome (RDS) being the most common cause (almost 90%) while in the late preterm and term infants, transient tachypnea of newborn (TTN) is the predominant cause (68%).[2]

Table 7.1: Causes of respiratory distress
Upper Airway Obstruction
Choanal atresia
Nasal stenosis
Pierre Robin sequence
Laryngeal stenosis or atresia
Hemangioma
Vocal cord paralysis
Vascular rings
Tracheobronchial stenosis
Masses
Cleft palate
Nasal stuffiness
Pulmonary Diseases
Respiratory distress syndrome (RDS)
Transient tachypnea of the newborn (TTN)
Aspiration (including meconium aspiration syndrome; MAS)
Pneumonia
Pneumothorax
Pneumomediastinum
Primary pulmonary hypertension
Tracheoesophageal fistula (TEF)
Pulmonary hemorrhage
Pulmonary hypoplasia
Pulmonary agenesis
Cystic adenomatoid malformation
Pleural effusion
Chylothorax
Neoplasm
Bronchopulmonary sequestration
Pulmonary arteriovenous malformation
Pulmonary interstitial emphysema
Pulmonary edema
Congenital alveolar proteinosis
Congenital lobar emphysema

Contd...

Table 7.1: Causes of respiratory distress (Contd...)

Cardiac Diseases

Cyanotic congenital heart disease
Acyanotic congenital heart disease
Arrhythmia
Congestive cardiac failure
Pneumopericardium, pericardial effusion, pyopericardium
Cardiomyopathy

Thoracic Causes

Chest wall deformity
Mass

Metabolic Disorders

Hypoglycemia
Infant of a diabetic mother
Inborn errors of metabolism

Diaphragmatic Causes

Hernia
Paralysis

Neuromuscular Diseases

Central nervous system damage (birth trauma, hemorrhage)
Medication (maternal sedation, narcotic withdrawal)
Muscular disease (myasthenia gravis)
Intraventricular hemorrhage
Meningitis
Hypoxic-ischemic encephalopathy
Seizure disorder
Hydrocephalus
Infantile botulism
Spinal cord injury

Infectious Causes

Sepsis
Pneumonia (especially group B Streptococcus)

Hematological Causes

Anemia
Polycythemia
Abnormal hemoglobin

Miscellaneous Causes

Asphyxia
Acidosis

ASSESSMENT OF RESPIRATORY DISTRESS

Initial Assessment

Initial assessment of respiratory distress in the delivery room should be done to find out life-threatening conditions, which require immediate management such as inadequate or obstructed airway (gasping, choking, stridor) or circulatory collapse (bradycardia, hypotension, poor perfusion). If such features are present then emergency measures such as bag and mask ventilation or intubation should be carried out as necessary.[4]

History

A detailed history is important in assigning a cause to the respiratory distress in a given infant (Table 7.2).

General Examination

It should be done to identify any feature which may give a clue to the etiology such as dysmorphic features, anomalies,

Table 7.2: Relevant history in a neonate with respiratory distress[6]

Antenatal

Diabetes mellitus
Fever, UTI
Polyhydramnios/oligohydramnios
Rh isoimmunization
Antenatal steroids status

Intranatal

PPROM/PROM
Intrapartum fever/chorioamnionitis
Sedative use
Meconium stained liquor
Abnormal fetal monitoring
Instrumental delivery/birth trauma
Need for bag and mask ventilation

Postnatal

Gestational age
Shake test
Onset/course of respiratory distress
Radiological features

features of intrauterine growth restriction, single umbilical artery, scaphoid abdomen, drooling of saliva, etc.

Respiratory Rate

Respiratory rate (RR) should be counted for full one minute with a timer and when the baby is quiet.[3] A normal neonate has a RR of 40–60/min. RR above 60/min is considered as tachypnea. But at times, baby can have respiratory rates well below 60/min but with significant retractions or has apneic episodes interspersed, which may signify severe respiratory distress with impending respiratory failure.

Grunting

Infants develop an expiratory groaning noise called grunting when they have significant respiratory distress. Grunting happens when the infant attempts to keep the alveoli open to maintain the functional residual capacity (FRC) by partially closing the glottis during expiration.[4] Grunting generally disappears first when the baby starts improving but it can also disappear in a baby who is worsening because of exhaustion. Hence, it has to be assessed in the context of other features such as oxygen saturation, color and activity of the infant.

Stridor

Stridor is produced due to narrowing of the major airways. It is often inspiratory but can be expiratory or biphasic. Stridor can occur in newborn due to laryngomalacia, Pierre Robin sequence, etc.

Chest Retractions

Retractions have to be assessed in the suprasternal, intercostal, subcostal and xiphoid area. Retractions can be mild to severe depending on the severity of respiratory distress. Suprasternal recession more often suggests upper airway obstruction and may be a pointer toward upper airway anomaly in neonates. Intercostal retraction suggests alveolar involvement. Nasal flaring also has to be looked for when assessing for chest retractions.

Oxygen Saturation

Oxygen saturation has to be checked preferentially both preductal (right hand) and postductal (leg). A preductal-postductal difference of more than 5–10% indicates probable right-to-left shunt through patent ductus arteriosus (PDA) in the setting of persistent pulmonary hypertension of the newborn (PPHN).[7]

Respiratory System Examination

Respiratory system examination includes inspection of the chest for symmetry of chest movements bilaterally, auscultation for the symmetry of breath sound and for the presence of any adventitious sounds such as crepitations. When there is suspicion of pneumothorax, trans-illumination of the chest should be carried out.

SCORING THE SEVERITY OF RESPIRATORY DISTRESS

Scoring the respiratory distress is essential as it provides an objective way of assessing the severity, and also monitoring the score at regular intervals helps in deciding the course of the illness either improvement or deterioration. Silverman score[8] (Table 7.3) and Downe's score[9] (Table 7.4) are used to assess the severity of the respiratory distress.

Table 7.3: Silverman score

Feature	Score 0	Score 1	Score 2
Upper chest movement	Synchronous	Inspiratory lag	See-saw respiration
Lower chest retractions	None	Minimal	Marked
Xiphoid retractions	None	Minimal	Marked
Nasal flaring	None	Minimal	Marked
Grunting	None	Audible with stethoscope	Audible without stethoscope

Silverman Score

Upper Chest Movement

Upper chest movement is assessed by observing the synchrony of the movement with the abdomen. Upper chest is the part of the chest anterior to the mid axillary line. Synchronized movement of upper chest with abdomen is scored '0', while

Table 7.4: Downe's score

Feature	Score 0	Score 1	Score 2
Cyanosis	None	In room air/40% FiO$_2$	In 40% FiO$_2$
Retractions	None	Mild	Moderate to severe
Grunting	None	Audible with stethoscope	Audible without stethoscope
Air entry	Normal	Decreased	Barely audible
Respiratory rate	<60	60–80	>80 or apnea

Score: >4 = Clinical respiratory distress
   >7 = Impending respiratory failure

lag of upper chest behind the abdomen is scored as '1' and see-saw movement of the chest and abdomen as '2'.

Lower Chest Retractions

Lower chest retractions are assessed by observing the retractions between the ribs below the mid axillary line and is rated as none, minimal or marked.

Xiphoid Retractions

Similarly, retractions below the xiphoid process are rated as none, minimal or marked.

Nasal Flaring

Normally, there should be no nasal flaring. Minimal flaring is scored as '1' and marked flaring is scored as '2'.

Expiratory Grunting

Grunting that is audible with a stethoscope is scored '1', and grunting that is audible without using a stethoscope is scored 2. The higher the score, more severe is the respiratory distress.

A score greater than 7 indicates that the baby is in respiratory failure.

Hemodynamic Stability

Pulse rate, blood pressure and capillary refill time have to be monitored to identify hypoperfusion which can be secondary to prolonged hypoxemia.

COMPARATIVE STUDY OF COMMON CAUSES OF RESPIRATORY DISTRESS (Table 7.5)

Respiratory Distress Syndrome

RDS also called as hyaline membrane disease (HMD) is seen almost exclusively in preterm infants. The risk of RDS decreases with increasing gestational age: 60% of babies born at fewer than 28 weeks' gestation, 30% of babies born between 28 and 34 weeks' gestation, and fewer than 5% of babies born after 34 weeks' gestation develop RDS.[10] Other factors that increase the risk of RDS include male sex, maternal gestational diabetes, perinatal asphyxia, hypothermia and multiple gestations.

Table 7.5: Comparison of common causes of respiratory distress

Condition	Risk factors	Clinical course	Radiological features
Respiratory distress syndrome (RDS)	• Prematurity (usually <34 wks) • Lack of antenatal steroids • Infant of diabetic mother • Birth asphyxia, Rh isoimmunization	• Onset at or soon after birth • Progresses till 48 hrs, static for 48 hrs and improves later • FiO_2 requirement often more than 40%, surfactant modifies the typical course	• Low volume lungs • Fine reticulogranular pattern—ground glass appearance • Air bronchogram • White-out lungs
Transient tachypnea of newborn (TTN)	• Predominantly late preterm and term infants • Cesarean section • Maternal diabetes	• Onset at or soon after birth • Maximum severity at birth and improves gradually • FiO_2 requirement seldom more than 40%	• Hyperinflated lungs • Perihilar streaking • Fluid in minor fissure • Pleural effusion • Mild cardiomegaly
Early onset sepsis (EOS)/ pneumonia	PROM, chorioamnionitis, maternal fever, unclean vaginal examinations	• Onset at birth or delayed • May fail to improve with oxygen/CPAP	• Homogeneous/ Non-homogeneous opacities bilaterally
Meconium aspiration syndrome (MAS)	• Meconium stained amniotic fluid	• Onset may be at birth or delayed • Meconium staining of cord/skin • Hyperinflated chest • Features of PPHN	• Hyperinflated lungs • Coarse nodular/ fluffy opacities • Patchy atelectasis • Areas of overinflation

Antenatal steroids and prolonged rupture of membranes decrease the risk of RDS. RDS presents at the time of or soon after birth, and symptoms worsen over time. Shake test done from the gastric aspirate may be negative.[11]

The chest radiograph shows diffuse atelectasis and the classic "ground glass" appearance of the lung fields. Air bronchograms, which are air-filled bronchi superimposed on the relatively airless parenchyma of the lung tissue, are also seen commonly on chest radiograph.

Transient Tachypnea of Newborn (TTN)[12]

This is a self-limited disease. It occurs in approximately 11 per 1,000 live births and appears more often in boys, in infants delivered by cesarean section, and in infants who have perinatal asphyxia or maternal complications such as asthma, diabetes, analgesia or anesthesia during labor.[13,14] Respiratory morbidity in elective cesarean section is inversely related to gestational age: 73.8/1000 in the 37th week, 42.3/1000 in the 38th week and 17.8/1000 in the 39th week of gestation (*therefore, elective cesarean sections should be delayed until 39 to 40 wks*).[15]

Infants who have TTN present clinically with tachypnea and occasionally grunting and nasal flaring immediately after birth. Typically, arterial blood gases reveal respiratory acidosis and mild-to-moderate hypoxemia.[16]

Chest radiography reveals hyperinflation, perihilar streaking due to dilated lymphatics, increased interstitial markings, fluid in the interlobar fissures and occasionally pleural effusion and mild cardiomegaly.

TTN is generally a benign, self-limited disease that usually responds well to oxygen therapy. Mechanical ventilation is seldom needed, although many infants require nasal continuous positive airway pressure (nCPAP) support.

Infants whose disease is uncomplicated usually recover without long term pulmonary sequelae. Full recovery is expected within 1 to 5 days.

Meconium Aspiration Syndrome (MAS)

MAS is defined as respiratory distress in an infant born through meconium stained amniotic fluid whose symptoms cannot otherwise be explained. Approximately 13% of all live births are complicated by meconium stained amniotic fluid, and of these, 4–5% of infants develop MAS.[17]

Once aspirated, meconium can cause obstruction of the air passages, chemical pneumonitis with activation of several inflammatory mediators and inactivation of lung surfactant. The infant who has MAS may present with varying degrees of respiratory distress and is likely to have a "barrel chest" with audible rales or rhonchi on auscultation.

The chest radiograph usually shows patchy areas of atelectasis alternating with areas of overinflation. Pneumothorax may be seen in 10–20% of infants who have MAS.[18]

Pneumonia

Pneumonia may be acquired in utero during delivery (or perinatally) or postnatally in the nursery or at home.

Pneumonia present before 72 hours of life is a manifestation of early onset sepsis (EOS) and the risk factors include maternal fever, chorioamnionitis, prolonged rupture of membranes (PROM), unclean vaginal examination and prematurity.

Pneumonias that are acquired later present most often as systemic disease.

In neonatal pneumonia, the chest radiograph may reveal patchy infiltrates, but the findings may be similar to that of RDS.

Management includes oxygen therapy, ventilatory support, antibiotics and often vasopressor support such as dopamine and dobutamine.

Congenital Heart Disease (CHD)

Infants who have CHD may present with cyanosis or heart failure. Signs that are generally consistent with CHD include: visibly hyperactive precordial impulse, gallop rhythm, poor capillary refill, weak pulses, decreased or delayed pulses in lower extremities, hepatomegaly and abnormal vascularity or cardiomegaly on chest radiography.[19] A single second heart sound without "split" may be indicative of CHD. Nada's criteria can be applied to identify infants with congenital heart disease.

A neonate who has cyanosis without marked respiratory distress and an O_2 saturation of less than 85% in both room air and 100% oxygen likely has an intracardiac shunt.

If the O_2 saturation increases to more than 85% on 100% oxygen, a full hyperoxia test should be performed. The test consists of obtaining a baseline right radial (preductal) arterial blood gas measurement with the child breathing room air and repeating the measurement while the infant is receiving 100% O_2. Arterial PaO_2 measurement greater than 250 mmHg on 100% oxygen rules out cyanotic CHD, between 100 and 250 mmHg suggests cyanotic CHD with good mixing or pulmonary disease, and less than 100 mmHg suggests cyanotic CHD (or severe pulmonary hypertension). Echocardiography needs to be done to confirm the diagnosis.

MANAGEMENT OF RESPIRATORY DISTRESS

Investigations

Often the diagnosis requires appropriate history, clinical examination and a proper chest X-ray. Sepsis screen, blood cultures may be required when sepsis is suspected. CSF examination is warranted in the presence of clinical sepsis or positive blood culture. Other investigations specific to the suspected clinical condition such as CT thorax in case of suspected lung anomalies or echocardiography in PPHN or congenital heart disease may be required.

Treatment

The basic principles of treatment include
1. Supportive care
2. Respiratory support
3. Monitoring for and management of complications
4. Specific therapy

Supportive Care

This includes maintenance of thermo-neutral environment by caring the infant under radiant warmer or in incubator, ensuring normal blood glucose levels with intravenous fluids and monitoring the vital parameters such as heart rate, respiratory rate and scoring of the respiratory distress.

Respiratory Support

Respiratory support provided to the infant depends on many factors such as the gestation of the infant, hemodynamic stability, the underlying condition, the severity and the presence of complication, if any. The objective is to ensure adequate oxygenation and ventilation, and thereby decrease the work of breathing.

Supplemental Oxygen

Most often babies with conditions such as TTN or mild RDS may require only supplemental oxygen which is delivered through head box. The FiO_2 requirement of the baby has to be monitored at regular intervals so that any increase in requirement to maintain the SpO_2 in the optimal range can be identified early and thereby the worsening of the lung condition or consequent complications developing if any.

CPAP

Infants who fail to maintain adequate oxygenation on supplemental oxygen or those who have mild to moderate respiratory distress with Silverman or Downe's score of more than 4 will require CPAP. It may also be used in late preterm and term infants with TTN or pneumonia if tolerated (see AIIMS Protocol on CPAP).

Mechanical Ventilation

Infants who fail to maintain oxygenation and ventilation on CPAP will require mechanical ventilation. Mode of ventilation and the settings will vary based on the weight and gestation of the infant, the condition being treated and the existing unit policy. Those who fail conventional ventilation may require high frequency ventilation.

Inhaled Nitric Oxide Therapy

Infants with features suggestive of PPHN will require inhaled iNO if they meet the criteria.

Monitoring of Complications

Infants with respiratory distress need to be monitored for worsening of the distress, hemodynamic instability, features of PPHN, acute kidney injury due to hypoxia and complications due to mechanical ventilation, etc. If any such complications develop, they should be managed appropriately.

Specific Therapy

Specific treatment strategies include surfactant replacement therapy for RDS, antibiotics for EOS/pneumonia, surgical resection for lung malformations, etc.

REFERENCES

1. Mathai SS, Raju U, Kanitkar M, et al. Management of respiratory distress in the newborn. MJAFI 2007;63:269–72.

2. Rubaltelli FF, Dani C, Reali MF, et al. Acute neonatal respiratory distress in Italy: a one-year prospective study, Acta Paediatr 1998;87:1261–68.

3. NNPD working definitions. NNPD report 2002–03. NNPD network, ICMR; p 67.

4. Hany Aly. Respiratory disorders in the newborn: identification and diagnosis. Pediatrics in Review 2004;25;201.

5. Bonafe' L, Rubaltelli F. The incidence of acute neonatal respiratory disorders in Padova county: an epidemiological survey. Acta Paediatr 1996;85:1236–40.

6. Jackson JC. Respiratory distress in the preterm infant. In: Avery's diseases of the newborn. 9th edn. Eds; Gleason CA, Devaskar S, Elsevier Philadelphia 2012;p633–46.

7. Kinsella JP. Inhale nitric oxide in the term newborn. Early Human Development 2008;84:709–16.

8. Silverman WA, Andersen DH. A controlled clinical trial of effects of water mist on obstructive respiratory signs, death rate and necropsy findings among premature infants. Pediatrics 1956;17:1–10.

9. Downes JJ, Vidyasagar D, Boggs TR Jr, Morrow GM 3rd edn. Respiratory distress syndrome of newborn infants. I. New clinical scoring system (RDS score) with acid-base and blood-gas correlations. Clin Pediatr (Phila) 1970;9:325–31.

10. Warren JB, Anderson JM. Core concepts: respiratory distress syndrome. Neoreviews 2009;10;e351–61.

11. Kopelman AE, Matthew OP. Common respiratory disorders of the newborn. Pediatr Rev 1995;16:209–17.

12. Avery ME, Gatewood OB, Brumly G. Transient tachypnea of the newborn. Am J Dis Child 1966;111:380–5.

13. Haliday H, McClure G, Reid M. Transient tachypnoea of the newborn: two distinct clinical entities. Arch Dis Child. 1981;56:322–5.

14. Morrison JJ, Rennie JM, Milton PJ. Neonatal respiratory morbidity and mode of delivery at term: influence of timing of elective caesarean section. Br J Obstet Gynaecol 1995;102:101–6.

15. O'Brodovich H, Canessa C, Ueda J, et al. Expression of the epithelial Na^+ channel in the developing rat lung. Am J Physiol 1993;265:C491–6.

16. Dargaville PA, Copnell B. The epidemiology of meconium aspiration syndrome: incidence, risk factors, therapies and outcome. Pediatrics 2006;117:1712–21.

17. Vain NE, Szyld EG, Prudent LM, Wiswell TE, Aguilar AM, Vivas NI. Oropharyngeal and nasopharyngeal suctioning of meconium-stained neonates before delivery of their shoulders: multicentre, randomised controlled trial. Lancet 2004;364:597–602.

18. Parker TA, Kinsella JP. Respiratory failure in the term newborn. In: Avery's diseases of the newborn. 9th edn. Eds; Gleason CA, Devaskar S, Elsevier, Philadelphia 2012; p.647–57.

19. Weschler SB, Wernovsky G. Cardiac disorders. In: Cloherty JP, Eichenwald EC, Stark AR Eds. Manual of neonatal care. 6th edn. Lippincott William & Wilkins, USA 2011; p.388.

8 Bronchopulmonary Dysplasia

Bronchopulmonary dysplasia (BPD) occurs in preterm infants who require mechanical ventilation and/or oxygen therapy for a primary lung disorder. Though the incidence of BPD has largely remained unchanged over the years, the improved survival of more immature infants has led to increased number of infants with this disorder.[1] These infants are more likely to have persistent respiratory symptoms requiring frequent hospital admissions in the first two years after birth.

DEFINITION AND INCIDENCE

The lack of uniformity in the diagnostic criteria for BPD partly explains the wide variation in the reported incidence among different centers.[2] The initial diagnostic criteria mandated continuing oxygen dependency during the first 28 days of life with compatible clinical and radiographic findings to label an infant as having BPD.[3] The fact that many infants would have intervals in the first few weeks during which they do not require any supplemental oxygen signified the major drawback of this definition. Later, it was proposed to use the need for supplemental oxygen at 36 wk postmenstrual age (PMA) as the diagnostic criterion especially in preterm very low birth weight (VLBW) infants.[4] The later definition, used widely in clinical trials even now, has the limitation of spuriously labeling more mature infants (e.g. those born at 34–35 wk) as having BPD.

To address the inconsistencies in the diagnostic criteria, the US National Institute of Health (NIH) organized a consensus conference in 2000 which suggested a new definition by incorporating many elements of previous definitions of BPD. The suggestion was to use oxygen need for $\geq$28 days and at 36 wk PMA to identify different severity of BPD (Table 8.1).[5]

Since the criteria for supplemental oxygen might vary across the units, Walsh proposed a physiological definition called the "room air challenge" to define BPD.[6]

Table 8.1: Definition of BPD[5]

	Gestational age	
	< 32 wk	*≥ 32 wk*
Time point of assessment	36 wk PMA or discharge*	>28 days but <56 days postnatal age or discharge*
Treatment with oxygen	>21% for at least 28 days	>21% for at least 28 days
Mild	Breathing room air at 36 wk PMA or discharge*	Breathing room air at 56 days postnatal age or discharge*
Moderate	Need for <30% oxygen at 36 wk PMA or discharge*	Need for <30% oxygen at 56 days postnatal age or discharge*
Severe	Need for ≥ 30% oxygen and/or positive pressure (IMV/CPAP/HHFNC) at 36 wk PMA or discharge*	Need for ≥ 30% oxygen and/or positive pressure (IMV/CPAP/HHFNC) at 56 days postnatal age or discharge*

Whichever comes first (PMA: postmenstrual age; BPD: bronchopulmonary dysplasia; IMV: intermittent mandatory ventilation; CPAP: continuous positive airway pressure, HHFNC: humidified high flow nasal cannula)

Ehrenkranz et al validated the consensus definition in a cohort of preterm (<32 wks) extremely low birth weight (ELBW) infants and reported an incidence of 77% by the new criteria.[7] Recently, a longitudinal study of 1656 surviving infants born between 23 and 29 weeks gestation reported an increase in BPD rates from 47.8 to 57.8%.[8] Few reports are available from the centers in India; one study from Chandigarh found the incidence of BPD (defined as need for oxygen at or beyond 28 days of life) to be 50% and 9% in extremely low birth weight (ELBW) and VLBW infants, respectively.[9]

PATHOGENESIS

BPD has a multifactorial etiology; the major risk factors include prematurity, oxygen therapy, mechanical ventilation, infection, patent ductus arteriosus (PDA) and genetic predisposition.[10] By far, the most important factor in the pathogenesis of BPD is prematurity. Exposure of immature lungs to high O_2 concentrations and positive pressure ventilation results in oxidative stress and ventilator induced lung injury (barotrauma/volutrauma). The resulting injury and inflammation lead to abnormal reparative processes in the lung. This is compounded by inflammation resulting from infections (intra-uterine/postnatal infection) that occur commonly in these infants. PDA contributes further to this process by inducing pulmonary edema and vascular endothelial injury. Recently, genetic polymorphisms are also thought to play a role in the causation of BPD.[11]

PATHOLOGY: 'OLD' VERSUS 'NEW' BPD

The severe form of BPD ('old' BPD) seen in infants who received aggressive ventilation and were exposed to high inspired oxygen concentration from birth is rare nowadays. This form was characterized by severe morphological changes including emphysema, atelectasis, fibrosis, and marked epithelial metaplasia and smooth muscle hypertrophy in the airways and in the pulmonary vasculature.[12]

In contrast, the milder forms of BPD ('new' BPD) seen today occurs in infants covered with antenatal corticosteroids and having only mild respiratory distress requiring shorter duration (or even no) mechanical ventilation and/or oxygen therapy after birth. Pathologically, this form is characterized by a striking decrease in alveolar septation and impaired vascular development, changes more compatible with an arrest in lung development than with mechanical injury.[13] For example, in an infant born before 28 to 30 weeks' gestation, the lung would have developed only to the saccular stage with some alveolarization. Incomplete development of lung coupled with a variety of postnatal insults such as resuscitation with high pressures and FiO_2, hypoxemia, acidosis, excess fluid, PDA, infections and suboptimum nutrition set the stage for development of new BPD. An increasing role of growth factors (such as thyroid transcription factor 1 and VEGF in the sacculation, alveolarization and vasculogenesis of peripheral lung) and epigenetics (such as SP-Bi4 deletion, polymorphism in genes coding pro- and anti-inflammatory cytokines) is being recognized in the pathogenesis of new BPD.[14]

Clinical and Radiological Features

Respiratory signs in infants with BPD include fast but shallow breathing, retractions and paradoxical breathing. Rales and rhonchi are usually heard on auscultation.

Radiographic features of 'old' and 'new' BPD are quite different, not surprising given the vastly different pathologic findings. 'Old' BPD, as originally described by Northway, had four distinct stages: stage 1, consistent with hyaline membrane disease; stage 2, opaque lung fields with air bronchograms due to areas of atelectasis alternating with emphysema; stage 3, small radiolucent fields; and stage 4, hyperinflated lungs with generalized cystic areas and dense fibrotic strands.[12] In contrast, infants with new BPD show only haziness reflecting diffuse loss of lung volume or increased lung fluid. Occasionally they have dense areas of segmental or lobar atelectasis or pneumonic infiltrates, but they do not show severe overinflation.

MANAGEMENT OF BPD

Given the multitude of factors that contribute to the pathogenesis of bronchopulmonary dysplasia, it is not surprising that there is no 'magic bullet' for its prevention and/or treatment. Indeed, the best bet for prevention of BPD would be to prevent preterm births itself, an implausible option as of now.

Prevention

Prevention requires a multidisciplinary approach starting right from the antenatal period.

Before Birth

Use of antenatal steroids in mothers at risk for delivering a premature infant reduces the incidence of neonatal deaths and RDS but *does not* reduce the incidence of BPD. This could arguably be due to increased survival of very immature infants who are at high risk of BPD or because of the inability to detect a real protective effect.[15] Antenatal thyrotropin-releasing hormone (TRH) is not effective in prevention of BPD.[16]

After Birth

Given that no *'ideal'* pharmacological agents are available for prevention of BPD, attention has now shifted to 'optimal' ventilatory strategies that would prevent/reduce lung injury and permit adequate lung development.

VENTILATORY STRATEGIES

Resuscitation in the Delivery Room

Clearance of fetal lung and airway fluid at birth is dependent on amiloride sensitive sodium channels which absorb sodium and drag water along due to osmotic forces from the lung lumen into the interstitium. This process is also facilitated by sustained lung inflations, which subserve to establish the functional residual capacity (FRC). One study showed that early establishment of FRC by giving at least two such inflations with a peak inspiratory pressure of around 20–25 cm H_2O and inspiratory time (Ti) of 10 seconds could significantly reduce later BPD.[17] The approach, though promising, needs to be evaluated in large trials before implementing in routine clinical practice.

Continuous Positive Airway Pressure (CPAP)

Early initiation of nasal CPAP has been shown to reduce the need for intubation and mechanical ventilation. Since one of the major risk factors for BPD is the need for mechanical ventilation, use of early CPAP should logically reduce its incidence. Numerous studies, mostly non-randomized, have reported the benefits of early CPAP in minimizing the need for mechanical ventilation and the incidence of BPD.[18] Surprisingly, few randomized controlled trials are available till date in this regard. Recently, a multi-centric study on CPAP *versus* intubation and ventilation at 5 minutes of age in infants born at 25–28 weeks' gestation found significant reduction in the need for oxygen at 28 days of life although this benefit did not extend to the need for oxygen at 36 weeks PMA.[19] Another multi-center trial randomized infants born between 24 and 27 weeks of gestation to intubation and surfactant treatment (within 1 hour after birth) or to CPAP initiated in the delivery room. The trial did not find any significant difference in death or bronchopulmonary dysplasia but reported a significant reduction in the use of postnatal corticosteroids for BPD in the enrolled infants.[20] It should be noted that *prophylactic* CPAP does not offer any benefit when compared to early use of CPAP.[21]

A recent multi-center randomized trial found no difference in the incidence of BPD between the three approaches used for the initial respiratory management of preterm neonates: prophylactic surfactant followed by a period of mechanical ventilation, prophylactic surfactant with rapid extubation to nasal CPAP or initial management with CPAP and selective surfactant treatment.[22] It appears that early use of CPAP might even mitigate the need for surfactant therapy in at least some neonates.

Nasal Intermittent Positive Pressure Ventilation (NIPPV)

NIPPV is a method of augmenting NCPAP by delivering ventilator breaths via the nasal prongs. It is thought to improve the tidal and minute volumes and decrease the inspiratory effort required by neonates as compared to nCPAP. When used as primary support in RDS, NIPPV does reduce the need for reintubation in the first 72 hours but has no effect on BPD.[23] In the post-extubation setting, a trend towards reduction in the rates of BPD was observed with NIPPV (typical RR 0.73; 95% CI 0.49, 1.07).[24]

Patient-triggered Ventilation (PTV)

Patient-triggered modes (SIMV, assist-control and pressure support ventilation) improve the infant-ventilator asynchrony; this should theoretically reduce the risk of VILI. The Cochrane review concluded that though PTV is associated with shorter duration of ventilation, it does not reduce the incidence of BPD.[25]

High Frequency Ventilation (HFV)

Animal studies indicate that HFV could lead to less lung injury when compared to conventional ventilation. However, randomized controlled trials comparing elective use of HFV with conventional ventilation in preterm infants have yielded conflicting results.

A recent meta-analysis that included 17 RCTs of conventional *versus* HFV found no significant difference in the incidence of BPD. Therefore, elective use of HFV cannot be recommended for preterm infants with RDS.[26]

Volume Targeted Ventilation (VTV)

The observation that volutrauma and not barotrauma is the primary determinant of VILI has enthused neonatologists to use volume controlled/targeted modes of ventilation in place of conventional pressure controlled modes. The Cochrane review that included 12 RCTs found a significant reduction in the combined outcome of death or bronchopulmonary dysplasia (RR 0.73 [95% CI 0.57–0.93]; NNT 8 [95% CI 5–33]).[27] However, as pointed out by the reviewers, these studies were conducted by researchers with expertise in these modes.[27] Given the different modes of VTV and the selection of associated parameters in different ventilators, careful education of health personnel is important in units considering the use of VTV.

Permissive Hypercapnia

Retrospective studies have suggested that hypocapnia that occurs during assisted ventilation is an independent risk factor for BPD. Subsequently, 'minimal ventilation' using smaller tidal volumes/less peak inflation pressures while accepting mild hypercapnia ($PaCO_2$ 45–55 mmHg) was studied in preterm infants. The Cochrane review that included two trials found no reduction in the incidence of death or BPD at 36 weeks PMA (RR 0.94, 95% CI 0.78, 1.15).[28] One of these two trials, however, reported a significant reduction in the incidence of BPD in the 501 to 750 gram subgroup.

Permissive Hypoxemia

Exposure to high oxygen concentration has long been recognized as an important factor in the pathogenesis of BPD. Preterm infants are more vulnerable to the harmful effects of free oxygen radicals. Surprisingly, there are few data to suggest either the optimal oxygen level required or the optimum target range for oxygen saturations (SpO_2) in these infants.

Observational studies suggest that in comparison with the more liberal oxygen therapy, the restrictive approach of accepting lower oxygen saturation values is associated with decreased incidences of BPD and ROP. Two RCTs have been conducted to examine if it is better to aim for high oxygen saturation in infants who are more than a few weeks old:

BOOST-trial and STOP-ROP trial.[29,30] Both these studies indicated that maintaining higher oxygen saturation (>95%) is associated with increased need for oxygen at 36 wks PMA and greater use of postnatal steroids and diuretics in premature infants (when compared to maintaining lower oxygen saturation of 89–94%). Recently, a large multi-center trial compared the target ranges of oxygen saturation of 85–89% or 91–95% among 1316 infants who were born between 24 weeks 0 days and 27 weeks 6 days of gestation. It reported that the lower target range of oxygenation (85–89%) resulted in an *increase* in mortality and a substantial decrease in severe retinopathy among survivors.[31] The results of the interim analysis of another large multi-center trial (BOOST II) also showed a higher mortality at 36 wks in the lower saturation target group.[32] It is expected that the primary outcomes of disability-free survival of these trials (anticipated in 2014) would help make the final recommendation on the 'optimal' oxygenation in preterm infants.

FLUIDS AND NUTRITION

Fluid Restriction

Anecdotal data indicate that relative fluid restriction reduces incidence of BPD in preterm infants. The Cochrane systematic review of studies on fluid restriction has found a significant benefit in NEC and PDA, but no significant reduction in BPD (Bell Cochrane 2008).[33] Moreover, what represents fluid restriction in VLBW infants is not definitely known. Hence, no definite recommendation can be made regarding fluid restriction as a strategy for reducing the incidence of BPD.

Nutrition

Nutrition plays an important role in lung development and maturation. Aggressive parenteral nutrition and early enteral feeding may help decrease the incidence of BPD in VLBW infants.[34] Ideally, nutritional management should begin from day one of life to minimize the respiratory morbidities. The initial management should meet the estimated fluid, protein and energy needs. Since enteral feeding is often delayed in these infants due to gastrointestinal immaturity, parenteral nutrition with proteins and lipids should be initiated as soon as possible after birth. It should be continued until daily oral intake reaches at least 130 mL/kg. Only expressed breast milk is to be used for enteral feeding. Fortifying breast milk with human milk fortifier (HMF) will make up for its deficiencies of protein and minerals like calcium and phosphorus. If fluids need to be restricted, addition of fat such as medium chain triglyceride (MCT) oil or glucose polymers will help in achieving the adequate growth.

The role of specific nutrients (e.g. inositol, vitamin E, selenium, glutamine, etc. except for vitamin A), however, remains speculative till now.

PHARMACOLOGICAL STRATEGIES

Exogenous Surfactant

Prophylactic surfactant therapy in infants born before 30 wks of gestation has not been shown to reduce the incidence of BPD. However, surfactant treatment for established RDS (*rescue therapy*) in infants born at or after 30 wks gestation is associated with significant reduction in the incidence of BPD.[35] Interestingly, a new technique of minimally invasive surfactant delivery using a thin vascular catheter inserted into the trachea resulted in a lesser need for mechanical ventilation and BPD as compared to traditional intubation and intralaryngeal installation.[36]

Vitamin A

Vitamin A is essential for maintaining the integrity of respiratory tract epithelial cells. Very preterm infants are relatively deficient in vitamin A, which has been shown to be associated with BPD. A large RCT of 807 infants with a birth weight of less than 1000 g has shown that a large dose of intramuscular vitamin A (5000 units three times a wk for 4 wks from birth) decreases the risk of BPD (OR 0.89; 95% CI 0.8–0.99).[37] A meta-analysis of seven RCTs has also confirmed this finding.[38]

We use intramuscular vitamin A in the above said dose for ELBW infants with respiratory distress requiring supplemental oxygen or mechanical ventilation at 24 hours of age.

Methylxanthines

Xanthines such as caffeine and aminophylline have been routinely used for prevention/treatment of apnea and for facilitation of extubation in premature infants. Recently, a large RCT that used caffeine for these indications in infants with birth weights of 500–1250 g has shown a significant decrease in the incidence of BPD. The authors attributed this rather unexpected finding to reduced duration of mechanical ventilation in the caffeine treated group.[39] One should, however, be cautious in extrapolating the beneficial effects of caffeine to aminophylline, the commonly used methylxanthine in most units of the country.

We use either caffeine or aminophylline after extubation and for treatment of apnea of prematurity in all preterm VLBW infants.

Indomethacin/Ibuprofen Therapy for PDA

Patent ductus arteriosus is one of the major risk factors for BPD. Hence, prevention or treatment of PDA should ideally reduce its risk. However, prophylactic use of indomethacin in very low birth weight infants has failed to show any reduction in the incidence of BPD despite a significant reduction in the incidence of PDA.[40] Similar results are obtained with ibuprofen, another drug used for closure of PDA.[41] In contrast, treatment of symptomatic PDA could possibly reduce the incidence of BPD.[42]

Postnatal Steroids

Given that inflammation plays a central role in the pathogenesis of BPD, steroids were thought to be a natural choice for its management. However, this therapy has turned out to be the most controversial area of care following reports of adverse neurodevelopmental outcomes.

The postnatal steroid use can be broadly categorized into early (less than 7 days) and late (at or after 8 days) regimes. Use of early postnatal steroid (dexamethasone/hydrocortisone) showed a significant decline in oxygen dependency both at 28 days and 36 weeks PCA. However, there are important concerns regarding the short-term (hyperglycemia, gastro-intestinal perforation, poor somatic growth, hypertrophic cardiomyopathy) as well as long-term adverse effects (neuro-developmental outcomes including cerebral palsy).[43] Late steroid therapy also reduces oxygen dependency at 28 days and 36 weeks PMA with an increased risk of hyperglycemia, glycosuria and hypertension as well as severe ROP.[44] One systematic review found that infants who received steroids (either early or late regimen) were twice as likely to develop cerebral palsy as the control infants.[45]

In view of these findings, routine *early* use of high-dose steroids is not recommended at present. Considering the fact that no other treatment options have proved to be consistently beneficial in preventing BPD, some centers still recommend use of steroids at lower doses and for shorter duration in extremely preterm infants who are dependent on mechanical ventilation even after the first week of life.

We use steroids occasionally in ELBW infants who continue to be on mechanical ventilation even after 10–14 days of life (3-day course using low dose dexamethasone).[46]

Inhaled steroids thought to reduce the adverse effects associated with systemic administration have not been shown to be beneficial either for prevention or for treatment.[47]

iNO Therapy

Animal studies have shown that iNO therapy, in addition to causing pulmonary vasodilatation also reduces lung inflammation and promotes lung growth. Unfortunately, most clinical studies in preterm infants with severe respiratory failure have not demonstrated any reduction in the risk of death or BPD with iNO.[48] Recently, two large RCTs conducted in this regard indicate that iNO therapy might be beneficial in a select group of preterm infants.[49,50] However, one should remember that the appropriate dose, timing, duration and more importantly, the subgroup of infants who are likely to benefit with this mode of therapy have not yet been clearly defined. Moreover, the prohibitive cost of iNO therapy precludes its use on a routine basis.

Diuretic Therapy

Diuretics help by increasing the reabsorption of fluid from the lungs. Though studies have shown beneficial effects in lung physiology, no such effects were observed in mortality or the incidence of BPD. Given the potential risks involved with long-term therapy, chronic use of furosemide or any other diuretics cannot be recommended now. However, diuretics can be used sparingly if there are clinical/radiographic features of pulmonary edema in an infant with evolving or established BPD.[51]

Occasionally, we use furosemide 0.5–1 mg/kg/day in infants with features suggestive of excess lung fluid; we stop after 24–48 hours if no improvement is noted in the clinical condition.

Mast Cell Stabilizers

Cromolyn sodium has been shown to decrease neutrophil migration and activation thus minimizing inflammation in the lungs. Two trials that have studied the possible role of cromolyn for prevention and treatment of BPD have not shown any benefit.[52]

Bronchodilators

They have not been found to be useful for prevention of BPD. [53]

Emerging Therapies

Preterm infants are susceptible to oxidant injury because they are deficient in antioxidant enzymes. Hence, antioxidants such as superoxide dismutase (SOD) promise to be an exciting strategy for prevention of BPD. A randomized trial that enrolled around 300 infants proved the safe nature of the drug CuZnSOD, but did not find any difference in the primary outcome of BPD at 36 wk PMA. Interestingly, SOD treated infants had fewer episodes of respiratory illness at 1 year of age suggesting that the drug could prevent long-term lung injury caused by reactive oxygen species.[54] Further studies are needed to define its exact role in the management of BPD.

Other antioxidants/free radical scavengers like vitamins C and E, allopurinol, N-acetylcysteine have not been proved to be useful till now.

The options available for prevention and their current status are summarized in Table 8.2.

Table 8.2: BPD-preventive strategies and their current status

Strategies	Proven benefit	Promising (needs more studies)	Probably beneficial (effects ±)	No benefit
Ventilatory	Volume targeted ventilation	NIPPV Permissive hypercapnia Sustained inflations	Early CPAP Patient triggered modes, permissive hypoxemia	High frequency ventilation
Fluids and nutrition	—	Aggressive early enteral and parenteral nutrition	Fluid restriction	
Pharmacological	Early rescue surfactant Caffeine Intramuscular vitamin A Postnatal steroids (but harmful as well)	Superoxide dismutase	Antenatal steroids iNO therapy, diuretics	Antenatal TRH Prophylactic surfactant Prophylactic indomethacin/ ibuprofen Inhaled steroids, bronchodilators, mast cell stabilizers

(NIPPV: nasal intermittent positive pressure ventilation; CPAP: continuous positive airway pressure; iNO: inhaled nitric oxide; TRH: thyrotropin releasing hormone)

TREATMENT OF EVOLVING/ESTABLISHED BPD

There are extremely limited data from clinical trials on which to base optimal ventilatory management in established BPD. The major goal is to maintain adequate gas exchange with as minimal support as possible. CPAP and NIPPV should be attempted as much as possible. For infants on ventilator, the settings should be titrated keeping in mind the rapidly changing pulmonary mechanics (increasing airway resistance as well as improving compliance). Often, slow rates with long Ti are needed as the disease progresses. Some neonates with marked variability in compliance and resistance may benefit from volume targeted ventilation. Similarly, PTV may be useful in infants who 'fight the ventilator'.[55] Accepting relatively high $PaCO_2$ (45–55 mmHg provided that pH >7.25) and slightly low saturations (88–93%) would help in minimizing the ventilator settings and thus help in early extubation (Table 8.3).

Table 8.3: Management of evolving or established BPD[#]

	Evolving BPD (2–4 wk age)	Established BPD (>4 wk age)

Ventilatory strategies	• Minimizing ventilatory support (e.g. using nCPAP whenever possible)
	• Tolerating slightly higher $PaCO_2$ (45–55 mmHg provided pH >7.25)
	• Target SpO_2 : 88–93%
	• If on IMV:
	  – Use PTV if possible
	  – Slow rates (25–40/min)
	  – Moderate PEEP (4–5 cm H_2O)
	  – Moderate Ti (0.35–0.45 sec)
	  – Low tidal volume (3–6 mL/kg)
	  – Early extubation to CPAP
		• Minimizing ventilatory support
		• Tolerating higher $PaCO_2$ (55–60 mmHg provided pH >7.25)
		• Target SpO_2 : 90 to 95%
		• If on IMV:
		  – Use PTV if possible
		  – Slow rates (20–40/min)
		  – Moderate PEEP (4–8 cm H_2O)
		  – Longer Ti (0.4–0.7 sec)
		  – Larger tidal volume (5–8 mL/kg)

Pharmacological strategies	• Methylxanthines to facilitate extubation
	• Steroids:* Consider in ELBW infants on ventilator support even after 10–14 days of age
	• Specific management:
	  – Diuretics for features of pulmonary edema
	  – Bronchodilators for bronchospasm
		• Steroids:* Individualize based on the clinical condition
		• Specific management:
		  – Bronchodilators for bronchospasm
		  – Sedation and muscle relaxation for 'BPD spells'

Others	• Nutrition:
	  – Increase daily calorie intake to 120 to 150 kcal/kg/d
	  – Give expressed breast milk fortified with HMF
	  – Use fat supplementation (e.g. MCT oil), if needed, for providing additional calories
	  – Give multivitamin supplements to meet RDA
		• Same as for evolving BPD

[#] *Modified with permission from Reference 55 *Could result in potentially harmful effects including adverse neurodevelopmental outcomes; counsel parents before initiation of therapy (nCPAP: nasal continuous positive airway pressure; IMV: intermittent mandatory ventilation; PTV: patient triggered ventilation; PEEP: positive end expiratory pressure; Ti:inspiratory time; HMF: human milk fortifier; MCT: medium chain triglycerides; RDA: recommended dietary allowance)*

Antenatal period	≤ Antenatal steroids (2 doses of betamethasone 24 hrs apart)
At birth	Avoid excessive pressure during resuscitation (use appropriate size bag for BMV)

Birth to 24 hrs

≤ Fluids: 60–80 mL/kg/d
≤ Nutrition: Oral feeds-breast milk (MEN/full feeds) to be initiated in stable infants
≤ Early CPAP
≤ If on ventilator:
  ○ Early rescue surfactant as indicated
  ○ **Settings:** fast rates (50–60/min), moderate PEEP (4–5 cm H_2O), short Ti (0.25–0.4 s)
  ○ **Target values**-SpO_2: 90–95%; $PaCO_2$ 45–55 mmHg; pH: 7.25–7.35
  ○ Early extubation to CPAP

24 hrs to 1 wk

≤ Fluids: daily increment of 15-20 mL/kg/d to reach a maximum of 150 mL/kg/d by day 7
≤ Nutrition:
  ○ Parenteral: TPN for ELBW infants till full enteral feeds are achieved
  ○ Enteral: Gradually increase feed volume by 20–30 mL/kg/d if accepting well; give only breast milk; fortify with HMF after reaching 100 mL/kg/d
≤ If on ventilator:
  ○ **Settings** and **target values** as above
  ○ Extubate to CPAP if possible
  ○ Methylxanthines to facilitate extubation
≤ For ELBW infants on oxygen or ventilator support at 24 hrs: **Inj. vitamin A** 5000 units IM thrice wkly for 4 wk

1 to 4 wk

≤ Fluids: 150 to 160 mL/kg/d
≤ Nutrition: Fortify breast milk with HMF; add more calories if needed
≤ If on ventilator:
  ○ Settings and target values as in Table 8.3
  ○ Extubate to CPAP as early as possible
≤ Diuretics/steroids/bronchodilators as indicated (seeTable 8.3)

> 4 wk

≤ Fluids: 150 to 160 mL/kg/d
≤ Nutrition: Fortify breast milk with HMF; add more calories if needed
≤ If on ventilator:
  ○ Settings and target values as in Table 8.3
  ○ Extubate to CPAP as early as possible
≤ Sedatives/steroids/bronchodilators as indicated (seeTable 8.3)

(BMV, bag and mask ventilation; CPAP, continuous positive airway pressure; PEEP, positive end expiratory pressure; MEN, minimal enteral nutrition; ELBW, extremely low birth weight infants; TPN, total parenteral nutrition; HMF, human milk fortifier; PTV, patient triggered ventilation; Ti, inspiratory time)

Fig. 8.1: Summarizes the steps of prevention and treatment of BPD (starting from the antenatal period until the time of discharge) in a preterm VLBW infant

The role of drugs in evolving/established BPD is minimal except in select group of infants (Table 8.3). Most of the drugs used have already been discussed under prevention of BPD. Diuretics and bronchodilators can be used if the clinical condition warrants but should be stopped if no response occurs within 24–48 hours of initiation of therapy. This is especially important in case of diuretic therapy. One should weigh the risk-benefit ratio before initiating steroids for an infant with established BPD. Infants with 'BPD spells' (sudden episodes of deterioration due to marked expiratory airflow limitation) may require sedation and muscle relaxation to reduce agitation.

Infants developing BPD require 20–40% more calories than their age-matched healthy controls. Their caloric requirement varies from 120 to 150 kcal/kg/day. This can be achieved by fortifying breast milk with human milk fortifier (HMF) or infant formula. For infants who require more calories, fat supplementation (e.g. MCT oil) is preferable to adding carbohydrates because of the less pronounced effects on CO_2 levels (see Table 8.3).[34]

Summary of steps to prevent and manage BPD is provided in Fig. 8.1.

REFERENCES

1. Smith VC, Zupancic JA, McCormick MC, Croen LA, Greene J, Escobar GJ, Richardson DK. Trends in severe BPD rates between 1994 and 2002. J Pediatr 2005;146:469–73.
2. Bancalari E, Claure N. Definitions and diagnostic criteria for bronchopulmonary dysplasia. Semin Perinatol 2006;30:164–70.
3. Bancalari E, Abdenour GE, Feller R, Gannon J. Bronchopulmonary dysplasia: clinical presentation. J Pediatr 1979;95:819–23.
4. Shennan AT, Dunn MS, Ohlsson A, Lennox K, Hoskins EM. Abnormal pulmonary outcomes in premature infants: prediction from oxygen requirement in the neonatal period. Pediatrics 1988;82:527–32.
5. Jobe AH, Bancalari E. Bronchopulmonary dysplasia. Am J Respir Crit Care Med 2001;163:1723–9.
6. Walsh MC, Wilson-Costello D, Zadell A, et al: Safety, reliability and validity of a physiologic definition of bronchopulmonary dysplasia. J Perinatol 2003;23:451–6.
7. Ehrenkranz RA, Walsh MC, Vohr BR, Jobe AH, Wright LL, Fanaroff AA, Wrage LA, Poole K; National Institutes of Child

Health and Human Development Neonatal Research Network. Validation of the National Institutes of Health, consensus definition of bronchopulmonary dysplasia. Pediatrics 2005;116: 1353–60.

8. Chong E, Greenspan J, Kirkby S, Culhane J, Dysart K. Changing use of surfactant over 6 years and its relationship to chronic lung disease. Pediatrics. 2008 Oct;122(4):e917–21.

9. Narang A, Kumar P, Kumar R. Chronic lung disease in neonates: emerging problem in India. Indian Pediatr 2002;39:158–62.

10. Kinsella JP, Greenough A, Abman SH. Bronchopulmonary dysplasia. Lancet 2006;29;367:1421–31.

11. Makri V, Hospes B, Stoll-Becker S, Borkhardt A, Gortner L. Polymorphisms of surfactant protein B encoding gene: modifiers of the course of neonatal respiratory distress. Eur J Pediatr 2002; 161:604–08.

12. Northway WH Jr, Rosan RC, Porter DY: Pulmonary disease following respiratory therapy of hyaline-membrane disease. Bronchopulmonary dysplasia. N Engl J Med 1967;276:357.

13. Jobe AH. The New BPD: an arrest of lung development. Pediatr Res 1999;46:641–3.

14. Merritt TA, Deming DD, Boynton BR. The 'new' broncho-pulmonary dysplasia: challenges and commentary. Semin Fetal Neonatal Med 2009 Dec;14(6):345–57.

15. Crowley PA. Antenatal corticosteroid therapy: a meta-analysis of the randomized trials, 1972 to 1994. Am J Obstet Gynecol 1995; 173:322–35.

16. Crowther CA, Alfi revic Z, Haslam RR. Thyrotrophin releasing hormone added to corticosteroids for women at risk of preterm birth for preventing neonatal respiratory disease. Cochrane Database Syst Rev 2004;2:CD000019.

17. Te Pas AB, Walther FJ. A randomized, controlled trial of delivery-room respiratory management in very preterm infants. Pediatrics. 2007 Aug;120(2):322–9.

18. Avery ME, Tooley WH, Keller JB, Hurd SS, Bryan MH, Cotton RB, et al. Is chronic lung disease in low birth weight infants preventable? A survey of eight centers. Pediatrics 1987;79:26–30.

19. Morley CJ, Davis PG, Doyle LW, Brion LP, Hascoet JM, Carlin JB; COIN Trial Investigators. Nasal CPAP or intubation at birth for very preterm infants. N Engl J Med 2008;14;358:700–8.

20. Finer NN, Carlo WA, Walsh MC, Rich W, Gantz MG, Laptook AR, et al. SUPPORT Study Group of the Eunice Kennedy Shriver NICHD Neonatal Research Network. Early CPAP *versus*

surfactant in extremely preterm infants. N Engl J Med. 2010 May 27;362(21):1970–9.

21. Subramaniam P, Henderson-Smart DJ, Davis PG. Prophylactic nasal continuous positive airways pressure for preventing morbidity and mortality in very preterm infants. Cochrane Database of Systematic Reviews 2005, Issue 3. Art. No.: CD001243.

22. Dunn MS, Kaempf J, de Klerk A, de Klerk R, Reilly M, Howard D, et al. Randomized trial comparing 3 approaches to the initial respiratory management of preterm neonates. Pediatrics. 2011 Nov;128(5):e1069–76.

23. Meneses J, Bhandari V, Alves JG. Nasal intermittent positive-pressure ventilation *versus* nasal continuous positive airway pressure for preterm infants with respiratory distress syndrome: a systematic review and meta-analysis. Arch Pediatr Adolesc Med. 2012 Apr;166(4):372–6.

24. Davis PG, Lemyre B, De Paoli AG. Nasal intermittent positive pressure ventilation (NIPPV) *versus* nasal continuous positive airway pressure (NCPAP) for preterm neonates after extubation. Cochrane Database of Systematic Reviews 2001;3:CD003212.

25. Greenough A, Dimitriou G, Prendergast M, Milner AD. Synchronized mechanical ventilation for respiratory support in newborn infants. Cochrane Database of Systematic Reviews 2008;3:CD000456.

26. Thome UH, Carlo WA, Pohlandt F. Ventilation strategies and outcome in randomised trials of high frequency ventilation. Arch Dis Child. 2005;90:F466–73.

27. Wheeler K, Klingenberg C, McCallion N, Morley CJ, Davis PG. Volume-targeted *versus* pressure-limited ventilation in the neonate. Cochrane Database of Systematic Reviews 2010; (11):CD003666.

28. Woodgate PG, Davies MW. Permissive hypercapnia for the prevention of morbidity and mortality in mechanically ventilated newborn infants. Cochrane Database of Systematic Reviews 2001; (2):CD002061.

29. Askie LM, Henderson-Smart DJ, Irwig L, Simpson JM. Oxygen-saturation targets and outcomes in extremely preterm infants. N Engl J Med 2003;4;349:959–67.

30. Supplemental Therapeutic Oxygen for Prethreshold Retinopathy of Prematurity (STOP-ROP), a randomized, controlled trial. I: primary outcomes. Pediatrics. 2000;105:295–310.

31. Carlo WA, Finer NN, Walsh MC, Rich W, Gantz MG, Laptook AR, et al. SUPPORT Study Group of the Eunice Kennedy Shriver

NICHD Neonatal Research Network. Target ranges of oxygen saturation in extremely preterm infants. N Engl J Med. 2010 May 27;362(21):1959–69.

32. Stenson B, Brocklehurst P, Tarnow-Mordi W. Increased 36-Week Survival with High Oxygen Saturation Target in Extremely Preterm Infants. N Engl J Med 2011 Apr 28;364(17):1680–81.

33. Bell EF, Acarregui MJ. Restricted *versus* liberal water intake for preventing morbidity and mortality in preterm infants. Cochrane Database Syst Rev 2008 Jan 23;(1):CD000503.

34. Biniwale MA, Ehrenkranz RA. The role of nutrition in the prevention and management of bronchopulmonary dysplasia. Semin Perinatol 2006;30:200–8.

35. Engle WA; American Academy of Pediatrics Committee on Fetus and Newborn. Surfactant-replacement therapy for respiratory distress in the preterm and term neonate. Pediatrics 2008;121: 419–32.

36. Göpel W, Kribs A, Ziegler A, Laux R, Hoehn T, Wieg C, et al. Avoidance of mechanical ventilation by surfactant treatment of spontaneously breathing preterm infants (AMV): an open-label, randomised, controlled trial. Lancet. 2011 Nov 5;378(9803): 1627–34.

37. Tyson JE, Wright LL, Oh W, Kennedy KA, Mele L, Ehrenkranz RA, Stoll BJ, Lemons JA, Stevenson DK, Bauer CR, Korones SB, Fanaroff AA. Vitamin A supplementation for extremely-low-birth-weight infants. National Institute of Child Health and Human Development Neonatal Research Network. N Engl J Med 1999;340:1962–8.

38. Darlow BA, Graham PJ. Vitamin A supplementation for preventing morbidity and mortality in very low birth weight infants. Cochrane Database Syst Rev 2002;4:CD000501.

39. Schmidt B, Roberts RS, Davis P, Doyle LW, Barrington KJ, Ohlsson A, et al. Caffeine for Apnea of Prematurity Trial Group. Caffeine therapy for apnoea of prematurity. N Engl J Med 2006;354: 2112–21.

40. Schmidt B, Davis P, Moddemann D, Ohlsson A, Roberts RS, Saigal S, et al; Trial of Indomethacin Prophylaxis in Preterms (TIPP) Investigators. Long-term effects of indomethacin prophylaxis in extremely low-birth-weight infants. N Engl J Med 2001;344: 1966–72.

41. Shah SS, Ohlsson A. Ibuprofen for the prevention of patent ductus arteriosus in preterm and/or low birth weight infants. Cochrane Database Syst Rev 2006;(1):CD004213.

42. Clyman RI. Recommendations for the postnatal use of indomethacin: an analysis of four separate treatment strategies. J Pediatr 1996;128:601–7.

43. Halliday HL, Ehrenkranz RA, Doyle LW. Early (<8 days) postnatal corticosteroids for preventing chronic lung disease in preterm infants. Cochrane Database Syst Rev 2010 Jan 20;(1):CD00114644.

44. Onland W, Offringa M, van Kaam A. Late (>7 days) inhalation corticosteroids to reduce bronchopulmonary dysplasia in preterm infants. Cochrane Database Syst Rev. 2012 Apr 18;4:CD002311.

45. Barrington KJ. The adverse neuro-developmental effects of postnatal steroids in the preterm infant: a systematic review of RCTs. BMC Pediatrics 2001;1:1–14.

46. Sankar MJ, Deorari AK. Postnatal corticosteroids for chronic lung disease (CLD). Indian Pediatr 2007;44:531–9.

47. Shah V, Ohlsson A, Halliday HL, Dunn MS. Early administration of inhaled corticosteroids for preventing chronic lung disease in ventilated very low birth weight preterm neonates (Cochrane Review). Cochrane Database Syst Rev 2000;2:CD001969.

48. Barrington KJ, Finer NN. Inhaled nitric oxide for respiratory failure in preterm infants. Cochrane Database Syst Rev; 2006:CD000509.

49. Kinsella JP, Cutter GR, Walsh WF, Gerstmann DR, Bose CL, et al. Early inhaled nitric oxide therapy in premature newborns with respiratory failure. N Engl J Med 2006;355:354–64.

50. Ballard RA, Truog WE, Cnaan A, Martin RJ, Ballard PJ, et al. Inhaled nitric oxide in preterm infants undergoing mechanical ventilation. N Engl J Med 2006;355:343–53.

51. Baveja R, Christou H. Pharmacological strategies in the prevention and management of bronchopulmonary dysplasia. Semin Perinatol 2006;30:209–18.

52. Ng GY, Ohlsson A. Cromolyn sodium for the prevention of chronic lung disease in preterm infants. Cochrane Database Syst Rev. 2001;(2):CD003059.

53. Ng GY, da S, Ohlsson A. Bronchodilators for the prevention and treatment of chronic lung disease in preterm infants. Cochrane Database Syst Rev 2001;(3):CD003214.A.

54. Davis JM, Parad RB, Michele T, et al. Pulmonary outcome at one year corrected age in premature infants treated at birth with recombinant CuZn superoxide dismutase. Pediatrics 2003;111:469–76.

55. Ambalavanan N, Carlo WA. Ventilatory strategies in the prevention and management of bronchopulmonary dysplasia. Semin Perinatol 2006;30:192–9.

9 Apnea

About 30–45% of preterm babies exhibit a periodic breathing pattern characterized by three or more respiratory pauses of greater than 3 seconds duration. Periodic breathing is a normal event in preterm infants, reflective of immaturity of respiratory control system in these infants and does not merit any treatment. In contrast, apnea is a pathological cessation of breathing that results in hemodynamic disturbances and hence merits treatment.

DEFINITION

Apnea is defined as cessation of breathing for longer than 20 sec or for shorter duration in presence of bradycardia and/or change in skin color (pallor or cyanosis).[1]

INCIDENCE

Apnea is a common manifestation of many neonatal diseases. It is usually related to immaturity of the central nervous system in preterm infants and called as apnea of prematurity (AoP). It can occur secondary to many other diseases.

The incidence of AoP is inversely proportional to gestational age. It varies from 10% in infants born at gestation of 34 weeks or more than 60% in infants born at less than 28 weeks of gestation.[1]

ETIOLOGY OF APNEA[2,3]

Apnea of Prematurity

It is related to immaturity of the central nervous system. This condition usually presents after 1–2 days of life (the detection may be delayed by the presence of ventilatory support in the initial few days of life) and within the first 7 days.

Apnea occurring beyond the period of 1–2 days to 7 days of life is generally secondary to a variety of causes.

Secondary Causes

Secondary causes of apnea include:

a. Temperature instability: Hypothermia and hyperthermia
b. Neurological: Intracranial infections, intracranial hemorrhage, seizures, perinatal asphyxia, placental transfer of narcotics, magnesium sulphate or general anesthetics.
c. Pulmonary: Respiratory distress syndrome (RDS), pneumonia, pulmonary hemorrhage, obstructive airway lesion, pneumothorax, hypoxemia, hypercarbia, tracheal occlusion by neck flexion.
d. Cardiac: Congenital cyanotic heart disease, hypo/hypertension, congestive heart failure, patent ductus arteriosus.
e. Gastrointestinal: Gastroesophageal reflux, abdominal distension.
f. Hematological: Anemia
g. Infections: Sepsis, pneumonia, meningitis, necrotizing enterocolitis
h. Metabolic: Acidosis, hypoglycemia, hypocalcemia, hyponatremia, hypernatremia

---
Practical Tips

AoP is a diagnosis of exclusion and should be considered only after secondary causes of apnea have been excluded. Common causes of secondary apnea include sepsis, pneumonia, asphyxia, temperature instability and anemia.

TYPES OF APNEA[4]

a. Central apnea (40%): Central apnea is characterized by total cessation of inspiratory efforts with no evidence of obstruction.
b. Obstructive apnea (10%): In obstructed apnea, the infant tries to breathe against an obstructed upper airway, resulting in chest wall motion without airflow throughout the entire apneic episode.
c. Mixed apnea (50%): Mixed apnea consists of obstructed respiratory efforts usually following central pauses.

The source of obstruction in preterm babies is generally abnormal neck position (undue flexion or extension) and/or secretions. Other sources of obstruction are uncommon.

Monitoring

All babies less than 35 weeks gestation should be monitored for at least in the first week of life or until absence of apneic episodes for at least 7 days. Infants greater than 34 weeks gestation should be monitored if they are sick.

MANAGEMENT OF APNEA

Emergency Treatment

The neonate should be checked for bradycardia, cyanosis and airway obstruction. The neck should be positioned in slight extension and oropharynx gently suctioned, if required. Most apneic spells respond to tactile stimulation. Oxygen by head box or nasal cannula is provided if the infant is hypoxic (maintain saturation between 90 and 95%). If the neonate continues to remain apneic and does not respond to tactile stimulation, positive pressure ventilation (PPV) should be initiated.

Clinical Examination

After stabilization, the infant should be evaluated for possible underlying cause(s). History should be reviewed for secondary causes such as perinatal asphyxia, maternal drugs, neonatal sepsis and feed intolerance. The infant should be examined for temperature instability, hypotension, pallor, cardiac murmur for PDA and poor perfusion. Onset of apnea within the first 7 days in a premature infant (gestation < 34 weeks) in absence of any secondary cause is likely to be AoP.

Investigations

Affected neonates should be subjected to following investigations, on individualized basis, to exclude common secondary causes of apnea: blood glucose, hematocrit, electrolytes, sepsis work up, chest X-ray, ultrasound head and other investigations depending on the history and physical examination (Table 9.1).

PREVENTION

- Nurse the infant in thermoneutral environment (servo-controlled radiant warmer or incubator) to avoid fluctuation in body temperature.

Table 9.1: Investigations to rule out secondary causes of apnea

Causes of apnea	Clinical features	Investigations
Sepsis, pneumonia, meningitis	Lethargy, decreased feeding, fast breathing, retraction, brady/tachycardia, shock	Sepsis workup, chest X-ray
Patent ductus arteriosus	Tachycardia, bounding pulses, hyperkinetic precordium, murmur, increased requirement for respiratory support	Chest X-ray, echo-cardiography
Intraventricular bleed	Sudden onset of pallor, shock, deranged sensorium	Cranial ultrasono-graphy
Metabolic: Hypoglycemia, hypocalcemia, hypo-natremia	Jitteriness, poor feeding, seizures	Measurement of blood sugar, serum calcium or electro-lyte levels
Anemia	Pallor, history of increased blood letting	Hb level
Polycythemia	Plethora, dullness, jitteriness, feed intolerance	Hb level

- Maintain head and neck in neutral position by using appropriate shoulder roll, if required.
- Maintain the patency of upper airway by gently removing the secretions, if present, avoiding vigorous nasal suctioning or prolonged use of nasogastric (NG) tubes. NG tubes are known to increase airway resistance. Orogastric tube is preferable.
- Maintain oxygen saturation in range on 90–95% by appropriate use of supplemental oxygen. Hyperoxia should be avoided. Saturation should be monitored by continuous pulse oximetry.

General Measures

- Maintain airway, breathing and circulation.
- Avoid vigorous suctioning of oropharynx.
- Avoid oral feeds in case of repeated episodes requiring BMV. Decreasing the volume of bolus feeding may be considered by giving it more frequently.
- Maintain environmental temperature to lower end of thermoneutral range and avoid large swings.

Specific Measures

Methylxanthines

Methylxanthines (MX) has been the mainstay of pharmaco-therapy of AoP. *MX therapy is not indicated for secondary causes of apnea.*

MX increases minute ventilation, improves CO_2 sensitivity, decreases hypoxic depression of breathing, enhances diaphragmatic contractility and decreases periodic breathing. The major mechanism of action is through competitive antagonism of adenosine receptors. A recent Cochrane review of the use of MX concluded that these are effective in reducing the number of apneic attacks and the use of mechanical ventilation in two to seven days after starting treatment.[5]

Adverse effects include tachycardia, jitteriness, irritability, feed intolerance, vomiting and hyperglycemia.

There are two drugs in MX group that are available for treating AoP—caffeine and aminophylline (theophylline). The efficacy of both the drugs is similar but caffeine has lesser side effects and better dosage convenience as it requires once a day administration as compared to dosing of three times a day of aminophylline. A recent multi-centric trial showed that caffeine therapy in infants below 30 weeks reduces bronchopulmonary dysplasia and patent ductus arteriosus.[6]

MX therapy for AoP is indicated in the following circumstances:

a. When apneic episodes are frequent
b. If the baby requires PPV for apnea that is unresponsive to tactile stimulation
c. Before extubating an infant <30 weeks' gestation

Current evidence does not support the use of prophylactic MX therapy for AoP.[7]

Caffeine needs to be given as a loading dose of 20 mg/kg followed in 24 hours by 5 to 8 mg/kg per dose, administered once every 24 hours. The loading dose of intravenous aminophylline is 5 to 6 mg/kg, followed by 1.5 to 3 mg/kg every 8 to 12 hours. Oral formulation of both the drugs can be used in place of intravenous formulation once the infant is stable and tolerating oral feeds.[8] Recommended therapeutic levels are 5 to 10 g/mL for aminophylline and 8 to 20 g/mL for caffeine.

MX therapy should be continued till 34 weeks corrected gestational age and stopped thereafter if no episode of apnea has occurred in the last 7 days. Caffeine or aminophylline initiated in order to facilitate extubation may be stopped after 5 to 7 days of therapy.[9]

MX therapy should be discontinued at least 1 to 2 weeks prior to discharge, a guideline that is especially relevant for caffeine because of its longer half-life. The infant should not be discharged until MX has been stopped.

What is Evidence?

The 'caffeine therapy for apnea of prematurity (CAP)' trial[6] has shown that infants <30 weeks treated with caffeine have lower risk of:
- Need for supplemental oxygen at a postmenstrual age of 36 weeks (adjusted OR: 0.63; 95% CI 0.52 to 0.76)
- Earlier discontinuation of respiratory support

Doxapram[10-12]

The evidence for efficacy and safety of doxapram therapy for treating AoP is limited. Moreover, doxapram is associated with serious side effects and hence, it *should not be employed* in treating babies with AoP.

CONTINUOUS POSITIVE AIRWAY PRESSURE

Continuous positive airway pressure (CPAP) is usually administered using nasal prongs (nasal CPAP) when clinically significant episodes persist despite optimal MX therapy.[13] At CPAP level of 5 cm of water, infants with AoP will have fewer episodes. This reduction is primarily related to significant reduction in episodes of obstructive and mixed apneas and the effect has been attributed to splinting of the upper airways by the positive airway pressure.

NASAL INTERMITTENT POSITIVE PRESSURE VENTILATION

Infants with AoP and not responsive to MX and CPAP therapy can be given a trial of nasal intermittent positive pressure ventilation (nIPPV). nIPPV may improve patency of the upper airway by creating intermittently elevated pharyngeal pressure. This intermittent inflation of the pharynx may activate respiratory drive, by Head's paradoxical reflex, where lung inflation provokes an augmented inspiratory reflex. This results in resumption of breathing in infants with apnea following cycling of the ventilator.

What is Evidence?

A Cochrane review has shown the beneficial effect of nIPPV for treating preterm infants with apnea that are frequent or severe. Its use appears to reduce the frequency of apneas more effectively than nCPAP. It showed a greater reduction in frequency of apneas (events/hr) with nIPPV as compared to nCPAP [WMD –1.19 (–2.31, –0.07)].[14]

MECHANICAL VENTILATION

The infant should be ventilated if both pharmacotherapy and CPAP have been tried and significant apneas continue to occur. If the lungs are normal, the infant should be ventilated at minimum pressures (peak inspiratory pressure of 10–12 cm of water and positive end expiratory pressure of 3–5 cm of water), low rate (20–25 per minute), short Ti (0.35–0.40 seconds) and low FiO_2 (0.3–0.5).

Persistent Apnea

Apneic episodes may persist beyond 37 to 40 weeks in some infants, especially those born before 28 weeks of gestation. MX therapy should be continued if apneic episodes continue to occur beyond 34 weeks of PMA. The neonate should be re-evaluated for secondary causes of apnea especially neurological problems and gastroesophageal reflux. As home monitoring is not feasible in low resource settings, the infants would require NICU care until drugs can be weaned and stopped.

Sudden Infant Death Syndrome (SIDS) and Apnea

AoP is not found to be an independent risk factor for SIDS. Only 2–4% of patients with SIDS have a history of AoP.

Neurodevelopmental Outcome

Most reports have found little evidence of any neurodevelopmental risk directly attributed to a history of AoP. Precisely measured predischarge apnea related to AoP, however, has been reported to be predictive of lower developmental indices at two years.[3]

REFERENCES

1. Hunt CE. Apnea and sudden infant death syndrome. In: Kligman RM, Neider ML, Super DM (Eds). Practical strategies in pediatric diagnosis and therapy. Philadelphia: WB Saunders 1996;135–47.

2. Bhatia J. Current options in the management of apnea of prematurity. Clin Pediatr 2000;39:327–36.

3. Thompson MW, Hunt CE. In Avery's Neonatology Pathophysiology and Management of the Newborn, 6th edn. MacDonald MG, Mullett MD, Seshia MMK (Eds). Lippincott Williams & Wilkins, Philadelphia, 2005;p. 539–45.

4. Martin RJ, Abu-Shaweesh, Baird TM. Pathophysiologic Mechanisms Underlying Apnea of Prematurity. NeoReviews 2002;3(4):e59.

5. Henderson-Smart DJ, De Paoli AG. Methylxanthine treatment for apnea in preterm infants. Cochrane Database Syst Rev 2010.

6. Schmidt B, Roberts PS, Davis P, Doyle LW, Barrington KJ, Ohlsson A, Caffeine for Apnea of Prematurity Trial Group et al. Caffeine therapy for apnea of prematurity. N Engl J Med 2006; 354:2112–21.

7. Henderson-Smart DJ, De Paoli AG. Prophylactic methylxanthine for prevention of apnoea in preterm infants. Cochrane Database Syst Rev 2012.

8. Martin RJ, Abu-Shaweesh, Baird TM. Clinical Associations, Treatment and Outcome of Apnea of Prematurity. NeoReviews 2002;3:e66.

9. Miller MJ, Martin RJ. Apnea of prematurity. Clin Perinatol 1992; 19:789–808.

10. Henderson-Smart DJ, Steer PA. Doxapram treatment for apnea in preterm infants. Cochrane Database Syst Rev 2012.

11. Gauda EB, Martin RJ. Control of breathing. In Avery's diseases of the newborn. 9th edn. Gleason CA, Devaskar SU (Eds). Elsevier Saunders, Philadelphia, 2012;p. 584–97.

12. Jardine DS, Rogers K. Relationship of benzyl alcohol to kernicterus, intraventricular hemorrhage, and mortality in premature infants. Pediatrics 1988;83:721.

13. Henderson-Smart DJ, Subramanian P, Davis PG. Continuous positive airway pressure *versus* theophylline for apnea in preterm infants. Cochrane Database Syst Rev 2009.

14. Lemyre B, Davis PG, De Paoli AG. Nasal intermittent positive pressure ventilation (NIPPV) *versus* nasal continuous positive airway pressure (NCPAP) for apnea of prematurity. Cochrane Database Syst Rev 2008.

Gastrointestinal Disorders

V

10   Jaundice

Jaundice is the most common morbidity in the first week of life, occurring in 60% of term and 80% of preterm newborns. It is the most common cause of re-admission after discharge from birth hospitalization.[1]

Jaundice in neonates is visible in skin and eyes when total serum bilirubin (TSB) concentration exceeds 5 to 7 mg/dL. In contrast, adults have jaundice visible in eyes (but not in skin) when TSB concentration exceeds 2 mg/dL. Increased TSB concentration in neonate results from varying contributions of three mechanisms namely, increased production from degradation of red cells, decreased clearance by the immature hepatic mechanisms and re-absorption by enterohepatic circulation (EHC).

High serum bilirubin levels carry a risk of causing neurological impairment. In most cases, jaundice is benign and no intervention is required. Approximately 5–10% of them have clinically significant jaundice that require treatment to lower serum bilirubin levels in order to prevent bilirubin brain damage.

PHYSIOLOGICAL VERSUS PATHOLOGICAL JAUNDICE

Jaundice attributable to physiological immaturity of neonates to handle increased bilirubin production is termed as 'physiological jaundice'. Visible jaundice usually appears between 24 and 72 hours of age. TSB level usually rises in term infants to a peak level of 12 to 15 mg/dL by 3 days of age and then falls. In preterm infants, the peak level occurs on the 3 to 7 days of age and TSB can rise over 15 mg/dL. It may take weeks before the TSB levels fall under 2 mg/dL in both term and preterm infants.

'Pathological jaundice' is said to be present when TSB concentrations are not in 'physiological jaundice' range, which is defined arbitrarily as more than 5 mg/dL on first day, 10 mg/dL on second day and 12–13 mg/dL thereafter in term neonates.[2] Any TSB value of 17 mg/dL or more should be regarded as pathologic and should be evaluated for the cause and possible intervention, such as phototherapy.[3]

It may be noted that the differentiation between 'pathological' and 'physiological' is rather arbitrary, and is not clearly defined. Presence of one or more of the following conditions would qualify a neonate to have pathological jaundice:[2]

1. Visible jaundice in first 24 hours of life. *However, slight jaundice on face at the end of first day (i.e. 18 to 24 hrs) is common and can be considered physiological.*
2. Presence of jaundice on arms and legs on day 2
3. Yellow palms and soles anytime
4. Serum bilirubin concentration increasing more than 0.2 mg/dL/hour or more than 5 mg/dL in 24 hours
5. If TSB concentration is more than 95th centile as per age-specific bilirubin nomogram
6. Signs of acute bilirubin encephalopathy or kernicterus
7. Direct bilirubin more than 1.5 to 2 mg/dL at any age
8. Clinical jaundice persisting beyond 2 weeks in term and 3 weeks in preterm neonates

CAUSES OF PATHOLOGICAL JAUNDICE

Common causes of pathological jaundice include:
1. Hemolysis: Blood group incompatibility such as those of ABO, Rh and minor groups, enzyme deficiencies such as G6PD deficiency, autoimmune hemolytic anemia
2. Decreased conjugation due to liver enzyme immaturity
3. Increased enterohepatic circulation such as lack of adequate enteral feeding that includes insufficient breastfeeding or the infant not being fed because of illness, GI obstruction
4. Extravasated blood: Cephalhematoma, extensive bruising, etc.

CLINICAL ASSESSMENT

- The parents should be counselled regarding benign nature of jaundice in most neonates, and for the need to be watchful and seek help if baby appears too yellow. The parents should be explained about how to see for jaundice in babies (in natural light and without any yellow background).

- Visual inspection of jaundice (Panel 1) is believed to be unreliable, but if it is performed properly (i.e. examining a naked baby in bright natural light and in absence of yellow background), it has reasonable accuracy particularly when TSB is less than 12 to 14 mg/dL or so. Absence of jaundice on visual inspection reliably excludes the jaundice. At higher TSBs, visual inspection is unreliable and therefore, TSB should be measured to ascertain the level of jaundice.[4]

- All neonates should be examined at every opportunity but not lesser than every 12 hr until first 3 to 5 days of life for jaundice. The babies discharged from the hospital earlier than 48 to 72 hours should be seen again after 48 to 72 hours of discharge.

- The neonates at higher risk of jaundice should be identified at birth and kept under enhanced surveillance for occurrence and progression of jaundice. These infants include[5]:
  Gestation <38 wk
  - Previous baby with significant jaundice
  - Visible jaundice in first 24 hrs
  - Age-specific TSB level being above 95th centile (if measured)

- Inadequacy of breastfeeding is a common cause of exaggerated jaundice during initial few days (breastfeeding jaundice). Breastfeeding problems such as improper positioning and attachment, cracked or sore nipple, engorgement, perceived inadequacy of milk production are very common and require intense and sustained support from health professionals caring for mothers and babies. Breastfeeding support must include, in addition to providing adequate information, *actual helping* the mothers to learn proper positioning and attachment, and adequate measures to address breastfeeding problems.

Panel 1: Visual Inspection

1. Examine the baby in bright natural light. Alternatively, the baby can be examined in white fluorescent light. Make sure there is no yellow or off white background.
2. Make sure the baby is naked.
3. Examine blanched skin and gums or sclerae.
4. Note the extent of jaundice (Kramer's rule)[6]
   - Face   5–7 mg/dL
   - Chest   8–10 mg/dL
   - Lower abdomen/thigh   12–15 mg/dL
   - Soles/Palms   >15 mg/dL
5. *Depth of jaundice (degree of yellowness) should be carefully noted* as it is an important indicator of level of jaundice, though it does not figure out in Kramer's rule.

   A deep yellow staining (even in absence of yellow soles or palms) is often associated with severe jaundice and therefore TSB should be estimated in such circumstances.

MEASUREMENT OF SERUM BILIRUBIN

Transcutaneous Bilirubinometry (TcB)[4]

a. TcB is a useful adjunct to TSB measurement, and routine employment of TcB can reduce need for blood sampling by nearly 30%. However, current devices are costly and have a significant recurring cost of consumables such as disposable tips, etc.

b. TcB can be used in infants of 35 weeks or more of gestation after 24 hrs. TcB is unreliable in infants less than 35 weeks gestation and during initial 24 hrs of age. TcB has a good correlation with TSB at lower levels, but it becomes unreliable once TSB level goes beyond 14 mg/dL.

c. Hour specific TcB can be used for prediction of subsequent hyperbilirubinemia. TcB value below 50th centile for age would rule out the risk of subsequent hyperbilirubinemia with high probability (high negative predictive value).[7]

d. Trends in TcB values by measuring 12 hrs apart would have a better predictive value than a single value.[8]

   We routinely perform TcB measurement in infants of 35 wk or more gestation to screen for hyperbilirubinemia. A TcB value of greater than 12 to 14 mg/dL is confirmed by TSB measurement.

Indications of TSB Measurement

a. Jaundice in first 24 hours.

b. Beyond 24 hrs: If visually assessed, jaundice is likely to be more than 12 to 14 mg/dL (as visual assessment becomes unreliable) beyond this TSB level or approaching the phototherapy range *or* beyond.

c. If you are unsure about visual assessment.

d. During phototherapy, for monitoring progress and after phototherapy to check for rebound in select cases (such as those with hemolytic jaundice).

Frequency of TSB Measurement

It depends upon the underlying cause (hemolytic *versus* non-hemolytic) and severity of jaundice as well as host factors such as age and gestation.[9] In general, in non-hemolytic jaundice in term babies with TSB levels being below 20 to 22 mg/dL, TSB can be performed every 12 to 24 hrs depending upon age of the baby. As opposed to this, a baby with Rh isoimmunization would require TSB measurement every 6 to 8 hours during initial 24 to 48 hours or so.

Methods of TSB Measurement

a. Biochemical· High performance liquid chromatography (HPLC) remains the gold standard for estimation of TSB. However, this test is not universally available and laboratory estimation of TSB is usually performed by van den Bergh's reaction. It has marked inter laboratory variability with coefficient of variation up to 10–12% for TSB and over 20% for conjugated fraction.[10]

b. Micro method for TSB estimation: It is based on spectrophotometry and estimates TSB on a micro blood sample. It is useful in neonates as bilirubin is predominantly unconjugated.

APPROACH TO A JAUNDICED NEONATE

A stepwise approach should be employed for managing jaundice in neonates (Fig. 10.1).

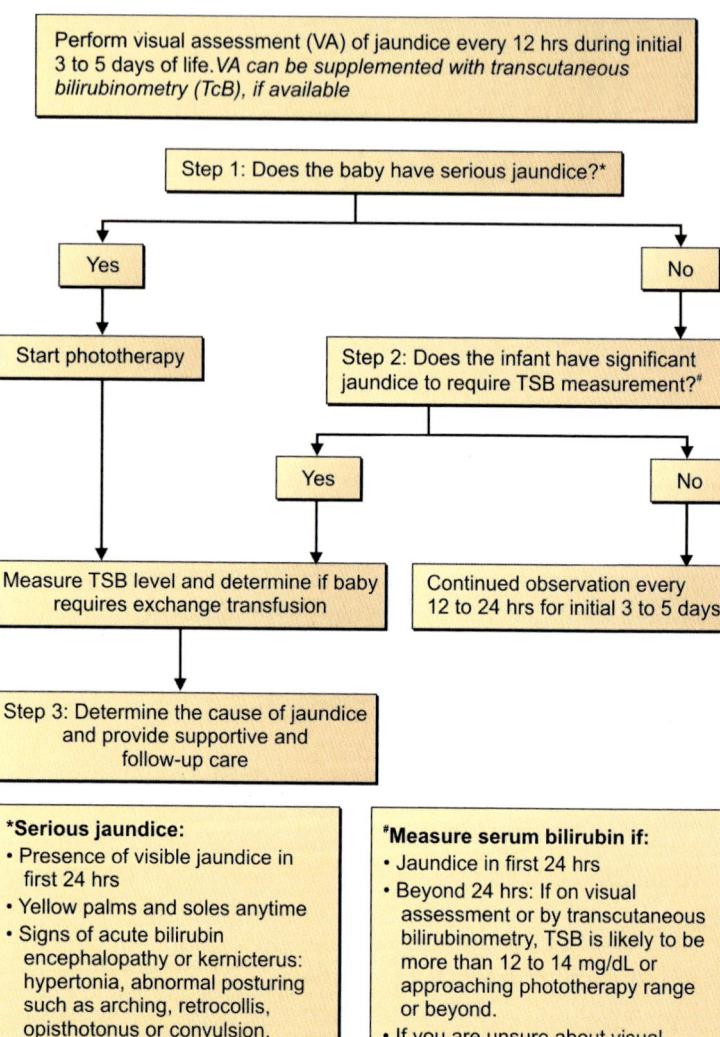

Fig 10.1: Approach to an infant with jaundice

All the neonates should be visually inspected for jaundice every 12 hrs during initial 3 to 5 days of life. TcB can be used as an aid for initial screening of infants. Visual assessment (when performed properly) and TcB have reasonable sensitivity for initial assessment of jaundice.

As a first step, serious jaundice should be ruled out. Phototherapy should be immediately initiated if the infant meets the criteria for serious jaundice. TSB should be determined subsequently in these infants to determine further course of action.

Note: Though recommended by AAP,[5] routine screening of all infants with TSB in order to predict the risk of subsequent hyperbilirubinemia has not been evaluated in Indian settings and therefore, cannot be recommended.

MANAGEMENT OF JAUNDICE

Infants Born at Gestation of 35 Weeks or More

American Academy of Paediatrics (AAP) criteria should be used for making decision regarding phototherapy or exchange transfusion in these infants.[5] AAP provides two age-specific nomograms—one each for phototherapy and exchange transfusion. The nomograms have lines for three different risk categories of neonates. These lines include one each for lower risk babies (38 wks or more and no risk factors), medium risk babies (38 wks or more with risk factors or 35–37 wks and without any risk factors) and higher risk babies (35–37 wks and with risk factors).

TSB value is taken for decision making and direct fraction should not be reduced from it. As a rough guide, phototherapy is initiated if TSB vales are at or higher than 10, 13, 15 and 18 mg/dL at 24, 48, 72 and 96 hours and beyond, respectively in babies at medium risk. The babies at lower and higher risk have their cut-offs at approximately 2 mg/dL higher or 2 mg/dL lower than those for medium risk babies, respectively.

Risk factors include presence of isoimmune hemolytic anemia, G6PD deficiency, asphyxia, temperature instability, hypothermia, sepsis, significant lethargy, acidosis and hypoalbuminemia.

Nomogram for exchange transfusion also has three risk categories of babies. Any baby showing signs of bilirubin encephalopathy such as hypertonia, retrocollis, convulsion, fever, etc. should receive exchange transfusion without any delay.

Preterm Babies

There are no consensus guidelines to employ phototherapy or exchange transfusion in preterm babies. The proposed TSB cut-offs for phototherapy and exchange transfusion are arbitrary and clinical judgement should be exercised before making a decision (Table 10.1).

Table 10.1: Phototherapy and exchange transfusion cut-offs for preterm babies (<35 wks)[9]

Post menstrual age (PMA; wk)	TSB (mg/dL) cut-offs for	
	Phototherapy	Exchange transfusion
<28 0/7	5–6	11–14
28 0/7– 29 6/7	6–8	12–14
30 0/7– 31 6/7	8–10	13–16
32 0/7– 33 6/7	10–12	15–18
34 0/7– 34 6/7	12–14	17–19

Reproduced with permission

Practical Tips

- Use postmenstrual age for phototherapy, for example, when a 29 0/7 weeks infant is 7 days old, use the TSB level for 30 0/7 weeks.
- Use the lower range of the indicated TSB levels for infants at greater risk for bilirubin toxicity (low gestation, low serum albumin levels <2.5 g/dL, rapidly rising TSB levels, suggesting hemolytic disease and sick babies).
- Infants are considered to be sick if they have acidosis (pH <7.15), blood culture positive sepsis in the prior 24 hrs, apnea and bradycardia requiring cardio-respiratory resuscitation (bagging and/or intubation) during the previous 24 hrs; hypotension requiring pressor treatment during the previous 24 hrs; and mechanical ventilation at the time of blood sampling.
- Recommendations for exchange transfusion apply to infants who are receiving intensive phototherapy to the maximal surface area but whose TSB levels continue to increase to the levels listed.
- For all infants, an exchange transfusion is recommended if the infant shows signs of acute bilirubin encephalopathy (hypertonia, arching, retrocollis, opisthotonos, high-pitched cry) although it is recognized that these signs rarely occur in VLBW infants.
- Use total bilirubin. Do not subtract direct-reacting or conjugated bilirubin from the total.
- Discontinue phototherapy when TSB is declining and is 1–2 mg/dL below the initiation level for the infant's postmenstrual age.

THERAPEUTIC OPTIONS

Phototherapy

Phototherapy (PTx) remains the mainstay of treating hyper-bilirubinemia in neonates. PTx is highly effective and carries an excellent safety track record of over 50 years. It acts by converting insoluble bilirubin (unconjugated) into soluble isomers that can be excreted in urine and feces. Many review articles have provided detailed discussion on phototherapy related issues. The bilirubin molecule isomerizes to harmless forms under blue-green light (460 to 490 nm); and the light sources having high irradiance in this particular wavelength range are more effective than the others.

Types of Phototherapy Lights

The phototherapy units available in the market have a variety of light sources that include fluorescent lamps of different colors (cool white, blue, green, blue-green or turquoise) and shapes (straight or U-shaped commonly referred as compact fluorescent lamps, i.e. CFL), halogen bulbs, high intensity light emitting diodes (LED) and fiberoptic light sources.

With easy availability and low cost in India, CFL phototherapy is being most commonly used device. Often, CFL devices have four blue and two white (for examination purpose) CFLs but this combination can be replaced with 6 blue CFLs in order to increase the irradiance output.

In the last couple of years, blue LED is making inroads in neonatal practice and has been found to be at least equally effective. LED has advantage of long life (up to 50,000 hrs) and is capable of delivering higher irradiance than CFL lamps.

Fiberoptic units can be used to provide undersurface photo-therapy in conjugation with overhead CFL/LED unit to enhance the efficacy of PTx but as a standalone source, fiber-optic unit is lesser effective than CFL/LED unit.

It is important that a plastic cover or shield be placed before phototherapy lamps to avoid accidental injury to the baby in case a lamp breaks.

Maximizing the Efficacy of Phototherapy

The irradiance of PTx lights should be periodically measured, and a minimum level of 30 $\mu W/cm^2/nm$ in the wavelength range of 460 to 490 nm must be ensured. As the irradiance varies at different points on the footprint of a unit, it should be measured at several points. The lamps should be changed if the lamps are flickering or ends are blackened and if irradiance falls below the specified level or as per the recommendation of manufacturers.

Expose maximal surface area of the baby. Avoid blocking the lights by any equipment (say radiant warmer), a large diaper or eye patch, a cap or hat, tape, dressing or electrode, etc. Ensure good hydration and nutrition of the baby. Make sure that light falls on the baby perpendicularly if the baby is in incubator. Minimize interruption of PTx during feeding sessions or procedures.

Administering Phototherapy

Make sure that ambient room temperature is optimum (25–28°C) to prevent hypothermia or hyperthermia in the baby. Remove all clothes of the baby except the diaper. Cover the baby's eyes with patches, ensuring that the patches do not block the baby's nostrils. Place the naked baby under the lights in a cot or bassinet if weight is more than 2 kg or in an incubator or radiant warmer if the baby is small (< 2 kg).

Keep the distance between baby and light 30 to 45 cm (or as per manufacturer recommendation).

Ensure optimum breastfeeding. Baby can be taken out for breastfeeding sessions and the eye patch can be removed for better mother–infant interaction. However, minimize interruption to enhance effectiveness of phototherapy. There is no need to supplement or replace breast milk with any other types of feed or fluid (e.g. breastmilk substitute, water, sugar water, etc.)

Monitoring and Stopping Phototherapy

Monitor temperature of the baby every 2 to 4 hrs. Measure TSB level every 12 to 24 hours.

Discontinue PTx once two TSB values 12 hrs apart fall below current age specific cut offs. The infant should be monitored clinically for rebound bilirubin rise within 24 hours after stopping phototherapy for babies with hemolytic disorders.

Role of Sunlight

Exposing the baby to sunlight does not help in treatment of jaundice and is associated with risk of sunburn and therefore should be avoided.

EXCHANGE TRANSFUSION

Double volume exchange transfusion (DVET) should be performed if the TSB levels reach to age specific cut-off for exchange transfusion or the infant shows signs of bilirubin encephalopathy irrespective of TSB levels.

Indications for DVET at birth in infants with Rh isoimmunization include:

1. Cord bilirubin is 5 mg/dL or more
2. Cord Hb is 10 g/dL or less

At birth, if a baby shows signs of hydrops or cardiac decompensation in presence of low PCV ($<35\%$), partial exchange transfusion with 50 mL/kg of packed cells should be done to quickly restore oxygen carrying capacity of blood.

The ET should be performed by pull and push technique using umbilical venous route. Umbilical catheter should be inserted just deep enough to get free flow of blood. Table 10.2 provides guidelines on type and volume of blood used in DVET.

S. No.	Condition	Type of blood
	Table 10.2: Type and volume of blood for exchange transfusion	
1	Rh isoimmunization	Rh negative and blood group 'O' or that of baby. Suspended in AB plasma. Cross-matched with baby's and mother's blood
2	ABO incompatibility	Rh compatible and blood group 'O' (*Not that of baby*). Suspended in AB plasma. Cross-matched with baby's and mother's blood
3	Other conditions (G6PD deficiency, non-hemolytic, other isoimmune hemolytic jaundice	Baby's group and Rh type cross-matched with baby's and mother's blood

- Volume of blood: Twice the blood volume of baby (total volume: 160 to 180 mL/kg)
- To prepare blood for DVET, mix two-thirds of packed cells and one-third of plasma.

Intravenous Immunoglobulins (IVIG)

IVIG reduces hemolysis and production of jaundice in isoimmune hemolytic anemia (Rh isoimmunization and ABO incompatibility) and thereby reduces the need for phototherapy and exchange transfusion.

IVIG administration can cause intestinal injury and necrotizing enterocolitis. Recent evidence has questioned the efficacy of IVIG. Due to evidence of GI injury and doubtful efficacy, we have discontinued the use of IVIG.

IV Hydration

Infants with severe hyperbilirubinemia and evidence of dehydration (e.g. excessive weight loss) should be given IV hydration. An extra fluid of 50 mL/kg of N/3 saline over 8 hr decreases the need for exchange transfusion.[11]

Other Agents

There is no proven evidence of benefit of drugs like phenobarbitone, clofibrate or steroids to prevent or treat hyperbilirubinemia in neonates and therefore, these agents should not be employed in treatment of jaundiced infants.

Prolonged Jaundice

There is no good definition of prolonged jaundice (PJ). Generally, persistence of significant jaundice for more than 2 weeks in term and more than 3 weeks in preterm babies is taken as PJ. Though, it is not uncommon to see persistence of mild jaundice in many infants for 4 to 6 weeks of age, most of these babies do well without any specific intervention or investigation.

The first and foremost step to manage an infant with PJ is to rule out cholestasis (Fig. 10.2). Yellow colored urine is a reasonable marker for cholestasis; however, the urine color could be normal during initial phase of cholestasis. For the practical purpose, an infant with PJ with normal colored urine can be considered to have unconjugated hyperbilirubinemia. If the infant has dark colored urine, the infant should be managed as per cholestasis guidelines.

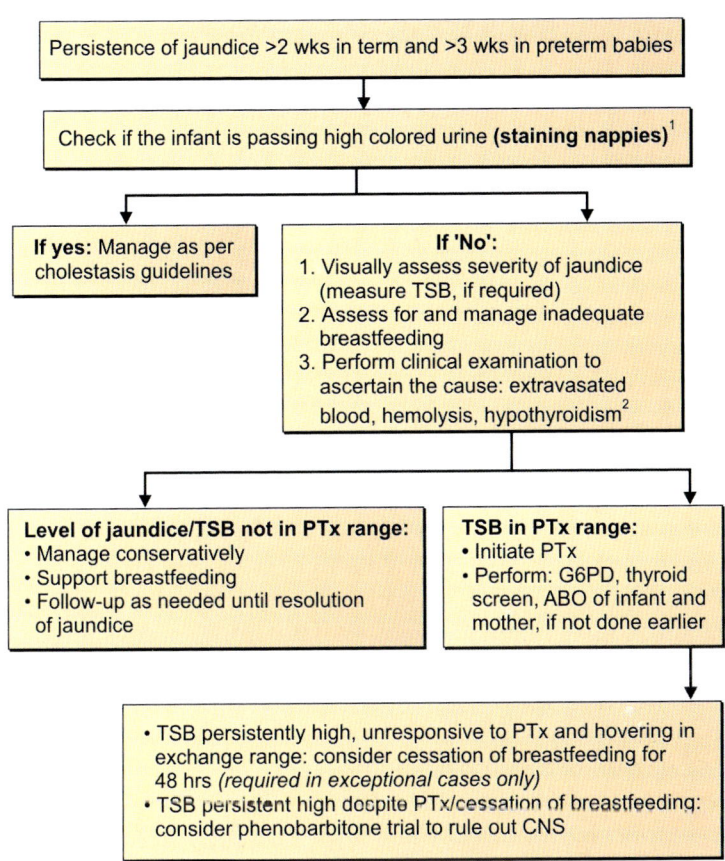

Persistence of jaundice >2 wks in term and >3 wks in preterm babies

↓

Check if the infant is passing high colored urine **(staining nappies)**[1]

If yes: Manage as per cholestasis guidelines

If 'No':
1. Visually assess severity of jaundice (measure TSB, if required)
2. Assess for and manage inadequate breastfeeding
3. Perform clinical examination to ascertain the cause: extravasated blood, hemolysis, hypothyroidism[2]

Level of jaundice/TSB not in PTx range:
• Manage conservatively
• Support breastfeeding
• Follow-up as needed until resolution of jaundice

TSB in PTx range:
• Initiate PTx
• Perform: G6PD, thyroid screen, ABO of infant and mother, if not done earlier

• TSB persistently high, unresponsive to PTx and hovering in exchange range: consider cessation of breastfeeding for 48 hrs *(required in exceptional cases only)*
• TSB persistent high despite PTx/cessation of breastfeeding: consider phenobarbitone trial to rule out CNS

[1]Thyroid screen can be considered at this stage; TSB: total serum bilirubin; CNS: Criggler-Najjar syndrome; PTx: photopherapy

Fig. 10.2: Approach to a neonate with prolonged jaundice

Infants with true PJ (unconjugated hyperbilirubinemia) should be assessed clinically for severity and possible cause of prolongation of jaundice (Table 10.3). If the clinical assessment of jaundice suggests TSB levels below phototherapy cut-offs for age (say <15 to 18 mg/dL in term infant), the infant may not be subjected to any unnecessary investigations. As many of these infants have PJ as a result of inadequate feeding, appropriate measures are taken to optimize breastfeeding. Thyroid screen can be considered in such infants at this stage

Table 10.3: Causes of prolonged jaundice

Common

1. Inadequacy of breastfeeding
2. Breast milk jaundice
3. Cholestasis
4. Continuing hemolysis, e.g. Rh, ABO and G6PD hemolysis

Rare

1. Extravasated blood, e.g. cephalhematoma
2. Hypothyroidism
3. Criggler-Najjar Syndrome
4. GI obstruction such as malrotation
5. Gilbert syndrome

if routine metabolic screen for hypothyroidism has not been carried out at birth.

If baby appears to have significant jaundice at this stage, TSB level should be performed and possible underlying cause should be looked for. In such infants, G6PD level, thyroid screen, ABO of infant and mother if not done earlier should be performed to delineate possible cause.

Infants having TSB in phototherapy range should be started on phototherapy. The adequacy of breastfeeding should be assessed by history, observation of breastfeeding session and degree of weight loss. Many of the mothers, even at this stage, have persisting breastfeeding problems such as poor attachment, sore nipple, etc.

Breast milk jaundice (BMJ) is relatively uncommon cause of jaundice. Inadequacy of breastfeeding is far more common than cause and therefore it should be carefully ruled out. BMJ is generally an innocuous entity and cessation of breastfeeding is generally not required. Infants with BMJ should be treated with phototherapy, if required. For a rare infant with TSB hovering in exchange range, a brief trial of interruption of breastfeeding can be considered. We have not stopped breast-feeding even for once for treatment of BMJ in last 15 years!

In an infant failing to respond to these measures, a diagnosis of CNS should be entertained. A trial of phenobarbitone can be considered to establish the diagnosis.

REFERENCES

1. Young Infants Clinical Signs Study Group. Clinical signs that predict severe illness in children under age 2 months: a multicentre study. Lancet 2008;371:135–42.

2. Madan A, Mac Mohan JR, Stevenson DK. Neonatal Hyper-bilirubinemia. In: Avery's Diseases of the Newborn. Eds: Taeush HW, Ballard RA, Gleason CA. 8th edn; WB Saunders, Philadelphia, 2005;p.1226–56.

3. Maisels MJ, Gifford K: Normal serum bilirubin levels in newborns and effect of breastfeeding. Pediatrics 1986;78:837–43.

4. Rennie J, Burman-Roy S, Murphy MS; Guideline Development Group. Neonatal jaundice: summary of NICE guidance. BMJ. 2010 May 19;340:c2409. doi:10.1136/bmj.c2409.

5. American Academy of Pediatrics Subcommittee on Hyper-bilirubinemia. Management of hyperbilirubinemia in the newborn infant 35 or more weeks of gestation. Pediatrics 2004;114:297–316.

6. Kramer LI. Advancement of dermal icterus in jaundiced newborn. Am J Dis Child 1969;118:454–8.

7. Kaur S, Chawla D, Pathak U, Jain S. Predischarge non-invasive risk assessment for prediction of significant hyperbilirubinemia in term and late preterm neonates. J Perinatol. 2011 Nov 17. doi: 10.1038/jp.2011;170.

8. Dalal SS, Mishra S, Agarwal R, Deorari AK, Paul V. Does measuring the changes in TcB value offer better prediction of Hyperbilirubinemia in healthy neonates? Pediatrics 2009;124: e851–7.

9. Halamek LP, Stevenson DK. Neonatal Jaundice. In Fanroff AA, Martin RJ (Eds): Neonatal Perinatal Medicine. Diseases of the fetus and infant. 7th edn. St Louis, Mosby Year Book 2002; p. 1335.

10. Van Imhoff DE, Dijk PH, Weykamp CW, Cobbaert CM, Hulzebos CV; BARTrial Study Group. Measurements of neonatal bilirubin and albumin concentrations: a need for improvement and quality control. Eur J Pediatr 2011;170:977–82.

11. Mehta S, Kumar P, Narang A. A randomized controlled trial of fluid supplementation in term neonates with severe hyper-bilirubinemia. J Pediatr 2005;147:781–5.

11 | Feeding of Low Birth Weight Neonates

Globally, about 18 million infants are born with a birth weight of <2500 g every year.[1] Though these low birth weight (LBW) infants constitute only about 14% of the total live births, they account for 60–80% of total neonatal deaths.[2] Most of these deaths can be prevented with extra attention to warmth, prevention of infections and more importantly optimal feeding.

Nutritional management influences immediate survival as well as subsequent growth and development of LBW infants. Simple interventions such as early initiation of breastfeeding and avoidance of pre-lacteal feeding have been shown to improve their survival in resource restricted settings.[3] Early nutrition could also influence the long-term neurodevelopmental outcomes; malnutrition at a vulnerable period of brain development has been shown to have deleterious effects in experimental animals.[4]

FEEDING OF LBW INFANTS: HOW IS IT DIFFERENT?

Term infants with normal birth weight require minimal assistance for feeding in the immediate postnatal period—they are able to feed directly from mothers' breast. In contrast, feeding of LBW infants is relatively difficult because of the following limitations:

1. Many LBW infants are born premature and have inadequate feeding skills; they might not be able to breastfeed and would require other methods of feeding such as spoon or gastric tube feeding.
2. They are prone to have significant illnesses which often preclude enteral feeding in the first few weeks of life.
3. Preterm very low birth infants (VLBW) have higher fluid requirements due to excessive insensible water loss.

4. Since intrauterine accretion of nutrients occurs mainly in the later part of the third trimester, VLBW infants (usually born before 32 weeks gestation) have low body stores at birth. Hence, they require supplementation of various nutrients. Even term LBW infants who are likely to be growth restricted need higher calories for 'catch-up' growth.

5. Because of the gut immaturity, they are more likely to experience feed intolerance necessitating adequate monitoring and treatment.

PROTOCOL FOR FEEDING LBW INFANTS

In this protocol, we would address the following issues in feeding the LBW infants:

1. How to decide the initial method of feeding in a given LBW infant?
2. For infants initiated on modes other than breastfeeding:
   a. How to progress to breastfeeding?
   b. What milk to be given?
   c. How much milk to be given?
3. What supplements are required?
4. How to assess the feeding adequacy and monitor the growth?
5. How to identify and manage feed intolerance?

DECIDING THE INITIAL METHOD OF FEEDING

It is essential to categorize LBW infants into two major groups – *sick* and *healthy* before deciding the method of feeding.

Sick Infants

This group constitutes infants with significant respiratory distress requiring assisted ventilation, shock requiring inotropic support, seizures, symptomatic hypoglycemia/hypocalcemia, electrolyte abnormalities, renal/cardiac failure, surgical conditions of gastrointestinal tract, necrotizing enterocolitis (NEC), hydrops, etc. These infants are usually started on intravenous (IV) fluids. Enteral feeds should be initiated as soon as they are hemodynamically stable.

It is important to realize that enteral feeding is important even in sick neonates. Oral feeds should not be delayed in them without any valid reason. Even infants with respiratory distress and/or on assisted ventilation can be started on enteral feeds once the acute phase is over and their color, saturation and perfusion have improved. Similarly, sepsis unless associated with shock/sclerema/NEC is not a contraindication for enteral feeding.

Healthy LBW Infants

Enteral feeding should be initiated immediately after birth in healthy infants with the appropriate feeding method determined by their gestation and oral feeding skills.

Maturation of Oral Feeding Skills

Breastfeeding requires effective sucking, swallowing and a proper coordination between suck/swallow and breathing. These complex skills mature with increasing gestation (Table 11.1).

Table 11.1: Maturation of oral feeding skills and the choice of initial feeding method in LBW infants[5]

Gestational age	Maturation of feeding skills	Initial feeding method
< 28 weeks	No proper sucking efforts No propulsive motility in the gut	Intravenous fluids
28–31 weeks	Sucking bursts develop No coordination between suck/ swallow and breathing	Oro-gastric (or nasogastric) tube feeding with occasional spoon/*paladai* feeding
32–34 weeks	Slightly mature sucking pattern Coordination between breathing and swallowing begins	Feeding by spoon/ *paladai*/cup
>34 weeks	Mature sucking pattern More coordination between breathing and swallowing	Breastfeeding

Initial Feeding Method

Traditionally, the initial feeding method in a LBW infant was decided based on the birth weight. This is not an ideal way because the feeding ability depends largely on gestation rather than the birth weight.

However, it is important to remember that *not all* infants born at a particular gestation would have same feeding skills.

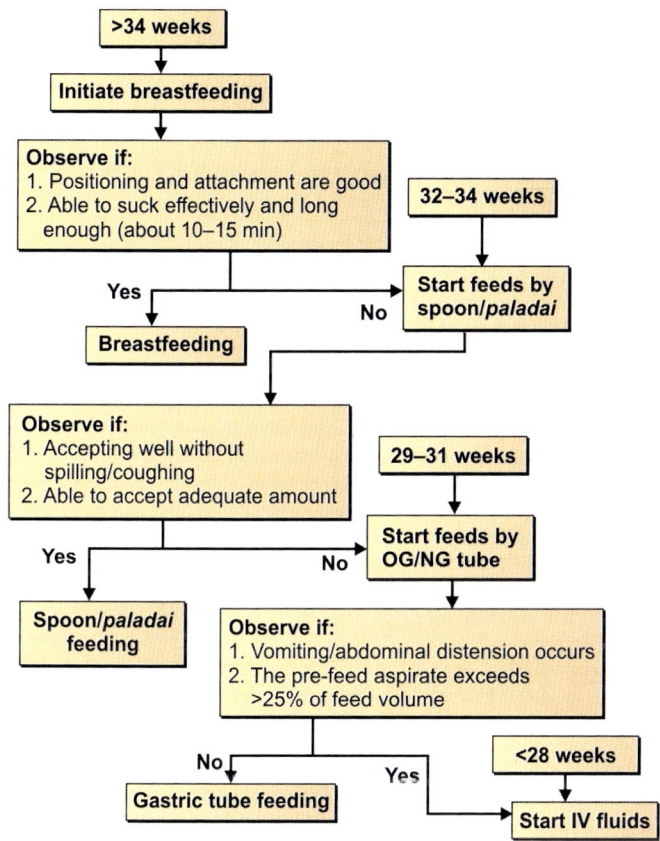

Fig. 11.1: Deciding the initial feeding method in LBW infants

Hence, the ideal method in a given infant would be to evaluate if the feeding skills expected for his/her gestation are present and then decide accordingly (Fig. 11.1).

All stable LBW infants, irrespective of their initial feeding method should be put on their mothers' breast. The immature sucking observed in preterm infants born before 34 weeks might not meet their daily fluid and nutritional requirements but helps in rapid maturation of their feeding skills and also improves the milk secretion in their mothers (*non-nutritive sucking*).

Spoon/Paladai Feeding

In our unit, we use paladai feeding in LBW infants who are not able to feed directly from the breast. The steps of paladai feeding are described in Panel 1.[6]

Panel 1: Steps of *Paladai* Feeding[6]

1. Place the infant in up-right posture on mother's lap.
2. Keep a cotton napkin around the neck to mop the spillage.
3. Take the required amount of expressed breast milk by using a clean syringe.
4. Fill the *paladai* with milk little short of the brim.
5. Hold the *paladai* from the sides (so that your fingers do not come into contact with the milk).
6. Place the *paladai* at the lips of the baby in the corner of the mouth and tip to pour a small amount of milk into the mouth.
7. Feed the infant slowly; he/she should actively swallow the milk.
8. Repeat the process until the required amount has been fed.
9. If the infant does not actively accept and swallow, try to arouse him/her with gentle stimulation.
10. While estimating the milk intake, deduct the amount of milk left in the cup and the amount of estimated spillage.
11. Wash the *paladai* with soap and water and then put in boiling water for 20 minutes to sterilize before next feed.

Intragastric Tube Feeding

The steps of intragastric tube feeding are given in *Panel 2*. Some of the controversial issues in gastric tube feeding are discussed below:

Nasogastric versus Orogastric Feeding

Physiological studies have shown that nasogastric (NG) tube increases the airway impedance and the work of breathing in very preterm infants.[7] Hence, orogastric tube feeding might be preferable in these infants. *We employ only orogastric tube feeding in our unit.*

Intermittent Bolus versus Continuous Intragastric Feeding

There are no differences in the time to reach full enteral feeding or somatic growth or the incidence of NEC between infants fed by intermittent bolus or continuous intragastric feeding.[8] Studies have shown that gastric emptying and duodenal motor responses are enhanced in infants given continuous intragastric feeding.[9] But a major disadvantage of this method is

Panel 2: Steps of Intragastric Tube Feeding[6]

1. Before starting a feed, check the position of the tube.
2. Remove the plunger of the syringe (ideally a sterile syringe should be used).
3. Connect the barrel of the syringe to the end of the gastric tube.
4. Pinch the tube and fill the barrel of the syringe with the required volume of milk.
5. Hold the tube with one hand, release the pinch and elevate the syringe barrel.
6. Let the milk run from the syringe through the gastric tube by gravity; *DO NOT force milk through the gastric tube by using the plunger of the syringe.*
7. Control the flow by altering the height of the syringe. Lowering the syringe slows the milk flow, raising the syringe makes the milk flow faster.
8. It should take about 10–15 minutes for the milk to flow into the infant's stomach.
9. Observe the infant during the entire gastric tube feed. Do not leave the infant unattended. Stop the tube feed if the infant shows any of the following signs: breathing difficulty, change in color/looks blue, becomes floppy and vomiting.
10. Cap the end of the gastric tube between feeds; if the infant is on CPAP, the tube is preferably left open after about half an hour.[11] Avoid flushing the tube with water or saline after giving feeds.

that the lipids in the milk tend to separate and stick to the syringe and tubes during continuous infusion resulting in significant loss of energy and fat content. *We use intermittent bolus feeding in our unit.*

Special Situations

Extremely low birth weight infants: They are usually started on parenteral nutrition from day one of life. Enteral feeds in the form of trophic feeding or minimal enteral nutrition (MEN) are initiated once the infant is hemodynamically stable. Further advancement is based on the infant's ability to tolerate the feeds.[10]

Severe IUGR with antenatally detected Doppler flow abnormalities: Fetuses with abnormal Doppler flow such as absent/reversed end diastolic flow (A/REDF) in the umbilical artery are likely to have had mesenteric ischemia *in utero.* After birth, they have a significant risk of developing feed intolerance and NEC.[11] The timing of initiation of oral feeds in these infants is controversial. We usually delay feeding until 48 hours of life in preterm (<35 weeks) infants with AEDF/REDF.

Infants on CPAP/ventilation: These infants can be started on orogastric (OG) tube feeds once they are hemodynamically stable. But it is important to leave the tube open intermittently to reduce gastric distension.

PROGRESSION OF ORAL FEEDS

All LBW infants, irrespective of their gestation and birth weight, should ultimately be able to feed directly from the mothers' breast. For preterm LBW infants started on IV fluids/OG tube/*paladai* feeding, the steps of progression to direct and exclusive breastfeeding are summarized in Fig. 11.2.

Term LBW infants started on IV fluids (because of their sickness) should be put on the breast once they are hemodynamically stable.

Choice of Milk for LBW Infants

All LBW infants, irrespective of their initial feeding method should receive ONLY breast milk. This can be ensured even in those infants who are fed by *paladai* or gastric tube by giving expressed breast milk (mother's own milk or human donor milk).

Expressed Breast Milk (EBM)

All preterm infants' mothers should be counseled and supported in expressing their own milk for feeding their infants. Expression should ideally be initiated within hours of delivery so that the infant gets the benefits of feeding colostrum. Thereafter, it should be done every 2–3 hrs so that the infant is exclusively breastfed. This would also help in maintaining the lactation in the mother. Expressed breast milk can be stored for about 6 hours at room temperature and for 24 hours in refrigerator.

The steps of breast milk expression are given in Panel 3. We counsel mothers for expression of breast milk soon after delivery by demonstration and by using posters and videos (available on our website: www.newbornwhocc.org).

Donor Human Milk

In centers where optimal milk banking facilities are available, donor human milk can be used. At present, only a few centers

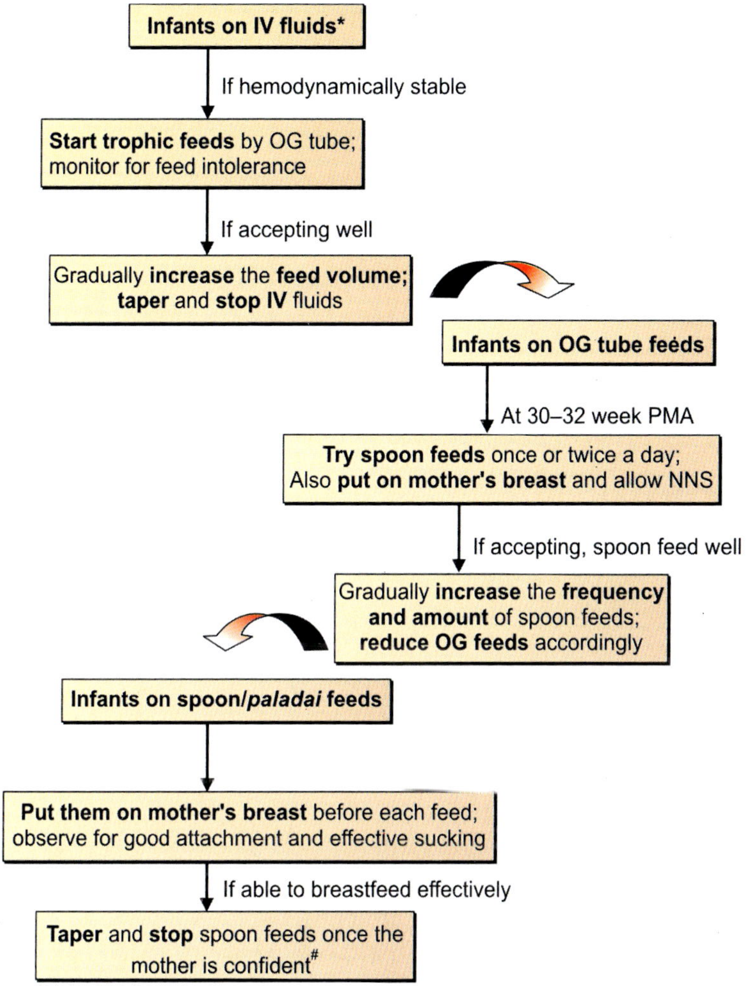

Infants on IV fluids*

If hemodynamically stable

Start trophic feeds by OG tube; monitor for feed intolerance

If accepting well

Gradually **increase** the **feed volume; taper** and **stop IV** fluids

Infants on OG tube feeds

At 30–32 week PMA

Try spoon feeds once or twice a day; Also **put on mother's breast** and allow NNS

If accepting, spoon feed well

Gradually **increase** the **frequency and amount** of spoon feeds; **reduce OG feeds** accordingly

Infants on spoon/*paladai* feeds

Put them on mother's breast before each feed; observe for good attachment and effective sucking

If able to breastfeed effectively

Taper and **stop** spoon feeds once the mother is confident[#]

(IV: intravenous; OG: orogastric tube; PMA: postmenstrual age; NNS: non-nutritive sucking)
*Term and near-term sick infants started on IV fluids can be initiated on breastfeeding once they are hemodynamically stable.
[#]Some infants may have to be given spoon feeding for some period even after they start accepting breastfeeding.

Fig. 11.2: Progression of oral feeding in preterm LBW infants

in India have standardized human milk banking facilities. Therefore, it is not a practical option in most Indian settings.

Panel 3: Steps of Expression of Breast Milk[6]

1. The mother should wash her hands thoroughly.
2. She should hold a clean wide mouthed container near her breast.
3. Ask her to gently massage the breast for 5–10 minutes before expressing the milk (using the pulp of two fingers or with knuckles of the fist in a circular motion towards the nipple as if kneading dough). Massage should not hurt her.
4. Ask her to put her thumb ABOVE the nipple and areola, and her first finger BELOW the areola opposite the thumb. She should support the breast with her other fingers.
5. Ask her to press her thumb and first finger slightly inward towards the chest wall.
6. She should press her breast behind the nipple and areola between her fingers and thumb. She must press on the lactiferous sinuses beneath the areola.
7. Press and release, press and release. This should not hurt-if it hurts, the technique is wrong. It may take some time before milk starts coming.
8. Ask her to press the areola in the same way from the SIDES to make sure that milk is expressed from all segments of the breast.
9. She should express one breast first till the milk flow slows; then express the other side; and then repeat both sides.
10. **Avoid** rubbing or sliding her fingers along the skin.
11. **Avoid** squeezing the nipple itself. Pressing or pulling the nipple cannot express the milk.

Special Situations

Sick mothers/contraindication to breastfeeding: In these rare circumstances, the options available are:
1. Formula feeds:
    (a) Preterm formula—in VLBW infants, and
    (b) Term formula—in infants weighing >1500 g at birth
2. Animal milk, e.g. cow's milk

Once the mother's condition becomes stable (or the contraindication to breastfeeding no longer exists), these infants should be started on exclusive breastfeeding.

How Much Milk to be Given

It is essential to calculate the fluid requirements and feed volumes for infants on *paladai*/gastric tube feeding.

Fluid Requirement

The daily fluid requirement is determined based on the estimated insensible water loss, other losses and urine output. Extreme preterm infants need more fluids in the initial weeks of life because of the high insensible water loss.

We usually start fluids at 80 mL and 60 mL/kg/day for infants birth weights of <1500 g and 1500–2499 g, respectively. Further requirements are calculated by daily estimation of weight loss/gain, urine output and specific gravity. The usual daily increment would be about 15–20 mL/kg/day so that by the end of first week, 150 mL/kg/day is reached in both the categories. We usually reach a maximum of 180 mL/kg/day by day 14 (for oral feeds; 150 mL/kg for IV fluids).[12]

Feed Volume

After estimating the fluid requirements, the individual feed volume to be given by OG tube or *paladai* (2-hrly/3-hrly) should be determined.

NUTRITIONAL SUPPLEMENTATION IN LBW INFANTS

LBW infants especially those who are born preterm require supplementation of various nutrients to meet their high demands.[13] The requirements of VLBW infants differ significantly from those with birth weights of 1500 to 2499 grams.

Supplementation in VLBW Infants

The infants who are usually born before 32 to 34 weeks gestation have inadequate body stores of most of the nutrients.[14] The amount of protein, energy, calcium, phosphorus, trace elements (iron, zinc) and vitamins (D, E and K) present in expressed breast milk is often unable to meet their high daily requirements (Table 11.2). Hence, these infants require multi-nutrient supplementation till they reach term gestation (40 weeks postmenstrual age). After this period, their requirements are similar to those infants with birth weights of 1500–2499 grams.

Multi-nutrient supplementation can be ensured by one of the following methods:

a. Supplementing individual nutrients, e.g. calcium, phosphorus and vitamins.

b. Fortification of expressed breast milk by using either human milk fortifiers (HMF) or preterm formula.

Supplementing breast milk with individual nutrients: The following nutrients have to be added to the expressed breast milk:

Table 11.2: Recommended dietary allowance (RDA) in preterm LBW infants and the estimated intakes with fortified and unfortified human milk

	RDA* (Units/kg/day)	Only expressed breast milk#	At daily intake of 180 mL/kg	
			EBM fortified with lactodex -HMF (4 g/100 mL)	EBM fortified with preterm formula (4 g/100 mL)
Energy (kcal)	110–135	117	144	153
Protein (g)	3.5–4.0	2.5	3.2	3.5
Carbohydrates (g)	11.6–13.2	11.6	16.8	15.4
Fat (g)	4.8–6.6	6.8	7.1	8.6
Calcium (mg)	120–140	43	223	104
Phosphate (mg)	0–90	22	112	56
Vitamin A (IU)	1330–3330	680	1228	788
Vitamin D (IU/day)	800–1000	3.5	140	36
Vitamin E (mg)	2.2–11	1.8	6.3	2.8
Vitamin B_6 (mcg)	45–300	25.7	116	43
Folic acid (mcg)	35–100	6	150	20
Zinc (mg)	1.1–2.0	0.6	0.88	0.9
Iron (mg)	2–3	0.2	0.2	0.9
Remarks		Deficient in protein, calcium, phosphorus and vitamins B_6 and D; zinc content is slightly less than the RDA	Deficient in protein, vitamins A and D, zinc, and iron	Deficient in calcium, phosphorus, vitamins, folic acid and B_6, zinc and iron; protein is slightly less

*ESPGHAN 2010[15]

Based on preterm mature milk

4 to 4.5 g/kg/day for ELBW infants

(RDA, recommended dietary allowance; EBM, expressed breast milk)

1. Calcium and phosphate supplements[a]
2. Vitamin A, B complex and zinc supplements[b]—usually in the form of multivitamin drops
3. Vitamin D_3 drops[c]
4. Folate drops[d]
5. Iron drops[e]

Since supplementation of minerals and vitamins would not meet the high protein requirements of these infants, this method is usually not preferred. If used, the supplements should be added at different times in the day to avoid undue increase in the osmolality.

Fortification with HMF: Fortification of expressed breast milk with HMF increases the nutrient content of the milk without compromising its other beneficial effects (such as reduction in NEC, infections, etc.). Experimental studies have shown that the use of fortified human milk results in net nutrient retention that approaches or is greater than expected intrauterine rates of accretion in preterm infants.[16] The Cochrane review on fortification found short-term improvement in weight gain, linear and head growth without any increase in adverse effects such as NEC.[17]

The standard preparations of human milk fortifiers (HMF) used in developed countries are not available in India. The only preparation available *(Lactodex-HMF, Raptakos, Brett and Co. Ltd;* ` *10/– per sachet)* has suboptimal quantities of vitamins A and D; also, it does not contain iron. Short of other options, it may still have to be used in VLBW infants. One study from Chandigarh has reported better growth with its use.[18] Recently another preparation (HIJAM; 1 g/sachet; Endocura Pharma) has been available in the market. The preparation has the advantage of having higher protein and vitamin D content. It is available in 1 g sachet which is the typical amount required to be added in one feed volume. The preparation has the disadvantage of higher cost and less pleasant taste.

---

[a] e.g. Syr. Ostocalcium (GlaxoSmithKline Co.), Syr. Ossopna-D (TTK Healthcare)
[b] e.g. Dexvita (Tridoss Co.), Visyneral-zinc drops (Lifeon Co.)
[c] e.g. Arbivit (Raptakos, Brett & Co.), Sunsips (Endura Co.)
[d] e.g. Folium (Speciality Meditech Co.), Folvite (Wyeth Lederle Co.)
[e] e.g. Ferrochelate (Albert David Co.), Tonoferon (East India Co.)

Table 11.3: Nutritional supplementation in preterm VLBW infants until 40 weeks PMA

Nutrients	Type of feeding			
	*Only expressed breast milk**	*EBM fortified with lactodex-HMF**	*EBM fortified with preterm formula*	
Calcium	Start calcium supplements (140–160 mg/kg/day) once the infant is on 100 mL/kg/day (e.g. *Syr. Ostocalcium at 8–10 mL/kg/d*)	Not needed	Start calcium supplements to meet the RDA once the infant is on 100 mL/kg/day (e.g. *Syr. Ostocalcium at 5–6 mL/kg/d*)	
Phosphorus	Start supplements (70–80 mg/kg/day) once the infant is on 100 mL/kg/day (e.g. *Syr. Ostocalcium at 8–10 mL/kg/d*)	Not needed	Start supplements to meet the RDA once the infant is on 100 mL/kg/day (e.g. *Syr. Ostocalcium at 5–6 mL/kg/d*)	
Zinc and vitamins A, B$_6$ etc.	Start multivitamin supplements once the infant is on 100 mL/kg/day (e.g. *Visyneral zinc/Dexvita* drops at 1.0 mL/day)	Start multivitamin supplements once the infant is on 100 mL/kg/day (e.g. *Visyneral zinc/Dexvita* drops at 1.0 mL/day)	Start multivitamin supplements once the infant is on 100 mL/kg/day (e.g. *Visyneral zinc/Dexvita* drops at 1.0 mL/day)	
Vitamin D	(Usually obtained from multivitamin drops and calcium supplements that contain vitamin D)	Start vitamin D3 drops once the infant is on 100 mL/kg/day (e.g. *Arbivit/Sunsips at 1.0 mL/day*)	*Start vitamin D$_3$ drops if the total intake is less than the RDA (e.g. Arbivit/Sunsips at 0.5 mL/day)*	
Folic acid	Start supplements once the infant is on 100 mL/kg/day (e.g. *Folvite/folium drops at 0.3 mL/day*)	Not needed (e.g. *Folvite/folium at 0.1 mL/day*)	Start supplements once the infant is on 100 mL/kg/day	
Iron	Start iron (2 mg/kg/d) at 4 weeks of life (e.g. *Tonoferon drops at 2 drops/kg/day*)	Start iron (2 mg/kg/d) at 4 weeks (e.g. *Tonoferon drops at 2 drops/kg/day*)	Start iron (2 mg/kg/d) at 4–6 weeks of life (e.g. *Tonoferon drops at 2 drops/kg/day*)	

(PMA: postmenstrual age; EBM: expressed breast milk; HMF: human milk fortifier)
Note: The examples quoted are only indicative; Readers are encouraged to use similar products of their choice.

The recommended dietary allowances (RDA) and the estimated intakes with fortified human milk are given in Table 11.2. *As seen from the table, VLBW infants on fortified breast milk would still require supplementation of vitamins A and D, zinc and iron.*

Fortification with preterm formula: The other option available for fortification is preterm formula (e.g. *Dexolac Special Care* [Wockhardt Co.], *Pre-Lactogen* [Nestle Co.]). The recommended concentration is **0.4 g per 10 mL** of breast milk. Though more economical than fortification by HMF, this method has two major drawbacks—(1) it is difficult to measure such small amounts of formula powder; and (2) the RDA of calcium, phosphorus, vitamin D, folic acid, etc. are not met even after fortification. While the former problem can be managed to a certain extent by using a small scoop of 1 g size for 25 mL of human milk, the latter needs to be circumvented by additional supplementation (Table 11.2).

The protocols for nutritional supplementation in VLBW infants until 40 weeks PMA and beyond are described in Tables 11.3 and 11.4.

We use HMF fortification for all preterm (<32 weeks) VLBW infants. It is started once they reach 100 mL/kg/day of enteral feeds in the dose recommended by the manufacturer (1 sachet per 50 mL of expressed breast milk). We start iron in the dose of 2 mg/kg/day at 2 weeks of age.

If HMF is unavailable, we use preterm formula (0.4 g/10 mL) for fortification. Since the intake of calcium, phosphorus, vit D, zinc and iron is low even after fortification with formula, we supplement these nutrients additionally (Table 11.4).

Table 11.4: Nutritional supplementation in preterm VLBW infants after 40 weeks PMA

Nutrients	Method of supplementation	Dose	Till when?
Vitamin D*	Vitamin D$_3$ drops	800–1000 IU/day	Till 1 year of age
Iron	Iron drops/syrup	2 mg/kg/day (maximum 15 mg/day)	Till 1 year of age

*Vitamin D is also present in multivitamin drops, cumulative intake is an image of 800–1000 IU/d.

We continue fortification till the infant reaches 40 weeks PMA or attains 2 kg (whichever, is later).

Supplementation for Infants with Birth Weights of 1500–2499 g

These infants who are more likely to be born at term or near term gestation (≥32 weeks) do not require multi-nutrient supplementation or fortification (HMF) of breast milk (cf. VLBW infants). However, vitamin D, iron and zinc might still have to be supplemented in them.

We supplement both vitamin D and iron in infants with birth weights of 1500–2499 grams; vitamin D (400 IU) is started at 2 weeks and iron (2 mg/kg/day) at 4 weeks of life; both are continued till 1 year of age (Table 11.5).

Table 11.5: Nutritional supplements for infants with birth weights of 1500–2499 g

Nutrients	Method of supplementation	Dose	When to start	Till when?
Vitamin D	Multivitamin drops/syrup	1 mL/day (so as to provide 400 IU/day of vitamin D)	2 weeks of age	Till 1 year of age
Iron	Iron drops/ syrup	2 mg/kg/day (maximum 15 mg/day)	4 weeks of age	Till 1 year of age

GROWTH MONITORING OF LBW INFANTS

Regular growth monitoring helps in assessing the nutritional status and adequacy of feeding; it also identifies those infants with inadequate weight gain.

All LBW infants (particularly < 2 kg) should be weighed daily till the time of discharge from the hospital. Other anthropometric parameters such as length and head circumference should be recorded weekly.

Both term and preterm LBW infants tend to lose weight (about 10% and 15%, respectively) in the first 7 days of life; they regain their birth weight by 10–14 days. Thereafter, the weight gain should be at least 15–20 g/kg/day till a weight of 2–2.5 kg is reached. After this, a gain of 20 to 30 g/day is considered appropriate.[19]

LBW infants should be discharged after:
– They reach 34 weeks gestation and are above 1400–1600 g and
– They show consistent weight gain for at least 3 consecutive . days.

Growth charts: Using a growth chart is a simple but effective way to monitor the growth. Serial plotting of weight and other anthropometric indicators in the growth chart allows the individual infant's growth to be compared with a reference standard. It helps in early identification of growth faltering in these infants.

Two types of growth charts are commonly used for growth monitoring in preterm infants: intrauterine and postnatal growth charts. Of these, the postnatal growth chart is preferred because it is a more realistic representation of the true postnatal growth (than an intrauterine growth chart) and also shows the initial weight loss that occurs in the first two weeks of life. The two postnatal charts that are most commonly used for growth monitoring of preterm VLBW infants are: Wright's and Ehrenkranz' charts.[20, 21] *We use both of them in our unit.*

Once the preterm LBW infants reach 40 weeks PMA, WHO MGRS growth charts are used for growth monitoring.

MANAGEMENT OF INADEQUATE WEIGHT GAIN

Inadequate weight gain is a common and pertinent problem in LBW infants. It starts from birth and continues after discharge resulting in failure to thrive and wasting in the first year of life. The common causes are summarized in Panel 4.

Management of inadequate weight gain consists of the following steps:
1. Proper counseling of mothers and ensuring adequate support for breastfeeding their infants; includes assessment of positioning/attachment, managing sore/flat nipple, etc.
2. Explaining the frequency and timing of both breastfeeding and spoon/*paladai* feeds: Infrequent feeding is one of the commonest causes of inadequate weight gain. Mothers should be properly counseled regarding the frequency and the importance of night feeds. A time-table where mother can fill the timing and amount of feeding is very helpful in ensuring frequent feeding.

Panel 4: Causes of Inadequate Weight Gain

1. Inadequate intake
   Breastfed infants:
   Incorrect feeding method (improper positioning/attachment)*
   Less frequent breastfeeding, not feeding in the night hours*
   Prematurely removing the baby from the breast (before the infant completes feeds)
   Infants on spoon/paladai feeds:
   Incorrect method of feeding* (e.g. excess spilling)
   Incorrect measurement/calculation
   Infrequent feeding
   Not fortifying the milk in VLBW infants
   Energy expenditure in infants who have difficulty in accepting spoon feeds
2. Increased demands
   Illnesses such as hypothermia/cold stress,* bronchopulmonary dysplasia
   Medications such as corticosteroids
3. Underlying disease/pathological conditions
   Anemia,* hyponatremia, late metabolic acidosis
   Late onset sepsis
   Feed intolerance and/or GER

---

* Common conditions
(EBM: expressed breast milk; GER: gastroesophageal reflux)

3. Giving EBM by spoon/*paladai* feeds after breastfeeding also helps in preterm infants who tire out easily while sucking from the breast.
4. Proper demonstration of the correct method of expression of milk and *paladai* feeding: It is important to observe how the mother gives *paladai* feeds; the technique and amount of spillage should be noted. This should be followed by a practical demonstration of the proper procedure.
5. Initiating fortification of breast milk when indicated.
6. Management of the underlying condition(s) such as anemia, feed intolerance, etc.
7. If these measures are not successful, increase either the
   a. Energy (calorie) content of milk by adding MCT oil, corn starch, etc. to EBM; infants on formula feeds can be given concentrated feeds (by reconstituting 1 scoop in 25 mL of water); OR
   b. Feed volume to 200 mL/kg/day.

INDICATORS OF FEED INTOLERANCE

The inability to tolerate enteral feedings in extremely premature infants is a major concern for the pediatrician/neonatologist caring for such infants. Often feed intolerance is the predominant factor affecting the duration of hospitalization in these infants.

There are no universally agreed-upon criteria to define feed intolerance in preterm infants.[17] Various clinical features that are usually considered to be the indicator(s) of feed intolerance are summarized in Panel 5.

Panel 5: Indicator(s) of Feed Intolerance[17]

Symptoms:
1. Vomiting (altered milk/bile or blood-stained)*
2. Systemic features: lethargy, apnea

Signs:
1. Abdominal distension (with or without visible bowel loops)*
2. Increased gastric residuals: >2 mL/kg or any change from previous pattern
3. Abdominal tenderness
4. Reduced or absent bowel sounds
5. Systemic signs: Cyanosis, bradycardia, etc.

* Common signs

Of these, vomiting, abdominal distension and increased gastric residual volume form the 'triad' for defining feed intolerance.

Vomiting: The characteristic of vomitus is important in assessing the cause while altered milk is usually innocuous, bile- or blood-stained vomiting should be thoroughly investigated.

Abdominal distension: It is essential to serially monitor the abdominal girth in all preterm LBW infants admitted in the ICU. This helps in early identification of feed intolerance and eliminates the need for routine gastric aspirate.

Gastric residual volume: It indicates the rapidity of gastric emptying. Since several factors (both systemic and local) influence the gastric emptying, the residual volume is a poor and non-specific indicator of feed intolerance. Measures to enhance the specificity such as quantifying the volume or using different cut-offs for defining feed intolerance have not been found to be much useful. Moreover, repeated gastric aspiration

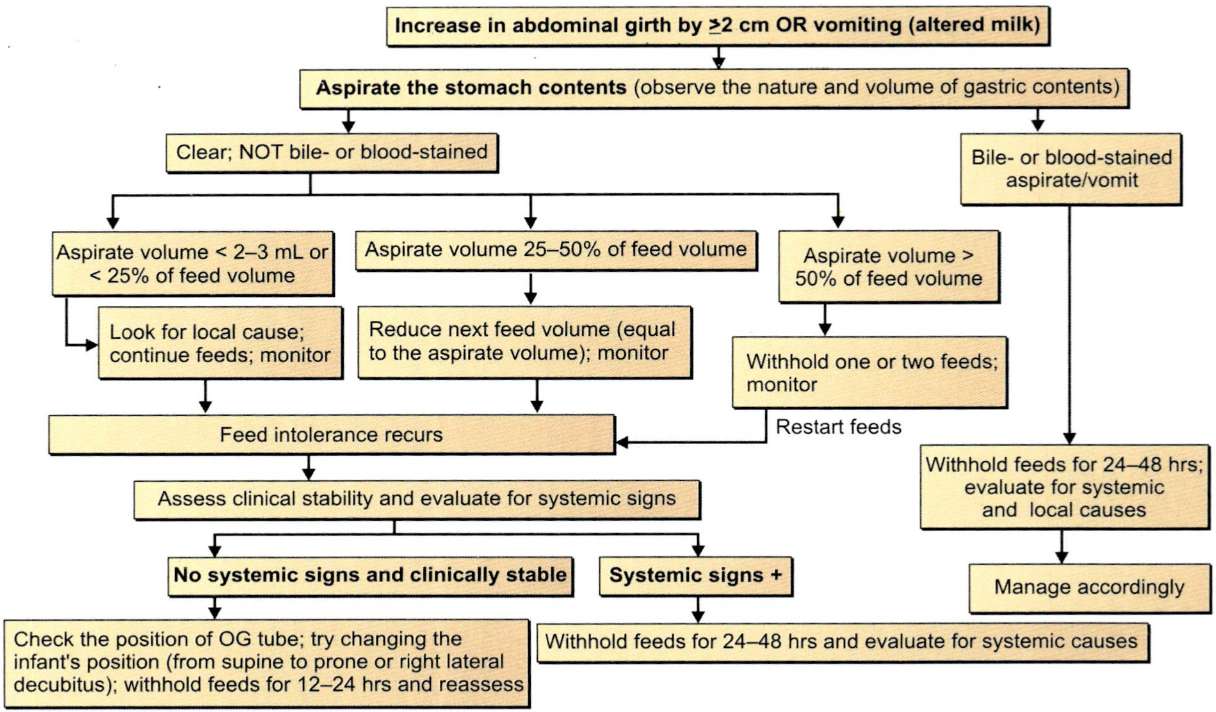

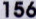

Fig. 11.3: Approach to feed intolerance in LBW infants

to look for residuals could injure the delicate mucosa aggravating the local pathology.

We monitor the abdominal girth every 2 hours in all preterm LBW infants admitted in the nursery. **We do not routinely aspirate the gastric contents before giving next feed.** It is done only if there is an increase in abdominal girth by ≥ 2 cm from the baseline.

MANAGEMENT OF FEED INTOLERANCE

The common factors attributed to feed intolerance in preterm infants are: immature intestinal motility, immaturity of digestive enzymes, underlying medical conditions such as sepsis, inappropriate feed volume and giving hyperosmolar medications/feedings, and importantly, necrotizing enterocolitis (NEC).

While issues such as feed volume and osmolality can be controlled to an extent, feed intolerance due to immaturity is rarely amenable to any intervention; conservative management till the gut attains full maturity is often the only option left.

The steps in evaluation and management of an infant with feed intolerance are given in Fig. 11.3.

REFERENCES

1. UNICEF. State of the World's Children 2005. New York: UNICEF, 2004.

2. Bang A, Reddy MH, Deshmukh MD. Child mortality in Maharashtra. Economic Political Weekly 2002;37:4947–65.

3. Edmond KM, Kirkwood BR, Tawiah CA, Agyei SO. Impact of early infant feeding practices on mortality in low birth weight infants from rural Ghana. J Perinatol. 2008 Mar 6. [Epub ahead of print]

4. Levitsky DA, Strupp BJ. Malnutrition and the brain: changing concepts, changing concerns. J Nutr 1995;125:S2212–20.

5. Omari TI, Rudolph CD. Gastrointestinal Motility. In: Polin RA and Fox WW (Eds). Fetal and Neonatal Physiology. 2nd edn. Philadelphia, WB Saunders Co 1998; p. 1125–38.

6. Anonymous. Feeding. In: Deorari AK, Paul VK, Scotland J, McMillan DD, Singhal N (Eds). Practical procedures for the newborn nursery. 2nd edn. New Delhi, Sagar Publishers 2003; p. 71–78.

7. Stocks J. Effect of nasogastric tubes on nasal resistance during infancy. Arch Dis Child 1980;55:17–21.

8. Premji SS, Chessell L. Continuous nasogastric milk feeding *versus* intermittent bolus milk feeding for premature infants less than 1500 grams. Cochrane Database of Systematic Reviews 2001, Issue 1. Art. No.: CD001819.

9. DeVille KT, Shulman RJ, Berseth CL. Slow infusion feeding enhances gastric emptying in preterm infants compared to bolus feeding. Clin Res 1993;41:787A.

10. Mishra S, Agarwal R, Jeevasankar M, Deorari AK, Paul VK. Minimal enteral nutrition. Indian J Pediatr 2008;75:267–9.

11. Dorling J, Kempley S, Leaf A. Feeding growth restricted preterm infants with abnormal antenatal Doppler results. Arch Dis Child Fetal Neonatal Ed 2005;90:F359–63.

12. Chawla D, Agarwal R, Deorari AK, Paul VK. Fluid and electrolyte management in term and preterm neonates. Indian J Pediatr. 2008;75:255–9.

13. Anonymous. Nutrition. In: Edmond K, Bahl R (Eds). Optimal feeding of low-birth-weight infants—Technical Review. World Health Organization 2006; p. 42.

14. Abrams SA. Abnormalities of serum calcium and magnesium. In: Cloherty JP, Eichenwald EC, Stark AR (Eds). Manual of Neonatal Care. 6th edn. Philadelphia: Lippincott Williams and Wilkins 2008; p. 558.

15. American Academy of Pediatrics Committee on Nutrition: Nutritional needs of preterm infants. In: Kleinman RE (Ezd): Pediatric Nutrition Handbook American Academy of Pediatrics. Elk Grove Village, IL, American Academy of Pediatrics, 2004; p. 23–54.

16. Schanler RJ, Garza C. Improved mineral balance in very low birth weight infants fed fortified human milk. J Pediatr 1987;112:452–6.

17. Kuschel CA, Harding JE. Multicomponent fortified human milk for promoting growth in preterm infants. Cochrane Database of Systematic Reviews 1998, Issue 4. Art. No.: CD000343.

18. Mukhopadhyay K, Narnag A, Mahajan R. Effect of human milk fortification inappropriate for gestation and small for gestation preterm babies: a randomized controlled trial. Indian Pediatr 2007 Apr;44(4):286–90.

19. Schanler RJ. Enteral nutrition for the high-risk neonate. In: Taeusch HW, Ballard RA, Gleason CA (Eds): Avery's Diseases of the Newborn, 8th edn. Philadelphia, Saunders 2005; p. 1043–60.

20. Wright K, Dawson JP, Fallis D, Vogt E, Lorch V. New postnatal growth grids for very low birth weight infants. Pediatrics 1993;91: 922–6.

21. Ehrenkranz RA, Younes N, Lemons JA, Fanaroff AA, Donovan EF, Wright LL, et al. Longitudinal growth of hospitalized very low birth weight infants. Pediatrics 1999;104:280–9.

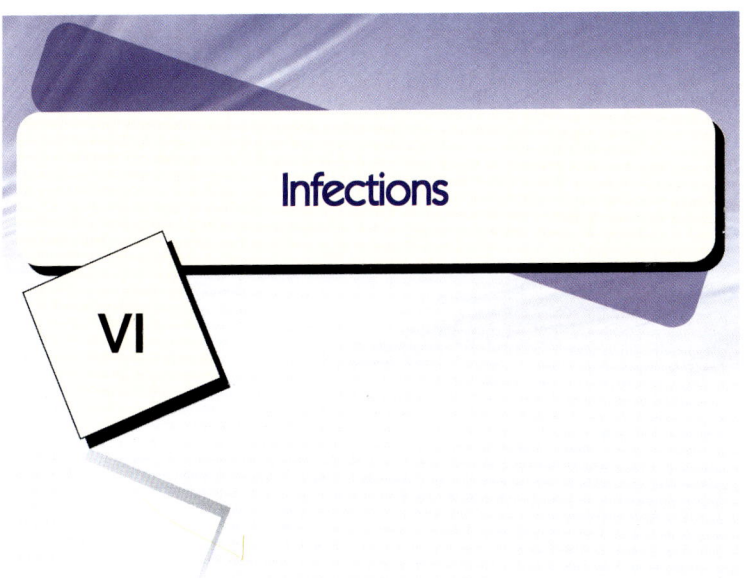

Infections

VI

Sepsis is the commonest cause of neonatal mortality; it is responsible for about 30–50% of the total neonatal deaths in developing countries.[1,2] It is estimated that up to 20% of neonates develop sepsis and approximately 1% die of sepsis related causes.[2] Sepsis related mortality is largely preventable with prevention of sepsis itself, timely recognition, rational antimicrobial therapy and aggressive supportive care.

DEFINITION

Neonatal sepsis is a clinical syndrome characterized by signs and symptoms of infection with or without accompanying bacteremia in the first month of life. It encompasses septicemia, meningitis, pneumonia, arthritis, osteomyelitis and urinary tract infections.

Superficial infections like conjunctivitis and oral thrush is not usually included under neonatal sepsis.

Epidemiology: Indian Data

The incidence of neonatal sepsis according to the data from National Neonatal Perinatal Database (NNPD) is 30 per 1000 live births.[3]

Among intramural births, *Klebsiella pneumoniae* was the most frequently isolated pathogen (32.5%), followed by *Staphylococcus aureus* (13.6%). Among extramural neonates (referred from community/other hospitals), *Klebsiella pneumoniae* was again the commonest organism (27%), followed by *Staphylococcus aureus* (15%) and *Pseudomonas* spp. (13%).[3]

CLASSIFICATION OF NEONATAL SEPSIS

Neonatal sepsis can be classified into two categories depending on the onset of symptoms:[4]

Early onset sepsis (EOS): It presents within the first 72 hours of life. In severe cases, the neonate may be symptomatic *at birth*. Infants with EOS usually present with respiratory distress and pneumonia. The source of infection is generally the maternal genital tract.

The following risk factors seem to be associated with an increased risk of early onset sepsis:[4, 5]
1. Low birth weight (<2500 grams) or prematurity
2. Febrile illness in the mother with evidence of bacterial infection within 2 weeks prior to delivery
3. Foul smelling liquor
4. Rupture of membranes >24 hours
5. Single unclean or >3 sterile vaginal examination(s) during labor
6. Prolonged labor (sum of 1st and 2nd stage of labor ≥ 24 hrs)
7. Perinatal asphyxia (Apgar score <4 at 1 minute)

Late onset sepsis (LOS): It usually presents after 72 hours of age. The infection in LOS is either hospital-acquired or community-acquired. Neonates usually present with septicemia, pneumonia or meningitis.[6,7] The risk factors of nosocomial sepsis include low birth weight, prematurity, admission in intensive care unit, mechanical ventilation, invasive procedures, central lines, administration of parenteral fluids and use of stock solutions.

Factors that increase the risk of community-acquired LOS include hygiene, poor cord care, bottle-feeding and prelacteal feeds. In contrast, breastfeeding helps in prevention of infections.

CLINICAL FEATURES OF NEONATAL SEPSIS

Non-specific Features

The earliest signs of sepsis are often subtle and non-specific; indeed, a high index of suspicion is needed for early diagnosis. This is more true in preterm infants. Neonates with sepsis may present with one or more of the following symptoms and signs: (a) Hypothermia or fever (former is more common in preterm low birth weight infants); (b) Lethargy, poor cry, refusal to suck; (c) Poor perfusion, prolonged capillary refill time; (d) Hypotonia, absent neonatal reflexes; (e) Brady/tachy-cardia; (f) Respiratory distress, apnea and gasping respiration; (g) Hypo/hyperglycemia; (h) Metabolic acidosis.

Specific Features Related to Various Systems

Central nervous system (CNS)	: Bulging anterior fontanelle, vacant stare, high-pitched cry, excessive irritability; stupor/coma, seizures, neck retraction. Presence of these features should raise a clinical suspicion of meningitis
Cardiac	: Hypotension, poor perfusion, shock
Gastrointestinal	: Feed intolerance, vomiting, diarrhea, abdominal distension, paralytic ileus, necrotizing enterocolitis (NEC)
Hepatic	: Hepatomegaly, direct hyperbilirubinemia (especially with urinary tract infections)
Renal	: Acute renal failure
Hematological	: Bleeding, petechiae, purpura
Skin changes	: Multiple pustules, abscess, sclerema, mottling, umbilical redness and discharge

INVESTIGATIONS

Since treatment should be initiated in a neonate suspected to have sepsis without any delay, only minimal and rapid investigations should be undertaken.[8]

Blood culture: It is the gold standard and should be performed in all cases of suspected sepsis prior to starting antibiotics. It is important to follow the proper procedure for collecting a blood culture.

The resident doctor/staff should wear sterile gloves prior to the procedure and prepare a patch of skin approximately 5 cm in diameter over the proposed venipuncture site. This area should be cleansed thoroughly with 70% isopropyl alcohol, followed by povidone-iodine and again by alcohol. The antiseptic agents should be applied in concentric circles moving outward from the centre. The skin should be allowed to dry in between antiseptic applications and before the sample is collected.

One mL blood should be adequate for a blood culture bottle containing 5–10 mL of culture media. Since samples collected from indwelling lines and catheters are contaminated, it should be preferably collected from a fresh venipuncture site. However, sample obtained from fresh cannulation is acceptable. The blood samples should be incubated for at least 72 hours before they are reported as sterile. It is now possible to detect bacterial growth within 12–24 hours using improved bacteriological techniques such as BACTEC and BACT/ALERT blood culture systems. These advanced techniques can detect bacteria at a concentration of 1–2 colony-forming unit (CFU) per mL.

Sepsis screen:[9,10] All neonates suspected to have sepsis should have a sepsis screen to corroborate the diagnosis. However, the decision to start antibiotics need not be conditional to sepsis screen result, if there is a strong clinical suspicion of sepsis.

The various components of the sepsis screen include total leukocyte count (TLC), absolute neutrophil count (ANC), immature to total (IT) neutrophil ratio, micro-erythrocyte sedimentation rate (ESR) and C reactive protein (CRP) (Table 12.1).

The ANC varies considerably in the immediate neonatal period and the normal reference ranges are available from Manroe's charts.[11] The lower limit for normal ANC begins at 1800/cmm at birth, rises to 7200/cmm at 12 hours of age and then declines and persists at 1800/cmm after 72 hours of age. For very low birth weight infants, the reference ranges are available from Mouzinho's charts.[12]

Presence of two abnormal parameters in a screen is associated with a sensitivity of 93–100%, specificity of 83%, positive and negative predictive values of 27% and 100%, respectively in detecting sepsis. Hence, if two (or more) parameters are abnormal, it should be considered as a positive screen and the neonate should be started on antibiotics. If the

Table 12.1: Sepsis screen

Components	Abnormal value
Total leukocyte count	$<5000/mm^3$
Absolute neutrophil count	Low counts as per Manroe chart[11] for term and Mouzinho's chart[12] for VLBW infants
Immature/total neutrophil	≥0.2
Micro-ESR	≥15 mm in 1st hour
C reactive protein (CRP)	≥1 mg/dL

(ESR: erythrocyte sedimentation rate)

screen is negative but clinical suspicion persists, it should be repeated in 12 hours. If the screen is still negative, sepsis can be excluded with reasonable certainty. However, the sepsis screen is less reliable in preterm infants and term infants during initial 48 hrs of life.

Lumbar puncture (LP): The incidence of meningitis in neonatal sepsis has varied from 0.3 to 3% in various studies.[3,6] The clinical features of septicemia and meningitis often overlap; it is quite possible to have meningitis along with septicemia *without* any specific symptomatology. This justifies performing LP in all neonates suspected to have LOS prior to starting antibiotics.

In EOS, lumbar puncture is indicated in the presence of a positive blood culture or if the clinical picture is consistent with septicemia. It is not indicated if antibiotics have been started solely due to the presence of risk factors.

Lumbar puncture could be postponed in a critically sick neonate. It should be performed once the clinical condition stabilizes. The cerebrospinal fluid characteristics are unique in the newborn period and normal values are given in Table 12.2.[13]

Radiology: Chest X-ray should be considered in the presence of respiratory distress or apnea. An abdominal X-ray is indicated in the presence of abdominal signs suggestive of necrotizing enterocolitis (NEC).

Urine culture: Urine cultures have a low yield and are not indicated routinely. However, neonates at risk for fungal sepsis, with urogenital malformation or vesicoureteral reflux or suspected of UTI (crying during micturition) should have a urine examination. Urine culture samples are obtained by suprapubic puncture, bladder catheterization or clean catch sample from midstream of urine.

Table 12.2: Normal cerebrospinal fluid examination in neonates[13]

CSF components	Normal range
Cells/mm^3	8 (0–30 cells)
PMN (%)	60%
CSF protein (mg/dL)	90 (20–170)
CSF glucose (mg/dL)	52 (34–119)
CSF/blood glucose (%)	51 (44–248)

(PMN: polymorphonuclear cells; CSF: cerebrospinal fluid)

UTI may be diagnosed in the presence of one of the following: (a) >10 WBC/mm^3 in a 10-mL centrifuged sample; (b) >10^4 organisms/mL in urine obtained by catheterization; and (c) any organism in urine obtained by suprapubic aspiration.

MANAGEMENT OF NEONATAL SEPSIS

Supportive

Adequate and proper supportive care is crucial. The baby should be nursed in a thermo-neutral environment taking care to avoid hypo/hyperthermia. Oxygen saturation should be maintained in the normal range; mechanical ventilation may have to be initiated if necessary. If the infant is hemodynamically unstable, intravenous fluids should be administered and the infant is to be monitored for hypo/hyperglycemia. Volume expansion with crystalloids/colloids and judicious use of inotropes. Packed red cells and fresh frozen plasma might have to be given in the event of anemia or bleeding diathesis.

Antimicrobial Therapy

There cannot be a single recommendation for the antibiotic regimen of neonatal sepsis for all settings. The choice of antibiotics depends on prevailing flora in a given unit and their antimicrobial sensitivity. This protocol does not provide a universal recommendation for all settings but lays down broad guidelines to make a rational choice of antibiotic combination. Decision to start antibiotics is based upon clinical features and/ or a positive septic screen (Fig. 12.1). However, duration of antibiotic therapy is dependent upon the presence of a positive blood culture and meningitis (Table 12.3).

Indications for Starting Antibiotics

The indications for starting antibiotics in neonates at risk of EOS include any one of the following:
a. Presence of ≥ 3 risk factors for early onset sepsis (*see above*)
b. Presence of foul smelling liquor
c. Presence of ≥ 2 antenatal risk factor(s) *and* a positive septic screen, and
d. Strong clinical suspicion of sepsis.

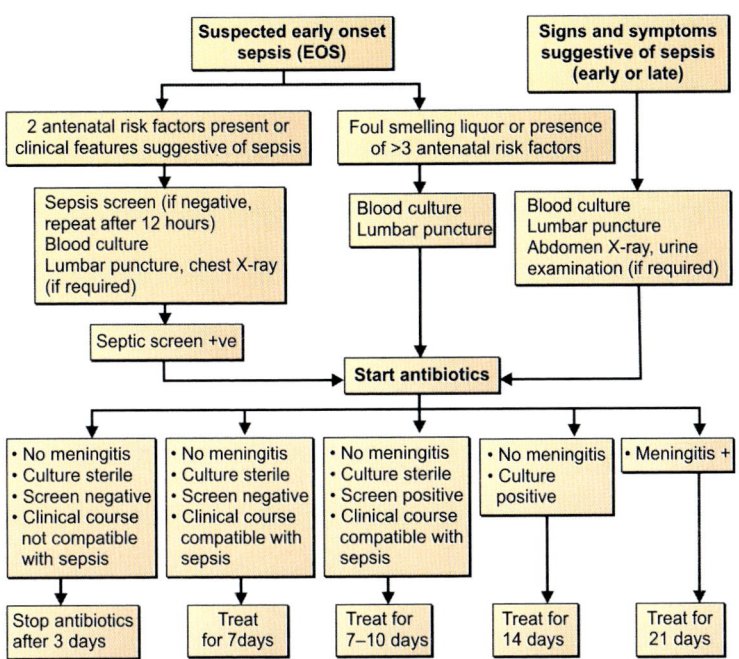

If no response is seen within 48–72 hours of starting treatment, a repeat blood culture should be obtained to determine appropriate choice and duration of antibiotic therapy. In symptomatic but otherwise reasonably stable babies, one can wait for the results of sepsis screen to rule out sepsis so as to avoid unnecessary use of antibiotics.

Fig. 12.1: Protocol for sepsis

Table 12.3: Duration of antibiotic therapy in neonatal sepsis

Diagnosis	Duration
Meningitis *(with or without positive blood/CSF culture)*	21 days
Blood **culture positive** but **no meningitis**	14 days
Culture **negative** sepsis **(screen positive** and *clinical course* **consistent with sepsis)**	7 to 10 days

The indications for starting antibiotics in LOS include:
a. Positive septic screen and/or
b. Strong clinical suspicion of sepsis.

Prophylactic antibiotics: We do not use prophylactic antibiotics in the following circumstances: infants on IV fluids/TPN, meconium aspiration syndrome and after exchange transfusion(s). An exchange transfusion conducted under strict asepsis (single use catheter, sterile gloves, removal of catheter after the procedure) does not increase the risk of sepsis and merit antibiotics.

Choice of antibiotics: Empirical antibiotic therapy should be unit-specific and determined by the prevalent spectrum of etiological agents and their antibiotic sensitivity pattern. Antibiotics once started should be modified according to the sensitivity reports (Table 12.4).

Table 12.4: Empirical choice of antibiotics for treatment of neonatal sepsis

	Sepsis and pneumonia	*Meningitis*
FIRST LINE (Resistant strains are less likely)	Ampicillin and gentamicin/amikacin	Add cefotaxime
SECOND LINE (Higher likelihood of resistant strains)	Cloxacillin/ciprofloxacin and netilmycin/amikacin	Add cefotaxime
THIRD LINE (Higher likelihood of resistant strains)	Piperacillin-tazobactam or cefoperazone-sulbactam and netilmycin/amikacin	Same Avoid ciprofloxacin

Consider vancomycin if MRSA is suspected.

The empirical choice of antibiotics is dependent upon the probable source of infection. For infections that are likely to be community-acquired where resistant strains are unlikely, a combination of ampicillin with gentamicin may be a good choice as first line therapy.

For infections that are acquired during hospital stay, resistant pathogens are likely and a combination of cloxacillin/cipro-floxacin with gentamicin or amikacin may be instituted. In nurseries where this combination is ineffective due to the presence of multiple resistant strains of Klebsiella spp. and other Gram-negative bacilli, a combination of a third generation cephalosporin (cefotaxime or ceftazidime) with amikacin may be appropriate. The 3rd generation cephalosporins have very good CSF penetration and are traditionally thought to have excellent antimicrobial activity against Gram-negative organisms. Hence, they are considered to be a good choice for the treatment of nosocomial infections and meningitis. However, recent reports suggest that at least 60–70% of the Gram-negative organisms are resistant to them.[14–16] Moreover, routine use of these antibiotics might increase the risk of infections with ESBL (extended spectrum beta-lactamase) positive organisms. Therefore, it is preferable to use antibiotics such as piperacillin-tazobactam or methicillin/vancomycin in units with high incidence of resistant strains.

A combination of piperacillin-tazobactam with amikacin should be considered if pseudomonas sepsis is suspected. Penicillin resistant *Staphylococcus aureus* should be treated with cloxacillin, nafcillin or methicillin. Addition of an aminoglycoside is useful in therapy against *Staphylococcus*. Methicillin resistant *Staphylococcus aureus* (MRSA) should be treated with a combination of ciprofloxacin or vancomycin with amikacin. Ciprofloxacin has excellent activity against Gram-negative organisms also; however, it does not have good CSF penetration. It may be used for the treatment of resistant Gram-negative bacteremia after excluding meningitis.

Reserve antibiotics: Newer antibiotics like aztreonam, meropenem and imipenem are also now available in the market. Aztreonam has excellent activity against Gram-negative organisms while meropenem is effective against most bacterial pathogens except methicillin resistant *Staphylococcus aureus* (MRSA) and enterococcus. Imipenem is generally avoided in neonates because of the reported increase in the incidence of seizures following its use. Empirical use of these antibiotics should be avoided; they should be reserved for situations where sensitivity of the isolated organism warrants its use.

In symptomatic but otherwise reasonably stable babies, one can wait for the results of sepsis screen so as to avoid unnecessary use of antibiotics.

Adjunctive Therapy

Exchange Transfusion (ET): Sadana et al[17] have evaluated the role of double volume exchange transfusion in septic neonates with sclerema and demonstrated a 50% reduction in sepsis related mortality in the treated group. We perform double-volume exchange transfusion with cross-matched fresh whole blood as adjunctive therapy in septic neonates with sclerema.

Intravenous Immunoglobulin (IVIG): Non-specific pooled IVIG has not been found to be useful.[18]

Granulocyte-Macrophage Colony Stimulating Factor (GM-CSF): This mode of treatment is still experimental.[19]

REFERENCES

1. Bang AT, Bang RA, Bactule SB, Reddy HM, Deshmukh MD. Effect of home-based neonatal care and management of sepsis on neonatal mortality: field trial in rural India. Lancet 1999;354:1955–61.

2. Stoll BJ. The global impact of neonatal infection. Clin Perinatol 1997;24:1–21.

3. Report of the National Neonatal Perinatal Database (National Neonatology Forum) 2002–03.

4. Singh M, Narang A, Bhakoo ON. Predictive perinatal score in the diagnosis of neonatal sepsis. J Trop Pediatr 1994 Dec;40(6):365–8.

5. Takkar VP, Bhakoo ON, Narang A. Scoring system for the prediction of early neonatal infections. Indian Pediatr 1974;11:597–600.

6. Baltimore RS. Neonatal nosocomial infections. Semin Perinatol 1998;22:25–32.

7. Wolach B. Neonatal sepsis: pathogenesis and supportive therapy. Semin Perinatol 1997;21:28–38.

8. Gerdes JS, Polin R. Early diagnosis and treatment of neonatal sepsis. Indian J Pediatr 1998;65:63–78.

9. Polinski C. The value of white blood cell count and differential in the prediction of neonatal sepsis. Neonatal Netw 1996;15:13–23.

10. Da Silva O, Ohlsson A, Kenyon C. Accuracy of leukocyte indices and C-reactive protein for diagnosis of neonatal sepsis: a critical review. Pediatr Infect Dis J 1995;14:362–6.

11. Manroe BL, Weinberg AG, Rosenfeld CR, Browne R. The neonatal blood count in health and disease. Reference values for neutrophilic cells. J Pediatr 1979;95:89–98.

12. Mouzinho A, Rosenfeld CR, Sanchez PJ, Risser R. Revised reference ranges for circulating neutrophils in very-low-birthweight neonates. Pediatrics 1994;94:76–82.

13. Sarff LD, Platt LH, McCracken GH Jr. Cerebrospinal fluid evaluation in neonates: Comparison of high-risk neonates with and without meningitis. J Pediatr 1976;88:473–7.

14. Upadhyay A, Aggarwal R, Kapil A, Singh S, Paul VK, Deorari AK. Profile of neonatal sepsis in a tertiary care neonatal unit from India: A retrospective study. Journal of Neonatology 2006;20:50–57.

15. Deorari Ashok K. For the Investigators of the National Neonatal Perinatal Database (NNPD). Changing pattern of bacteriologic profile in Neonatal Sepsis among intramural babies. Journal of Neonatology 2006;20:8–15.

16. Zaidi AK, Huskins WC, Thaver D, Bhutta ZA, Abbas Z, Goldmann DA. Hospital-acquired neonatal infections in developing countries. Lancet 2005;365:1175–88.

17. Sadana S, Mathur NB, Thakur A. Exchange transfusion in septic neonates with sclerema: effect on immunoglobulin and complement levels. Indian Pediatr 1997;34:20–5.

18. Jenson HB, Pollock HB. The role of intravenous immunoglobulin for the prevention and treatment of neonatal sepsis. Semin Perinatol 1998;22:50–63.

19. Goldman S, Ellis R, Dhar V, Cairo MS. Rationale and potential use of cytokines in the prevention and treatment of neonatal sepsis. Clin Perinatol 1998;25:699–710.

13   Perinatal HIV

The human immunodeficiency virus (HIV) pandemic is one of the most serious health crises the world faces today. In 2010, an estimated 390,000 children were newly infected with HIV with majority of transmission being perinatal. UNAIDS estimated that since 1995 more than 350,000 new HIV infections in children have been prevented due to ART for prophylaxis in pregnant women.[1] AIDS has killed more than 25 million people since 1981 and an estimated 35.3 (32.2–38.8) million people are now living with HIV, about 3.3 (3–3.7) million of whom are children.[2] In India, estimated 2.1 (1.7–2.6) million people are living with HIV infection as on year 2012. Adult prevalence of HIV infection in India is 0.3%.[2]

MODE OF TRANSMISSION

Most children living with HIV acquire the infection through mother-to-child transmission (MTCT). HIV infection can be transmitted from an infected mother to her fetus during pregnancy, delivery or by breastfeeding. HIV can be transmitted to the fetus as early as the first trimester of pregnancy. However, maternal transmission to the fetus occurs most commonly in the perinatal period. Perinatal transmission is an extremely important mode of transmission of HIV infection in developing countries.

Risk Factors for Perinatal HIV Transmission[3]

Viral factors: High viral load, non-syncytium inducing phenotype, HIV-1

Maternal factors: Advanced disease (low CD4 count, symptoms of AIDS), primary infection of mother during pregnancy, rupture of membranes more than four hours maternal bleeding, mother not on antiretroviral therapy, vaginal delivery, other sexually transmitted diseases, isolated HIV-1 infection.

Fetoplacental factors: Chorioamnionitis, placenta previa, first of twins, prematurity (increased peripartum transmission).

Infant factors: HLA concordance with mother

Postnatal factors: Breastfeeding, higher breast milk virus load, mastitis or maternal nipple lesions, maternal seroconversion during breastfeeding, infant having thrush at less than six month age (in breastfeeding infant).

Prevention of Perinatal HIV

- In the absence of any intervention, the risk of perinatal transmission is 15–30% in non-breastfeeding populations.[4]
- Breastfeeding by an infected mother increases the risk by 5–20% to a total of 20–45%.[5]
- The earlier evidence had shown that the risk of MTCT can be reduced to under 2% by interventions that include antiretroviral (ARV) prophylaxis given to women during pregnancy and labor and to the infant in the first 6 weeks of life, obstetrical interventions including elective cesarean delivery (prior to the onset of labor and rupture of membranes), and complete avoidance of breastfeeding.[6–8]
- However, in view of emerging evidence, the national guidelines for prevention of parent-to-child transmission of HIV, cesarean section in HIV positive pregnant women should be performed for obstetric indication only.[9] Mother-to-child transmission is increased by the prolonged rupture of membranes, multiple per vaginal examinations, assisted instrumental delivery (vacuum or forceps) and invasive fetal monitoring procedures (scalp/fetal blood monitoring). Hence, the membranes should not be artificially ruptured unless there is fetal distress or delay in progress of labor, repeated vaginal examinations minimized, any invasive procedure on the fetus be avoided and instrumental delivery should not be undertaken unless required in cases of fetal distress or significant maternal fatigue. Routine episiotomy is avoided as far as possible. Suctioning of the newborn should be avoided unless liquor is meconium stained.

ARV Regime for Treating Pregnant Women[9]

Earlier, ART regimen in pregnant and lactating mothers was complex in terms of different regimens for treatment and prophylaxis, need for CD4 measurements to determine treatment eligibility and type of regimen, changing antepartum-intrapartum-postpartum regimens and an expanded NVP prophylaxis in infants.

The recent guidelines have simplified the protocol by recommending an optimized, fixed dose combination ART regimen of tenofovir (TDF) + lamivudine (3TC) and efavirenz (EFV) to all pregnant and breastfeeding women. That provides programmatic and clinical benefits of ease of implementation, harmonized regimens with those for non-pregnant adults, increased coverage and better acceptance.[11]

- Pregnant women who are detected to be HIV infected during antenatal period should be initiated on ART (TDF –300 mg + 3TC–300 mg + EFV–600 mg) regardless of clinical stage or CD4 count. This fixed dose combination is recommended as first line ART in pregnant and breastfeeding women (including pregnant women in the first trimester of pregnancy and women of child bearing age). Lifelong ART is initiated as soon as possible including the entire breast-feeding period. The initiation of ART should not be delayed for want of CD4 test results.
- Alternate regimens are AZT+ 3TC+ EFV or AZT+ 3TC+ NVP or TDF+ 3TC+ NVP.
- Pregnant women already on ART for their own health should continue to receive whatever regimen she is stabilized on and is responding adequately, throughout pregnancy, labor, breastfeeding period and thereafter lifelong.

ARV Regime for Treating Infants Born to HIV Infected Women

- If mother received ART adequately and regularly in antenatal period:
  – Daily NVP prophylaxis at birth and continued for 6 weeks
- If mother presented directly in labor without adequate duration of ART (at least 24 wks) or did not receive any ART earlier:

– Daily *NVP prophylaxis at birth* (Table 13.1) *and continued for 12 weeks* (dose may be increased to 20 mg once daily after 6–8 weeks of age[16])

Table 13.1 Dose and duration of infant's daily NVP prophylaxis

Birth weight	NVP daily dose	NVP daily dose
<2000 gm	2 mg/kg once daily	0.2 mL/kg
2000–2500 gm	10 mg once daily	1 mL once a day
>2500 gm	15 mg once daily	1.5 mL once a day

Give first dose of NVP within 6 to 12 hours of delivery.

BREASTFEEDING[11]

- Breastfeeding is an important mode of transmission of HIV infection in developing countries. The risk of HIV infection via breastfeeding is highest in the early months of breast-feeding.[10] The goal is to maximize the HIV-free survival in infants.
- Factors that increase the likelihood of transmission include detectable levels of HIV in breast milk, the presence of mastitis and low maternal CD4 + T cell count.
- According to the updated guidelines for prevention of parent-to-child transmission (PPTCT) of HIV using multi-drug antiretroviral regimen in India,[9] infants should be given exclusive breastfeeds for the first six months followed by complementary feeds.
- Support exclusive breastfeeding for a minimum period of 6 months and continue breastfeeds in addition to complementary feeds for 1 year. After 1 year, breastfeeding should stop gradually within one month. Baby should undergo DNA PCR testing 6 weeks after cessation of breastfeeds.
- Exclusive replacement feeds may be started if the mother has died or has terminal illness or decides not to breastfeed despite adequate counseling. In such a case, commercial infant formula milk is given as a replacement feed when AFASS (**A**ffordable, **F**easible, **A**cceptable, **S**ustainable and **S**afe in the 2006 WHO recommendations on HIV and Infant Feeding) criteria are met. Replacement feeding should be given by katori spoon; bottle feeds should be avoided.
- Mixed feeding (feeding breastfeeds and replacement feeds) should not be given in the first 6 months.

POSTNATAL DIAGNOSIS OF HIV INFECTION[13]

Refer to Fig. 13.1

- In children younger than 18 months, diagnosis of HIV infection is based on a positive virological test at 6 weeks for HIV or its components (usually by HIV-DNA PCR). The diagnosis should be confirmed by a second test on a separate sample repeated at the earliest.[12]

- If an infant or child is breastfeeding, he or she remains at risk of acquiring HIV infection throughout the breastfeeding period. Virological assays to detect HIV infection should be conducted at least six weeks or more after the complete cessation of breastfeeding to rule out HIV infection.

- Positive antibody testing is not recommended for definitive or confirmatory diagnosis of HIV infection in children until 18 months of age.[13] Confirmation test for HIV has to be done at 18 months using three rapid tests for all babies.[9]

- Early infant diagnosis is now being offered in the national program by National AIDS Control Organization (NACO).

- For breastfeeding infants who have been diagnosed HIV positive, pediatric ART should be started and breastfeeding to be continued ideally until the baby is 2 years old.

Cotrimoxazole Prophylaxis

- Cotrimoxazole prophylaxis is recommended for all HIV-exposed infants under age 18 months starting at 4–6 weeks of age or when first seen and continued until HIV infection can be excluded.[14]

- Cotrimoxazole prophylaxis is also recommended for a breastfeeding child of any age, continued until HIV infection can be excluded following cessation of breastfeeding, with testing performed six weeks or more after breastfeeding was stopped.

- In children <6 month dose is 2.5 mL once a day (syrup trimethoprim 40 mg and sulphamethoxazole 200 mg/5 mL).

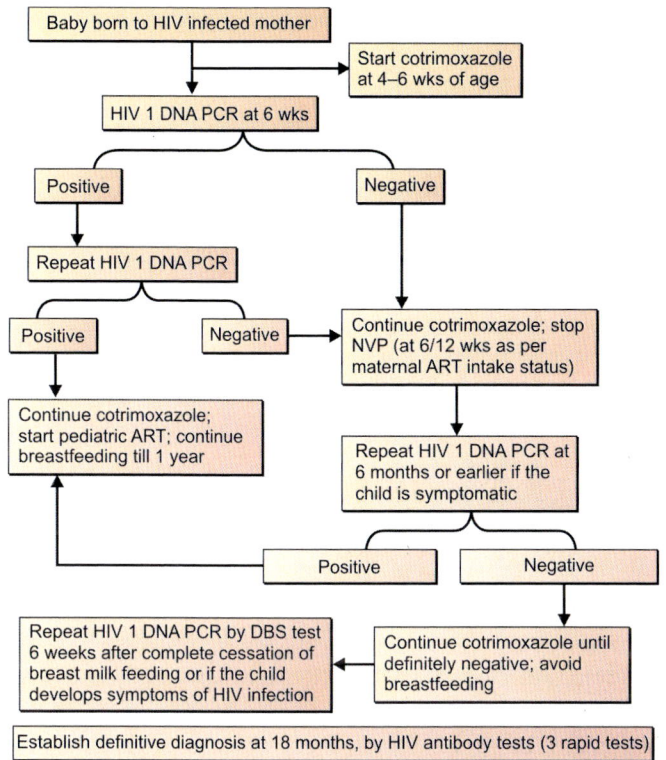

Fig. 13.1: Diagnostic algorithm for HIV-exposed infants less than 6 months

IMMUNIZATION

- HIV exposed or infected but asymptomatic children should receive all standard vaccines as per national schedule.[15,17]
- HIV infected children with immune suppression or symptoms should receive all standard vaccines *except* BCG, OPV and varicella vaccines.
- Consider HiB and pneumococcal vaccines in all HIV exposed children (irrespective of symptoms or CD4 count).

REFERENCES

1. UNAIDS/WHO. Global HIV/AIDS response. Epidemic update and health sector progress towards universal access. November, 2011.

2. UNAIDS Report on the Global AIDS. Epidemic–2013.

3. Havens P, Waters D. Management of the infant born to a mother with HIV infection. Pediatr Clin North Am 2004;51:909–37.

4. The Working Group on Mother-to-Child HIV. Transmission of rates of mother-to child transmission of HIV-1 in Africa, America and Europe: results from 13 perinatal studies. J Acquir Immune Defic Syndr 1995;8:506–10.

5. De Cock KM, Fowler MG, Mercier E, et al. Prevention of mother-to-child HIV transmission in resource-poor countries: translating research into policy and practice. JAMA 2000;283:1175–82.

6. Lallemant M, Jourdain G, Le Coeur S, et al. Single-dose perinatal nevirapine plus standard zidovudine to prevent mother-to-child transmission of HIV 1 in Thailand. N Engl J Med 2004;351: 217–28.

7. Thorne C, Patel D, Fiore S, Peckham C, Newell ML. Mother-to-child transmission of HIV infection in the era of highly active anti-retroviral therapy. Clinical Infectious Diseases 2005;40:458–65.

8. Magoni M, Bassani L, Okong P et al. Mode of infant feeding and HIV infection in children in a program for prevention of mother-to-child transmission in Uganda. AIDS 2005;19:433–7.

9. GOI, MOHFW. Updated guidelines for prevention of parent-to-child transmission (PPTCT) of HIV using multi drug antiretroviral regimen in India, Dec 2013.

10. Dunn DT, Tess BH, Rodrigues LC, Ades AE. Mother-to-child transmission of HIV: implications of variation in maternal infectivity. AIDS 1998;12:2211–6.

11. WHO. New guidance on prevention of mother-to-child transmission of HIV and infant feeding in the context of HIV, July 2010.

12. WHO. Consolidated guidelines on the use of antiretroviral drugs for treating and preventing HIV infection, Chapter 7: Clinical guidance across the continuum of care: antiretroviral therapy, 2013.

13. Chantry CJ, Cooper ER, Pelton SI, Zorilla C, Hillyer GV, Diaz C. Seroreversion in human immunodeficiency virus-exposed but uninfected infants. Pediatr Infect Dis J 1995;14:382–7.

14. WHO. Guidelines on cotrimoxazole prophylaxis for HIV-related infections among children, adolescents and adults in resource-limited settings recommendations for a public health approach. 2006.

15. Anonymous. Immunization in special circumstances. In: Shah RC, Shah NK, Kukreja S (Eds). IAP Guide Book on Immunization, Mumbai; IAP Committee on Immunization 2005–2006;52–54.

16. Coovadia HM, Brown ER, Fowler MG, Chipato T, Moodley D, Manji K, et al. Efficacy and safety of an extended nevirapine regimen in infant children of breastfeeding mothers with HIV-1 infection for prevention of postnatal HIV-1 transmission (HPTN 046): a randomized, double blind, placebo controlled trial. Lancet 2012 Jan 21;379(9812):221–8. doi:10.1016/S0140–6736(11) 61653-X.

17. IAP recommended immunization schedule 2013 for children aged 0–18 years.

INFANT BORN TO MOTHER WITH TUBERCULOSIS

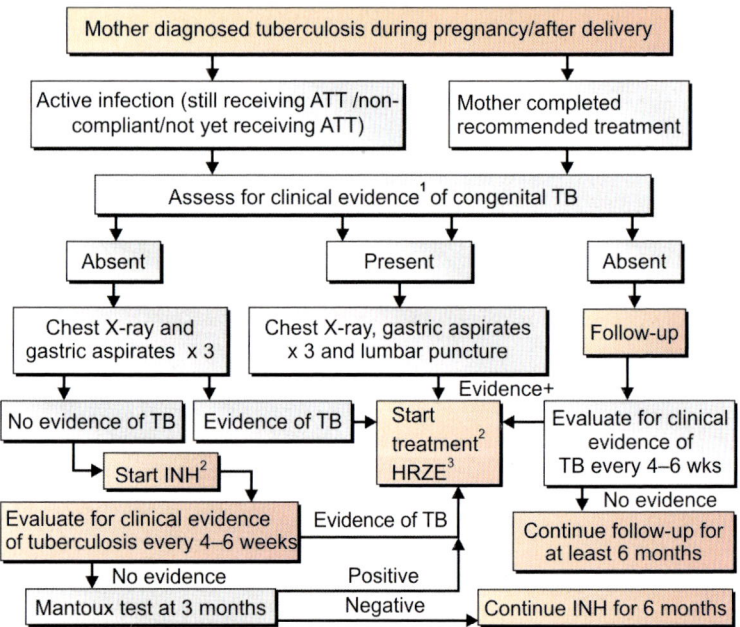

1. Clinical features of congenital TB: Respiratory distress, hepatosplenomegaly, lymphadenopathy, fever, poor feeding and poor weight gain.
2. Dose of INH: 10 mg/kg/day. Adjust the dose of ATT drugs at each postnatal visit according to weight. No need to give pyridoxine routinely.
3. If ethambutol is given in a dose of 20 mg/kg/day or lesser and for 2 months, the risk of optic neuritis is negligible.
4. Give BCG after completion of the INH course.
5. Reassure the mother that it is safe to breastfeed her baby.
6. Separation of mother and neonate is necessary only if mother is sick/non-adherent to treatment/ has MDR infection.

INFANT BORN TO MOTHER WITH SYPHILIS INFECTION (CDC 2010)

> Routine serological testing for syphilis (STS) must be undertaken in all women at first prenatal visit. In high risk cases, it should be repeated at 28 wk and delivery. Routine STS in neonates for screening purpose is not useful in view of high false negative rates

↓

> Mother with syphilis (reactive VDRL/RPR and confirmed by reactive TPHA/FTA-ABS)

↓

Evaluate the infant:
1. Adequacy of maternal treatment
2. Examination of the placenta or umbilical cord for any gross/microscopic pathology
3. Dark field microscopy of suspicious lesions or body fluids
4. Clinical examination of infant for evidence of syphilis (non-immune hydrops, jaundice, hepatosplenomegaly, rhinitis, skin rash, pseudoparalysis)
5. Quantitative VDRL/RPR (TPHA/FTA-ABS not required) on infant serum (cord blood unreliable)

S. No.	Scenario	Additional evaluation	Treatment
1.	**Proven/highly probable disease** • Physical abnormalities suggestive of congenital syphilis • VDRL/RPR: 4X higher titer than the mother's titer • Positive darkfield test of body fluid(s)	1. CSF (VDRL, cell, protein) 2. CBC, differential and platelet count 3. Other tests as clinically indicated (long-bone and chest X-rays, LFTs, head USG, ophthalmologic examination and auditory brainstem response)	Penicillin G (1 to 1.5 lakh units/kg/day) as 50,000 units/kg/dose IV for a total of 10 days • Every 12 hrs during first 7 days of life • Every 8 hrs thereafter **OR** Procaine penicillin G 50,000 units/kg/dose IM in a single daily dose for 10 days
2.	• Normal physical examination • VDRL/RPR ≤4X of maternal titer • Mother: Not treated/ inadequately treated/ treated with non-penicillin regimen/ treated <4 wks before delivery	Do	Do if complete evaluation not done or uncertain follow-up **OR** Benzathine penicillin G 50,000 units/kg/dose IM in a single dose if complete evaluation is normal and follow-up is certain

Contd...

Contd...

S. No.	Scenario	Additional evaluation	Treatment
3.	• Normal physical examination • VDRL/RPR ≤4X of maternal titer • Mother: Adequately treated during pregnancy and more than 4 wks before delivery and does not have any reinfection or relapse	No evaluation required	No treatment is required if follow-up is certain. **OR** Benzathine penicillin G 50,000 units/kg as a single IM injection might be considered, particularly if follow-up is uncertain.
4.	• Normal physical examination • VDRL/RPR titer ≤ 4X of maternal titer • Mother: Adequately treated before pregnancy and her VDRL/RPR titer remained low and stable before and during pregnancy and at delivery		

For more details: http://www.cdc.gov/std/treatment/2010/STD-Treatment-2010-RR5912.pdf

NEONATE BORN TO MOTHER WITH HEPATITIS B INFECTION

Neonate born to mother with hepatitis B infection
(prenatal testing of all pregnant women for HBsAg is recommended)

↓

At birth: Give hepatitis B vaccine along with HBIG (200 IU IM)
(preferably within 12 hrs but not later than 48 to 72 hrs of birth)

↓

Follow-up: Complete the HBV immunization as per schedule

The programs following 3 doses schedule:

- For infant < 2 kg: do not count birth dose and give three more doses

- For infant 2 kg or more: Give a total of three doses counting the birth dose

The programs following 4 doses schedule:

- It remains the same for all babies irrespective of BW

↓

Follow-up testing: Should be done at 9 to 18 months of age for anti-HBs and HbsAg

↓

Infants with anti-HBs 10 mIU/mL or more and HBsAg negative are immune: No action required	Infants with anti-HBs <10 mIU/mL and HBsAg negative: No HBV infection but fail to respond to immunization: Revaccination (3 doses)	Infants with anti-HBs negative and HBsAg positive has HBV infection; follow-up

- Risk of vertical transmission:
  - Mother HBsAg +ve but HBeAg –ve: 5–20%

    HBsAg +ve and HBeAg +ve: 70–90%
- No contraindication to breastfeeding
- Hepatitis B vaccine gives 90% of active immunity; Hepatitis B immune globulin gives additional 5–10% immunity. As HBIG is costly and has availability issues in India, giving vaccine alone may be good enough.
- 90% of infected infants become chronic carriers.

INFANT WITH MATERNAL TOXOPLASMOSIS

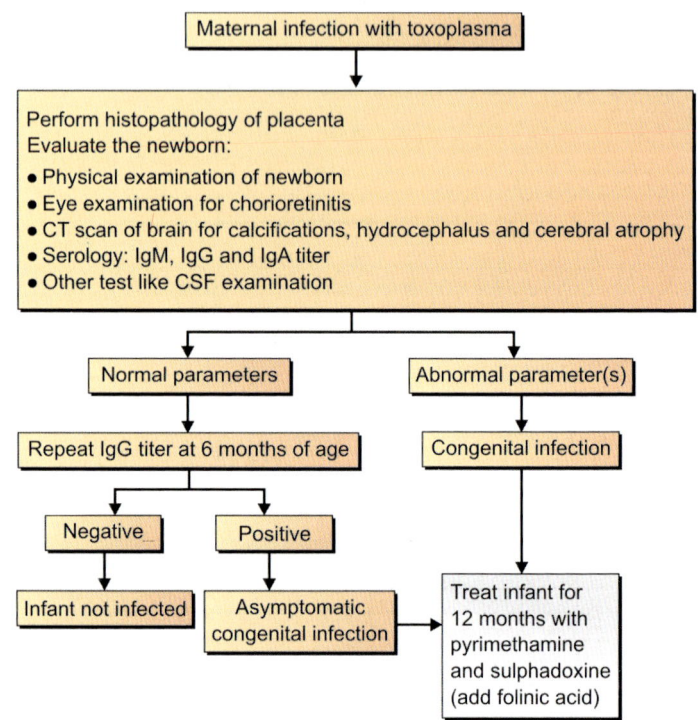

- For details on diagnosis of maternal infection: *http://www.dpd.cdc.gov/dpdx/ HTML/Frames/S-Z/Toxoplasmosis/body_Toxoplasmosis_serol1.htm*
- Majority of the infants are asymptomatic at birth. Clinical evidence include: hepatosplenomegaly, hydrocephalus, pneumonia, thrombocytopenia, lymphadenopathy, chorioretinitis, intracranial calcifications, myocarditis
- High incidence of long-term sequelae (e.g. chorioretinitis) in untreated infants even if asymptomatic at birth

MANAGEMENT OF AN INFANT OF MOTHER WITH VARICELLA INFECTION

Onset of maternal rash with respect to birth of baby (days)														
Day of life	←	−7	−6	−5	−4	−3	−2	−1	1	2	3	4	5	6	→
Likelihood of neonatal infection	Infant has protective antibodies **and** likelihood of severe disease is low			Infant does not have protective antibodies **and** likelihood of severe neonatal disease is high							Infant does not have protective antibodies **but** likelihood of severe neonatal disease is low				
Isolation	Do not separate baby from mother, continue breastfeeding, Isolate dyad from other infants			Separate mother and baby until maternal lesions have dried up and crusted* If baby develops rash: baby to stay with mother. Mother/baby with active vesicles isolated from other mothers and babies							Separate mother and baby until maternal lesions have dried up and crusted* If baby develops rash: baby to stay with mother. Mother/baby with active vesicles isolated from other mothers and babies				
Treatment	No VZIG Acyclovir if baby develops rash			VZIG within 72 hours of exposure *(not required if mother has zoster)* Consider acyclovir							No VZIG Acyclovir if baby develops rash				

Give expressed breast milk even if mother-infant dyad is separated. Breastfeeding allowed once mother is non-infectious.

- Dose of VZIG: 125 IU/kg IM
- If VZIG unavailable, give IVIG 400 mg/kg
- Incubation period of varicella is 10 to 21 days

Exposure of a hospitalized infant to health care provider with chickenpox
- All exposed susceptible patients should be discharged as soon as possible.
- All exposed susceptible patients who cannot be discharged should be placed in isolation from 10 to 21 days.
- Ascertain gestation of infant and take maternal history of chickenpox:
  - Infant <28 wks: VZIG regardless of maternal history of varicella
  - Infant 28 wks or more and preterm and no maternal history of chickenpox: VZIG
  - For healthy term infants: No VZIG

Metabolic and Hematological Disorders

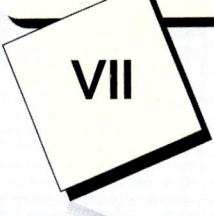

VII

Hypocalcemia

Calcium (Ca) is actively transferred from mother to fetus during last trimester, as demonstrated by a significantly higher level of total Ca concentration in cord blood as compared to maternal serum.[1] Parathyroid hormone (PTH) and calcitonin (CT) do not cross the placental barrier. PTH related peptide (PTHrP) is the main regulator of the positive Ca balance across the placenta. Serum Ca (SCa) in the fetus is 10 to 11 mg/dL at term (1 to 2 mg/dL higher as compared to mother).

After birth, the SCa levels in newborns depend on the PTH secretion, dietary calcium intake, renal calcium reabsorption, and skeletal calcium and vitamin D status. Hence, after delivery, SCa levels start decreasing (the rate and extent of decrease is inversely proportional to the gestation) and reaches a nadir of 7.5 to 8.5 mg/dL in healthy term babies by day 2 of life. This postnatal drop in SCa may be related to decreased PTH level, end organ unresponsiveness to PTH[2], abnormalities of vitamin D metabolism, hyperphosphatemia, hypomagnesemia and hypercalcitonemia, which occur by 12–24 hours of age.[3]

PTH levels increase gradually in the first 48 hours of life and normal levels of SCa are achieved by 3rd day of life.[4] The intestinal absorption and the renal processing of Ca mature by 2 to 4 weeks. This transition phase is responsible for the increased risk of early onset hypocalcemia in high-risk neonates.

DEFINITION

Hypocalcemia is defined by different tSCa and iSCa cut-offs for preterm and term infants (Penal 1).[6]

Panel 1: Definition of Hypocalcemia		
Gestation of infants	**Total serum calcium level**	**Ionic serum calcium level**
Preterm	<7 mg/dL (1.75 mmol/L)	<4 mg/dL (1 mmol/L)
Term	<8 mg/dL (2 mmol/L; total)	<4.8 mg/dL (1.2 mmol/L)

The SCa is usually reported in different units viz. mg/dL, mEq/L and mmol/L. The relationship between these units is related to the following equations:

$$mmol/L = [mg/dL \times 10] \div molecular\ wt$$
$$mEq/L = mmol/L \times valency$$

Since the molecular weight of Ca is 40 and the valence is +2, 1 mg/dL is equivalent to 0.25 mmol/L and to 0.5 mEq/L. Thus, values in mg/dL may be converted to molar units (mmol/L) by dividing it by 4.

CALCIUM HOMEOSTASIS IN NEWBORN

Body Ca exists in two major compartments: skeleton (99%) and extracellular fluid (1%). Ca in the extracellular fluid is present in three forms[5]:
- Bound to albumin (40%)
- Bound to anions like phosphorus, citrate, sulfate and lactate (10%), and
- Free ionized form (50%)

Ionized serum calcium (iSCa) is crucial for many biochemical processes including blood coagulation, neuromuscular excitability, cell membrane integrity and function, and cellular enzymatic and secretory activity.

Measurement of the total serum Ca (tSCa) concentration alone can be misleading because the relationship between tSCa and iSCa is not always linear. Correlation between two is poor when the serum albumin concentration is low and to a lesser degree, with disturbances in acid–base status, both of which occur frequently in premature or sick infants. With hypoalbuminemia, tSCa is low while iSCa is normal. Falsely low iSCa may be recorded in alkalosis and with heparin contamination of blood sample. In general, the tSCa falls by 0.8 mg/dL (0.2 mmol/L) for every 1.0 g/dL fall in the plasma albumin concentration.

Therefore, estimation of tSCa is a poor substitute for measuring the iSCa.

EARLY ONSET NEONATAL HYPOCALCEMIA (ENH)

This condition is fairly common and seen within the first 3 to 4 days of life in the following clinical settings (Table 15.1):

Table 15.1: Causes of early onset hypocalcemia

Prematurity
Pre-eclampsia
Infant of diabetic mother
Perinatal stress/asphyxia
Maternal intake of anticonvulsants (phenobarbitone, phenytoin sodium)
Maternal hyperparathyroidism
Iatrogenic (alkalosis, use of blood products, diuretics, phototherapy, lipid infusions, etc.)

Prematurity: This may be related to premature termination of transplacental supply, exaggeration of the postnatal drop to hypocalcemic levels, increased calcitonin and diminished target organ responsiveness to parathyroid hormone.

Infant of diabetic mother (gestational and insulin dependent): This may be related to increased Ca demands of a macrosomic baby.[7] Magnesium depletion in mothers with diabetes mellitus causes hypomagnesemic state in the fetus. This hypomagnesemia induces functional hypoparathyroidism and hypocalcemia in the infant. A high incidence of birth asphyxia and prematurity in infants of diabetic mothers are also contributing factors.

Perinatal asphyxia: Delayed introduction of feeds, increased calcitonin production, increased endogenous phosphate load, renal insufficiency and diminished parathyroid hormone secretion—all may contribute to hypocalcemia.

Maternal hyperparathyroidism: This causes intrauterine hypercalcemia suppressing the parathyroid activity in the fetus resulting in impaired parathyroid responsiveness to hypocalcemia after birth. Hypocalcemia may be severe and prolonged.

Intrauterine growth restriction (IUGR): Infants with IUGR may have hypocalcemia if they are born preterm and/or have had perinatal asphyxia. *IUGR or Small for gestational age (SGA) is generally not an independent risk factor for ENH.*

Maternal anti-convulsants: Intake of anti-convulsants like phenobarbitone and phenytoin alters the vitamin D metabolism. The infants of epileptic mothers may be at risk of neonatal hypocalcemia. It can be prevented by vitamin D supplementation to mothers.

Iatrogenic: Any condition causing alkalosis increases the binding of the calcium with albumin and causes decrease in iSCa.

There is no universal recommendation regarding routine screening of at-risk infants for ENH. However, the following categories of infants may be considered for the same:
  (a) Preterm infants born before 32 wks
  (b) Infants of diabetic mothers
  (c) Infants born after severe perinatal asphyxia defined as Apgar score < 4 at 1 minute of age

Time schedule for screening: at 24 and 48 hours of age risk babies.

CLINICAL PRESENTATION

Asymptomatic: ENH is usually asymptomatic unlike the late onset variety and is incidentally detected.

Symptomatic: The symptoms may be of neuromuscular irritability—myoclonic jerks, jitteriness, exaggerated startle and seizures. They may represent the cardiac involvement like tachycardia, heart failure, prolonged QT interval, decreased contractibility. More often they are non-specific and not related to the severity of hypocalcemia. Apnea, cyanosis, tachypnea, vomiting and laryngospasm are other symptoms that are noted.

Diagnosis

Laboratory: By measuring total or ionized serum calcium. Ionized calcium is the preferred mode for diagnosis of hypocalcemia.

ECG: QoTc > 0.22 seconds or QTc > 0.45 seconds

$$QTc = \frac{QT \text{ interval in seconds}}{\sqrt{R\text{-}R \text{ interval in seconds}}}$$

$$QoTc = \frac{QoT \text{ interval in seconds}}{\sqrt{R\text{-}R \text{ interval in seconds}}}$$

(QT interval is measured from origin of q wave to end of T wave on ECG; QoT is measured from origin of q wave to origin of T wave).

A diagnosis of hypocalcemia based only on ECG criteria is likely to yield a high false positive rate. Although these parameters have good correlation with hypocalcemia in low birth weight infants (sensitivity of 77% and specificity of 94.7%),[8] neonates suspected to have hypocalcemia by ECG criteria should have the diagnosis confirmed by measurement of serum calcium levels.

TREATMENT OF EARLY ONSET HYPOCALCEMIA

Patients at increased risk of hypocalcemia: Preterm infants ($\leq$ 32 weeks), sick infants of diabetic mothers and those with severe perinatal asphyxia should receive 40 mg/kg/day of elemental calcium (4 mL/kg/day of 10% calcium gluconate) for prevention of early onset hypocalcemia. However, there is no sufficient evidence for this practice. Infants tolerating oral feeds may receive this calcium orally every 6 hourly. Therapy should be continued for 3 days. Oral calcium preparations have high osmolality and should be avoided in babies at higher risk of necrotizing enterocolitis (Fig. 15.1).

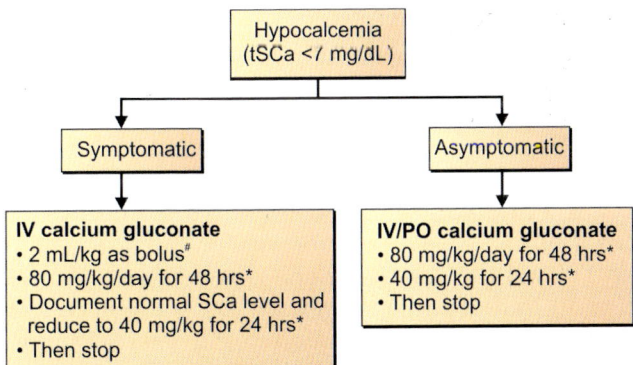

One mL of calcium gluconate contains 9 mg of elemental calcium
Diluted 1:1 in 5% dextrose and administered under cardiac monitoring
*Added to IV fluids and given as infusion. Take care of extravasation as that can result into skin sloughing. In case of asymptomatic ENH, the same can be given PO.

Fig. 15.1: Management of early neonatal hypocalcemia

Patients diagnosed to have asymptomatic hypocalcemia: Infants detected to have hypocalcemia on screening and who are otherwise asymptomatic should receive 80 mg/kg/day elemental calcium (8 mL/kg/day of 10% calcium gluconate) for 48 hours (Fig. 15.1). This may be tapered to 50% dose for another 24 hours and then discontinued. Neonates tolerating oral feeds may be treated with oral calcium (IV preparation may be used orally).

Patients diagnosed to have symptomatic hypocalcemia: These patients should receive a bolus dose of 2 mL/kg/dose diluted 1:1 with 5% dextrose over 10 minutes under cardiac monitoring. When there is severe hypocalcemia with poor cardiac function, calcium chloride 20 mg/kg may be given through a central line over 10–30 minutes (as chloride in comparison to gluconate does not require the metabolism by the liver for the release of free calcium). This should be followed by a continuous IV infusion of 80 mg/kg/day elemental calcium for 48 hours. Continuous infusion is preferred over IV bolus doses (1 mL/kg/dose every 6 hourly). Calcium infusion should be reduced to 50% of the original dose for the next 24 hours and then discontinued. The infusion may be replaced with oral calcium therapy on the last day. Normal calcium values should be documented at 48 hours before weaning the infusion.

All categories of hypocalcemia should be treated for at least 72 hours. Symptomatic hypocalcemia should be treated with a continuous infusion for at least 48 hours.

Precautions and Side Effects

Bradycardia and arrhythmia are known side effects of IV calcium boluses. Hence, bolus doses of calcium should be diluted 1:1 with 5% dextrose and given slowly (over 10 to 30 minutes) under cardiac monitoring. An umbilical venous catheter (UVC) may be used for administration of calcium only after ensuring that the tip is positioned in the inferior vena cava. Hepatic necrosis may occur if the tip of the UVC lies in a branch of the portal vein. Umbilical artery catheter (UAC) should never be used for giving calcium injections. Accidental injection into the UAC may result in arterial spasms and intestinal necrosis.

Skin and subcutaneous tissue necrosis may occur due to extravasation. Hence, IV sites where calcium is being infused should be checked frequently to monitor for extravasation.

Prolonged or Resistant Hypocalcemia

This condition should be considered in the following situations:
- Symptomatic hypocalcemia unresponsive to adequate doses of calcium therapy.
- Infants needing calcium supplements beyond 72 hours of age.
- Hypocalcemia presenting at the end of first week.

These infants should be investigated for causes of LNH (see below).

LATE ONSET NEONATAL HYPOCALCEMIA (LNH)

This condition is rare as compared to ENH. It usually presents at the end of first week of life. It is usually symptomatic in the form of neonatal tetany or seizures. This is usually caused by high phosphate intake (iatrogenic). The causes are listed in Table 15.2.

Table 15.2: Causes of late onset hypocalcemia

Increased phosphate load: cow milk, renal insufficiency

Hypomagnesemia

Vitamin D deficiency

Maternal vitamin D deficiency

Malabsorption

Renal insufficiency

Hepatobiliary disease

PTH resistance

Transient neonatal pseudohypoparathyroidism

Hypoparathyroidism
- *Primary:* Hypoplasia/aplasia (DiGeorge syndrome, CATCH 22 syndrome), activating mutations of the calcium sensing receptor (CSR)
- *Secondary:* Maternal hyperparathyroidism, metabolic syndromes (Kenny-Caffey syndrome, long-chain fatty acyl CoA dehydrogenase deficiency, Kearns-Sayre syndrome
- *Iatrogenic:* Citrated blood products, lipid infusion, bicarbonate therapy, loop diuretics, glucocorticosteriods, phosphate therapy, aminoglycosides (mainly gentamicin)

Alkalosis

Phototherapy

Examination

Such babies should have an examination with special emphasis on cataracts, hearing deficit and any evidence of basal ganglia involvement (movement disorder).

Investigations

Table 15.3 summarizes investigations to be considered in LNH or if the hypocalcemia does not respond to adequate doses of calcium.

Table 15.3: Investigations required in infants with persistent/late onset hypocalcemia

First line	Second line
Serum phosphate	Serum magnesium
Serum alkaline phosphatase (SAP)	Serum parathormone levels (PTH)
Liver function tests	Urine calcium creatinine ratio
Renal function tests	Maternal calcium, phosphate and
X-ray chest/wrist	alkaline phosphatase
Arterial pH	

If hypocalcemia is present with hyperphosphatemia and a normal renal function, hypoparathyroidism should be strongly suspected. (See Table 15.4 for interpretation of diagnostic investigation.)

Table 15.4: Interpretation of investigations

Disorder	Findings
Hypoparathyroidism	High : Phosphate Low : SAP, PTH, $1,25(OH)_2$, vitamin D_3
Pseudohypoparathyroidism	High : SAP, PTH, phosphate Low : $1,25(OH)_2$, vitamin D_3
Chronic renal failure	High : Phosphate, SAP, PTH, pH (acidotic), deranged RFT Low : $1,25(OH)_2$, vitamin D_3
Hypomagnesemia	High : PTH Low : Phosphate, Mg, $1,25(OH)_2$, vitamin D_3
VDDR I	High : SAP, PTH Low : Phosphate, $1,25(OH)_2$, vitamin D_3
VDDR II	High : SAP, $1,25(OH)_2$, vitamin D_3, PTH Low : Phosphate

TREATMENT OF LNH

The treatment of LNH is specific to etiology and may in certain diseases be lifelong.

1. *Hypomagnesemia:* Symptomatic hypocalcemia unresponsive to adequate doses of IV calcium therapy is usually due to hypomagnesemia. It may present either as ENH or later as LNH. The neonate should receive 2 doses of 0.2 mL/kg of 50% $MgSO_4$ injection, 12 hours apart, deep IM followed by a maintenance dose of 0.2 mL/kg/day of 50% $MgSO_4$, PO for 3 days.

2. *High phosphate load:* These infants have hyperphosphatemia with near normal calcium levels. This happens in situation of non-human milk feeding (containing high phosphate content). Exclusive breastfeeding should be encouraged and top feeding with cow's milk should be discontinued. Phosphate binding gels should be avoided.

3. *Hypoparathyroidism:*[9] These infants tend to be *hyperphosphatemic and hypocalcemic with normal renal function.* Elevated phosphate levels in the absence of exogenous phosphate load (cow's milk) and presence of normal renal functions indicates parathormone inefficiency.

   It is important to realize that if the phosphate level is very high then adding calcium may lead to calcium deposition and tissue damage. Thus, attempts should be made to reduce the phosphate (so as to keep the calcium and the phosphate product less than 55).[10] These neonates need supplementation with calcium (50 mg/kg/day in 3 divided doses) and $1,25(OH)_2$ vitamin D_3 (0.5–1 mg/day). Syrups with 125 mg and 250 mg per 5 mL of calcium are available. $1,25(OH)_2$ vitamin D_3 (calcitriol) is available as 0.25 mg capsules. Therapy may be stopped in hypocalcemia secondary to maternal hyperparathyroidism after 6 weeks.

4. *Vitamin D deficiency states:* These babies have hypocalcemia associated with hypophosphatemia due to an intact parathormone response on the kidneys. They benefit from Vitamin D_3 supplementation in a dose of 30–60 mg/kg/day.

Monitoring

The baby is monitored for the SCa and phosphate, 24 hours urinary calcium and calcium creatinine ratio. Try to keep the calcium in the lower range as defective distal tubular absorption leads to hypercalciuria and nephrocalcinosis.[11]

PROGNOSIS AND OUTCOME

Most cases of ENH resolve within 48–72 hours without any clinically significant sequelae.

LNH secondary to exogenous phosphate load and magnesium deficiency also responds well to phosphate restriction and magnesium repletion. When caused by hypoparathyroidism, hypocalcemia requires continued therapy with vitamin D metabolites and calcium salts. The period of therapy depends on the nature of the hypoparathyroidism which can be transient, last several weeks to months or be permanent.

REFERENCES

1. Schauberger CW, Pitkin RM, Maternal-perinatal calcium relationships. Obstet Gynecol 1979;53:74–6.

2. Linarelli LG, Bobik J, Bobik C. Newborn urinary cyclic AMP and developmental responsiveness to parathyroid hormone. Pediatrics 1972;50:14–23.

3. Hillman, Rajanasathit S, Slatopolsky E, Haddad JG. Serial measurements of serum calcium, magnesium, parathyroid hormone, calcitonin and 25-hydroxy-vitamin D in premature and term infants during the first week of life. Pediatr Res 1977;11: 789–44.

4. Salle BL, Delvin EE, Lapillonne A, Bishop NJ, Glorieux FH. Perinatal metabolism of vitamin D. Am J Clin Nutr 2000;71 (5 suppl):S1317–24.

5. Singh J, Moghal N, Pearce SH, Cheetham T. The investigation of hypocalcaemia and rickets. Arch Dis Child. May 2003;88(5): 403–7.

6. Oden J, Bourgeois M. Neonatal endocrinology. Indian J Pediatr 2000;67:217–23.

7. Schwartz R, Teramo KA. Effects of diabetic pregnancy on the fetus and newborn. Semin Perinatol 2000;24:120–35.

8. Nekvasil R, Stejskal J, Tuma A. Detection of early onset neonatal hypocalcemia in low birth weight infants by Q-Tc and Q-oTc interval measurement. Acta Paediatr Acad Sci Hung 1980; 21(4):203–10.

9. Marx SJ. Hyperparathyroid and hypoparathyroid disorders. N Engl J Med 2000;343:1863–75.

10. Sharma J, Bajpai A, Kabra M et al. Hypocalcemia–Clinical, biochemical, radiological profile and follow-up in a tertiary hospital in India. Indian Pediatrics 2002;39:276–282.

11. Rigo J, Curtis MD. Disorders of Calcium, Phosphorus and Magnesium Metabolism in Richard J Martin, Avory A Fanaroff, Michele C Walsh (Eds). Neonatal Perinatal Medicine—Diseases of the fetus and infant. 8th edn. Elsevier, Philadelphia, 2006; p.1508–14.

16 Polycythemia

Polycythemia or an increased hematocrit is associated with hyperviscosity of blood. As the blood viscosity increases, there is impairment of tissue perfusion and a tendency to form microthrombi. Significant damage may occur if these events occur in the cerebral cortex, kidneys and adrenal glands. Hence, this condition requires urgent diagnosis and prompt management.

The viscosity of blood is directly proportional to the hematocrit and plasma viscosity and inversely proportional to the deformability of red blood cells. Symptoms of hypo-perfusion correlate better with viscosity as compared to hematocrit. Viscosity is, however, difficult to measure bedside. Hyperviscosity is therefore suspected in the presence of an abnormally high hematocrit with or without suggestive symptoms.

Relationship between viscosity and hematocrit is almost linear up to a hematocrit of 65% and exponential thereafter.[1,2] The polycythemia-hyperviscosity syndrome is thus usually confined to infants with hematocrits of more than 65%; it is very rare with hematocrits of < 60%.

DEFINITION

A diagnosis of polycythemia is made in the presence of a venous hematocrit more than 65% or a venous hemoglobin concentration in excess of 22 g/dL. Hyperviscosity is defined as a viscosity greater than 14.6 centipoise at a shear rate of 11.5 per second.[3]

INCIDENCE

The incidence of polycythemia is 1.5–4% of all live births.[4,5] The incidence is higher among both small for gestational age (SGA) and large for gestational age (LGA) infants. The incidence of polycythemia is 15% among term SGA infants as compared to 2% in term AGA infants.[6]

Neonates born at high altitudes also have a higher incidence of polycythemia.[1] Maternal smoking is an important risk factor for polycythemia.[7] Term neonates born to mothers engaged in smoking during pregnancy are 2.5 times more likely to require a partial exchange transfusion for polycythemia than their counterparts of non-smoker mothers.[7] Infants born by cesarean section have a lower hematocrit values than those delivered vaginally.[8] Infants subjected to delayed cord clamping carry nearly four times greater risk of asymptomatic polycythemia.[9]

In the last 3 years, the incidence of polycythemia ranged from 0.95 to 1.5% in our centre.

PHYSIOLOGICAL CHANGES IN POSTNATAL LIFE

Significant changes take place in the hematocrit from birth through the first 24 to 48 hrs of life. The hematocrit peaks at 2 hrs of age and values up to 71% may be normal at this age.[10–11] It gradually declines to 68% by 6 hrs and usually stabilizes by 12 to 24 hrs. The initial rise in hematocrit is related to a transudation of fluid out of the intravascular space.

CLINICAL FEATURES OF POLYCYTHEMIA

Polycythemia can result in a wide range of symptoms involving several organ systems (Table 16.1). About 50% of neonates with polycythemia develop one or more symptoms. However, most of these symptoms are non-specific and may be related to the underlying conditions rather than due to polycythemia per se.

Screening for Polycythemia

Screening should be done for polycythemia in certain high-risk groups (Table 16.2).

Table 16.1: Clinical features ascribed to polycythemia and hyperviscosity

Central nervous system

Early: Hypotonia and sleepiness, irritability, jitteriness, seizures and infarcts
Late: Motor deficits, lower achievement and IQ scores

Metabolism

Hypoglycemia
Jaundice
Hypocalcemia

Heart and lungs

Tachycardia, tachypnea, respiratory distress
Cyanosis, plethora
Chest radiography: Cardiomegaly, pulmonary plethora
Echocardiography: Increased pulmonary resistance, decreased cardiac output

Gastrointestinal tract

Poor suck, vomiting
Feed intolerance—abdominal distension
Necrotizing enterocolitis

Kidneys

Oliguria (depending on blood volume)
Transient hypertension
Renal vein thrombosis

Hematology

Mild thrombocytopenia
Thrombosis (rare)

Miscellaneous

Peripheral gangrene
Priapism
Testicular infarction

Table 16.2: Screening for polycythemia

Eligible candidates

a. Small for gestational age (SGA) infants
b. Infants of diabetic mothers (IDM)
c. Large for gestational age (LGA) infants
d. Monochorionic twins especially the larger twin
e. Infants with morphological features of growth retardation such as many loose folds of skin around the buttocks and thighs, loss of subcutaneous fat, difference of HC and CC ≥ 3 cm

Schedule

2 hrs, 6 hrs, 12 hrs, 24 hrs, 48 hrs and 72 hrs of age

Method

Centrifuge venous blood in heparinized capillaries for 3 to 5 min @ 10000 to 15000 rpm

CAPILLARY VERSUS VENOUS HEMATOCRIT

Capillary hematocrit measurements are unreliable and highly subjected to variations in blood flow. Capillary hematocrit is significantly higher than venous hematocrit. This difference is even more apparent in infants receiving large placental transfusion.[12]

Practical Tip

Capillary samples may be used for screening, but all high values should be confirmed by a venous sample for the diagnosis of polycythemia.

METHODS OF HEMATOCRIT DETERMINATION

Two methods are available:
1. *Automated hematology analyzer:* This calculates the hematocrit from a direct measurement of mean cell volume and the hemoglobin.
2. *Micro-centrifuge:* Blood is collected in heparinized micro-capillaries (110 mm length and 1–2 mm internal diameter) and centrifuged at 10,000 to 15,000 rotations per minute (rpm) for 3–5 minutes. Plasma separates and the packed cell volume is measured to give the hematocrit.

An automated analyzer gives lower value as compared to hematocrit measured by the centrifugation method.[13] Most of the reported data on polycythemia is on centrifuged hematocrit.

MANAGEMENT OF POLYCYTHEMIA

Before a diagnosis of polycythemia is considered, it is mandatory to exclude dehydration. If the birth weight is known, re-weighing the baby and looking for excessive weight loss (more than 10–15%) would help in the diagnosis of dehydration. If this is present, it should be corrected by increasing fluid/feed intake. The hematocrit should be measured again after correction of dehydration. Once a diagnosis of polycythemia is made, associated metabolic problems including hypoglycemia should be excluded.

Management of polycythemia is dependent upon two factors (Fig. 16.1):
1. Presence of symptoms suggestive of polycythemia and/or
2. Absolute value of hematocrit

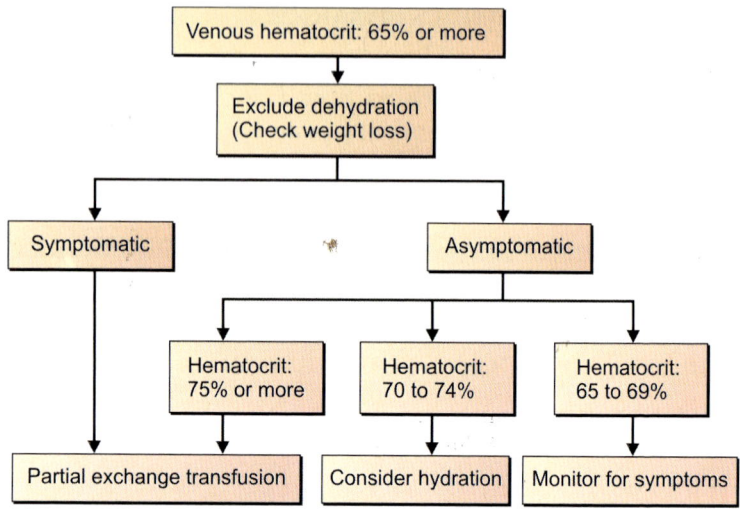

Fig. 16.1: Management algorithm of polycythemia

Symptomatic Polycythemia

The definitive treatment for polycythemia is to perform a partial exchange transfusion (PET). PET involves removing some of the blood volume and replacing it with normal saline so as to decrease the hematocrit to a target hematocrit of 55%. Following PET, symptoms like jitteriness may persist for 1–2 days despite the hematocrit being lowered to physiological ranges.

The volume of blood to be exchanged is given by the formula shown in Panel 1.

Panel 1: Volume to be Exchanged

$$= \frac{\text{Blood volume}^* \times (\text{observed hematocrit} - \text{desired hematocrit})}{\text{Observed hematocrit}}$$

Blood volume should be ideally found out from Rawlings chart.[14] As a rough guide, it is 80–90 mL/kg in term babies and 90–100 mL/kg in preterm babies.

For example, for a 35 wk gestation newborn weighing 2 kg (assume blood volume 90 mL/kg) and observed hematocrit of 75% and desired hematocrit of 55%, the amount of blood to be exchanged would be:

= 2*90* (75–55/75)

= 48 mL of blood to be exchanged with normal saline to bring hematocrit from 75% to 55%.

As a rough guide, the volume of blood to be exchanged is usually 20–25 mL/kg.

PET: Peripheral versus Umbilical Route

PET may be carried out via the peripheral or the central route.

In the former, blood is withdrawn from the peripheral arterial line and replaced simultaneously with saline via a peripheral venous line.

In the central route, blood can be withdrawn from umbilical venous catheter and saline replaced by a peripheral vein. Alternatively, in central route, the umbilical venous catheter may be used for both withdrawal of blood and replacement of saline (pull and push technique, similar to double volume exchange transfusion or the blood is withdrawn from umbilical arterial line and saline replaced from umbilical venous line.

The route of PET may influence infection rates, mesenteric artery flow abnormalities and NEC rates.[15,16]

PET: Choice of Exchange Fluid

Crystalloids such as normal saline (NS) or Ringer's lactate (RL) are preferred over colloids because they are less expensive and are easily available. Crystalloids produce nearly comparable reduction in hematocrit as colloids (Panel 2)[17,18] and do not have the risk of transfusion associated infections. Moreover, adult plasma has been shown to increase the blood viscosity when mixed with fetal erythrocytes.

We use only normal saline for partial exchange transfusion.

Panel 2: Choice of Exchange Fluid: What is Evidence?

A systematic review determined efficacy of crystalloid *versus* colloid solutions to identify the best fluid for PET:[17]
- Clinically unimportant difference in hematocrit favoring colloids than crystalloids:
  - at 2–6 hr: 2.3% (95% CI 1.3 to 3.3%)
  - at 24 hr: 1.7% (95% CI 0.8 to 2.7%)

Asymptomatic Polycythemia

The line of management in infants with asymptomatic polycythemia depends upon their hematocrit values.

1. *Hematocrit 75% or more:* These infants are usually managed with PET.
2. *Hematocrit between 70% and 74%:* Conservative management with hydration may be tried in these infants. An extra fluid/feeds of 20 mL/kg may be added to the daily fluid

requirements. The additional fluid intake may be ensured by either enteral (supervised feeding) or parenteral route (IV fluids). The rationale for this therapy is that fluid brings about hemodilution and the resultant decrease in viscosity.

3. *Hematocrit between 65% and 70%:* These babies need monitoring for any symptoms of polycythemia and re-estimation of hematocrit. Further management depends upon the repeat hematocrit values.

EVIDENCE FOR MANAGEMENT OF POLYCYTHEMIA

PET reverses the physiological abnormalities associated with the polycythemia–hyperviscosity syndrome. It improves capillary perfusion, cerebral blood flow and cardiac function. However, there is very little data to suggest that PET improves long-term outcome in patients with polycythemia. The latest Cochrane review (2010) concluded that there is no proven clinically significant short- or long-term benefit of PET in polycythemic newborn infants who are clinically well or who have minor symptoms related to hyperviscosity. PET may increase the risk of NEC (Panel 3).[19]

Panel 3: Partial Exchange Transfusion for Polycythemia: What is Evidence?
A Cochrane review (2010)[19] on this issue showed: • No effect on neonatal mortality (one study; RR 5.23, 95% CI 0.66, 41.26).   • No difference in developmental delay (4 low quality studies; RR 1.45, 95% CI 0.83 to 2.54).   • Increased risk of NEC in infants receiving PET (2 studies; RR 11.18, 95% CI 1.49, 83.64).   • No differences in short-term complications including hypoglycemia (two studies) and thrombocytopenia (one study).

However, as studies included in the review were of low quality, the large numbers of surviving infants were not assessed for developmental outcomes, and therefore, the true risks and benefit of PET is unclear. A recent study by Iris et al showed that restrictive management of polycythemia does not increase short-term complications.[20]

Given the uncertainty regarding the long-term outcomes, it is preferable to restrict PET in symptomatic infants with hematocrit of >65% and in asymptomatic neonates with hematocrit of >75%.

REFERENCES

1. Mackintosh TF, Walkar CH. Blood viscosity in the newborn. Arch Dis Child 1973;48:547–53.

2. Phibbs RH. Neonatal Polycythemia. In: Rudolph AB (Ed): Pediatrics, 16th edn. New York: Appleton Century Crofts, 1997; p. 179.

3. Ramamurthy RS, Brans WY. Neonatal Polycythemia I. Criteria for diagnosis and treatment. Pediatrics 1981;68:168–74.

4. Wirth FH, Goldberg KE, Lubchenco LO: Neonatal hyperviscosity I. Incidence. Pediatrics 1979;63:833–6.

5. Stevens K, Wirth FH. Incidence of neonatal hyperviscosity at sea level. Pediatrics 1980;97:118.

6. Bada HS, Korones SB, Pourcyrous M, et al. Asymptomatic syndrome of polycythemic hyperviscosity: effect of partial exchange transfusion. J Pediatr 1992;120:579–85.

7. Awonusonu FO, Pauly TH, Hutchison AA. Maternal smoking and partial exchange transfusion for neonatal polycythemia. Am J Perinatol 2002;19:349–54.

8. Lubetzky R, Ben-Shachar S, Mimouni FB, et al. Mode of delivery and neonatal hematocrit. Am J Perinatol 2000;17:163–5.

9. Hutton EK, Hassan ES. Late *versus* early clamping of the umbilical cord in full-term neonates: systematic review and meta-analysis of controlled trials. JAMA 2007;297:1241–52.

10. Shohat M, Merlob P, Reisner SH: Neonatal Polycythemia I. Early diagnosis and incidence relating to time of sampling. Pediatrics 1984;73:7–10.

11. Shohat M, Reisner SH, Mimouni F, et al. Neonatal polycythemia II. Definition related to time of sampling. Pediatrics 1984;73:11–3.

12. Oh W. Neonatal polycythemia and hyperviscosity. Pediatr Clin North Am 1986;33:523–32.

13. Goldberg K, Wirth FH, Hathaway WE, et al. Neonatal hyperviscosity II. Effect of partial exchange transfusion. Pediatrics 1982;69:419–25.

14. Rawlings JS, Pettett G, Wiswell TE, et al. Estimated blood volumes in polycythemic neonates as a function of birth weight. J Pediatr 1982;101:594–9.

15. Rodriguez-Balderrama I, Rodriguez-Juarez DA, Cisneros-Garcia N, et al. Comparison of 2 methods of partial exchange transfusion in newborns with polycythemia: peripheral-peripheral and central-peripheral. Bol Med Hosp Infant Mex 1993;50:633–8.

16. Hein HA, Lathrop SS. Partial exchange transfusion in term, polycythemic neonates: absence of association with severe gastrointestinal injury. Pediatrics 1987;80:75–8.

17. De Waal KA, Baerts W, Offringa M. Systematic review of the optimal fluid for dilutional exchange transfusion in neonatal polycythaemia. Arch Dis Child Fetal Neonatal 2006;91:F7–10.

18. Deorari AK, Paul VK, Shreshta L, Singh M. Symptomatic neonatal polycythemia: Comparison of partial exchange transfusion with saline *versus* plasma. Indian Pediatr 1995;32:1167–71.

19. Ozek E, Soll R, Schimmel MS. Partial exchange transfusion to prevent neurodevelopmental disability in infants with polycythemia. Cochrane Database Syst Rev 2010 Jan 20;(1):CD005089.

20. Morag I, Strauss T, Lubin D, Schushan-Eisen I, Kenet G, Kuint J. Restrictive management of neonatal Polycythemia. Am J Perinatol 2011;28:677–682.

There is no universal definition for hypoglycemia.[1] Various investigators have empirically recommended different blood glucose levels (BGLs) that should be maintained in neonatal period to prevent injury to the developing brain.[2,3] The "normal" range of blood glucose is variable and depends upon factors like birth-weight, gestational age, body stores, feeding status, availability of energy sources as well as the presence or absence of disease.[4,5] Further, there is no concrete evidence to show the causation of adverse long-term outcomes by a particular level or duration of hypoglycemia.[6] Hence, a consensus has been to evolve an "operational threshold" as definition.

DEFINITION

The operational threshold for hypoglycemia is defined as *the concentration of plasma or whole blood glucose at which clinicians should consider intervention, based on currently available evidence in literature.*[7] Operational threshold has been defined as BGL of less than 40 mg/dL (plasma glucose level less than 45 mg/dL).[8]

WHO defines hypoglycemia as BGL of less than 45 mg/dL (2.2 mmol/L).

Screening for Hypoglycemia

Screening for hypoglycemia is recommended in certain high risk infants (Table 17.1).

Time Schedule for Screening

There is a paucity of the literature that looks into optimal timing and the intervals of glucose monitoring. Lowest blood sugar

Table 17.1: Indication for routine blood glucose screening[9]

1. Infants <2000 grams
2. Infants ≤35 weeks
3. Small for gestational age infants (SGA): birth weight <10th percentile
4. Infant of diabetic mothers (IDM)
5. Large for gestational age (LGA) infants: birth weight >90th percentile*
6. Infants with Rh-hemolytic disease
7. Infants born to mothers receiving therapy with terbutaline/propranolol/lebatolol/oral hypoglycemic agents
8. Infants with morphological IUGR. This group includes neonates with birth weight between 10th to 25th and possibly up to 50th percentile, with features of fetal under-nutrition such as three or more loose skin folds in gluteal region, overall decreased subcutaneous fat and head circumference to chest circumference difference >than 3 cm.
9. Any sick neonate e.g. those with perinatal asphyxia, polycythemia, sepsis, shock, etc. during active phase of illness. The screening may be discontinued once their condition gets stabilized.
10. Infants on parenteral nutrition.

*LGA infants of constitutionally large parents may be exempted from routine screening.

values are seen at 2 hours of life. IDMs frequently experience asymptomatic hypoglycemia early viz. 1 to 2 hours and rarely beyond 12 hours (range 0.8 to 8.5 h), supporting need for early screening for this population.[10] However, preterm and SGA may be at highest risk up to 36 h (range 0.8 to 34.2 h).[11]

Some SGA and preterm infants may develop hypoglycemia when feeding is not established. Based on these assumptions and current knowledge, Table 17.2 elaborates the schedule and frequency of monitoring in different situations.

Table 17.2: Schedule of blood glucose monitoring

Category of infants	Time schedule
1. At risk neonates (SN 1–8 in Table 17.1)	2, 6, 12, 24, 48 and 72 hrs
2. Sick infants (infants with sepsis, asphyxia, shock during active phase of illness. Once the underlying condition is under control, frequency of screening can be reduced or omitted)	Every 6–8 hrs (individualize as needed)
3. Stable VLBW infants on parenteral nutrition	Initial 72 hrs: every 6 to 8 hrs After 72 hrs: once a day

Infants exhibiting signs compatible with hypoglycemia at any time also need to be investigated.

Education and Counseling of Caregivers regarding the Screening

Parents should be told that their infant is at-risk and therefore requires blood tests at regular intervals. This will ensure appropriate parental participation in monitoring and allay fears if further interventions are required.

Infants in whom Screening is not Required

Screening for hypoglycemia is not recommended in term healthy breastfed appropriate for gestational age (AGA) infants. However, term infants with poor feeding, presence of inadequate lactation or presence of cold stress may be considered for screening.

METHOD OF BLOOD GLUCOSE LEVEL ESTIMATION

- *Point of care (POC) reagent strips (Glucose oxidase method):* Though widely used, glucose estimation by this method is unreliable especially at levels where therapeutic intervention is required such as BGL 40 to 50 mg/dL (high false positivity for hypoglycemia). They are useful for screening purpose but low values should be confirmed by proper laboratory analysis. However, treatment of hypoglycemia may be initiated based on the results of the reagent strips.

  It is important to consider the variations between capillary and venous, blood and plasma, and immediate and stored samples (whole blood sugar value is 10–15% less than that of plasma value; the BGL can fall by 14 to 18 mg/dL per hour in samples that await analysis).[12] Arterial samples have slightly higher value as compared to venous or capillary samples.

  The first generation strips focused on change in color by enzymatic reaction on application of blood drop. The color can be read by naked eye or by reflectance meters. However, the results get affected by hematocrit values, acidosis, presence of bilirubin, etc.

- The newer generation glucose reagent strips generate a current on reaction of glucose with enzymes such as glucose oxidase or glucose dehydrogenase. The amount of current is proportional to amount of sugar present in plasma.

Though these second generation glucose readers are more accurate than the previous version but still are not reliable. Any abnormal BGLs by this technique must be confirmed by standard laboratory methods.

- *Laboratory diagnosis*: This is the most accurate method. In the laboratory, glucose can be measured by either the *glucose oxidase* (calorimetric) method or by the *glucose electrode method (as used in blood gas and electrolyte analyzer machine)*. Blood samples should be analyzed quickly to avoid erroneously low glucose levels.

CLINICAL SIGNS ASSOCIATED WITH HYPOGLYCEMIA

- *Asymptomatic:* It is well known that low BGL may not manifest clinically and be totally asymptomatic. There is considerable controversy in regard to the need for treatment of the infants with low BGLs but without any symptoms.[13,14]
- *Symptomatic:* A smaller proportion of infants with hypoglycemia can be symptomatic. Clinical signs of hypoglycemia are variable and may include stupor, jitteriness, tremors, apathy, episodes of cyanosis, convulsions, intermittent apneic spells or tachypnea, weak and high pitched cry, limpness and lethargy, difficulty in feeding and eye rolling. Episodes of sweating, sudden pallor, hypothermia and cardiac arrest have also been reported.

Diagnosis

- *Asymptomatic hypoglycemia* is said to be present when BGL is less than 40 mg/dL (confirmed by laboratory estimation) and the infant does not manifest with any clinical features.
- *Symptomatic hypoglycemia* should be diagnosed if hypoglycemia (BGL is less than 40 mg/dL) coexists with clinical symptoms. Neonates generally present with nonspecific signs that result from a variety of illnesses. Therefore, the affected infant should be carefully evaluated for all possible causes.

  If clinical signs attributable to hypoglycemia persist despite intravenous glucose, then other causes of persistent/resistant hypoglycemia should be explored.

MANAGEMENT OF ASYMPTOMATIC HYPOGLYCEMIA

Table 17.3 summarizes management of an infant with asymptomatic hypoglycemia.

Table 17.3: Management of infants with asymptomatic hypoglycemia

BGL 20–40 mg/dL	Trial of oral feeds (expressed breast milk or formula) and repeat blood test after 1 hour.
	1. If repeat BGL is ≥40 mg/dL, two hourly feeds are ensured with 6 hourly monitoring of BGL for 48 hrs. The target blood glucose value is 50 to 120 mg/dL.
	2. If repeat blood sugar is <40 mg/dL, IV dextrose is started and further management is as for symptomatic hypoglycemia.
BGL levels <20 mg/dL	IV dextrose (6 mg/kg/min) Subsequent management as for symptomatic hypoglycemia.

ORAL FEEDS

Direct breastfeeding is the best option for trial of an oral feed. If the infant is unable to suck, expressed breast milk may be given. Breast milk promotes ketogenesis (ketones are important alternate sources for the brain along with other sources such as pyruvate, free fatty acids, glycerol and amino acids). If breast milk is not available, then formula feeds may be given.

Some of the randomized clinical trials in SGA[15] and appropriate-for-gestational age[16] infant found that the sugar or sucrose fortified milk (5 g sugar per 100 mL milk) raises blood glucose and prevents hypoglycemia. Such supplementation may be tried in the asymptomatic neonates with blood sugar levels between 20 and 40 mg/dL. However, this practice carries a potential to compromise breastfeeding rates and therefore, one should be prudent in exercising this option.

MANAGEMENT OF SYMPTOMATIC HYPOGLYCEMIA

All symptomatic infants should be treated with IV fluids (Fig. 17.1).

For symptomatic hypoglycemia including seizures, a bolus of 2 mL/kg of 10% dextrose (200 mg/kg) should be given. This mini-bolus helps to rapidly correct BGL.[14] The bolus should be followed by continuous glucose infusion at an initial rate of 6–8 mg/kg/min. BGL should be checked after 30 to 60 min and then every 6 hour until blood sugar is >50 mg/dL.

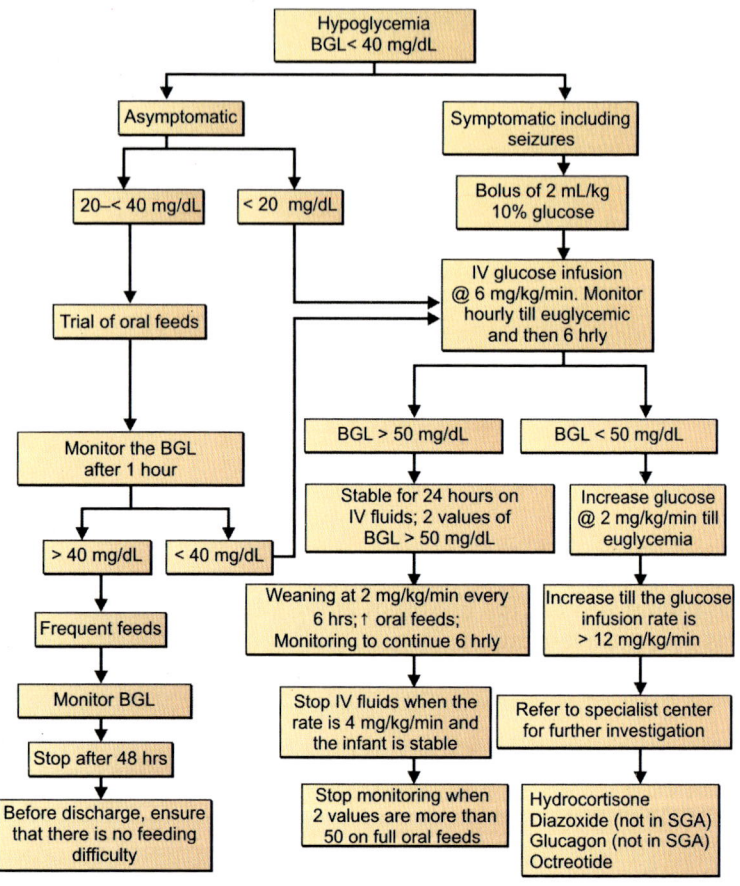

Fig. 17.1: Algorithm for management of neonatal hypoglycemia

If BGL stays below 40 mg/dL despite bolus and glucose infusion, glucose infusion rate (GIR) should be increased in steps of 2 mg/kg/min every 15 to 30 min until a maximum of 12 mg/kg/min.

After 24 hours of IV glucose therapy, once two or more consecutive BGLs are > 50 mg/dL, the infusion can be tapered off at the rate of 2 mg/kg/min every 6 hours with BGL monitoring. Tapering has to be accompanied by concomitant increase in oral feeds. Once a rate of 4 mg/kg/min of glucose infusion is achieved and oral intake is adequate and the BGLs are consistently > 50 mg/dL, the infusion can be stopped.

It is important to ensure continuous glucose infusion preferably using an infusion pump and without any interruption. Do not stop glucose infusion abruptly as severe rebound hypoglycemia may occur. Avoid using more than 12.5% dextrose infusion through a peripheral vein due to the risk of thrombophlebitis.

Practical Tip

If there is persistent hypoglycemia, check the intravenous line for functioning. Also recheck the intravenous fluid preparation and infusion rate.

RECURRENT/RESISTANT HYPOGLYCEMIA

This condition should be considered when either the infant has recurrent episodes of hypoglycemia or if he fails to maintain normal BGL despite a GIR of 12 mg/kg/min or required IV glucose for greater than 7 days. High levels of glucose infusion may be needed in the infants to achieve euglycemia. These infants must be investigated for underlying cause (Table 17.4).

Besides increasing GIR for resistant hypoglycemia, certain drugs may be tried. Before administration of drugs, take the samples to investigate the cause (Table 17.5). Drugs that are used include the following:

Table 17.4: Important causes of resistant hypoglycemia

Congenital hypopituitarism
Adrenal insufficiency
Hyperinsulinemic states
Galactosemia
Glycogen storage disorders
Maple syrup urine disease
Mitochondrial disorders
Fatty acid oxidation defect

Table 17.5: Investigations to be done in resistant hypoglycemia

Serum insulin levels
Serum cortisol levels
Growth hormone levels
Blood ammonia
Blood lactate levels
Urine ketones and reducing substances
Urine and sugar aminoacidogram
Free fatty acid levels
Galactose 1 phosphate uridyl transferase levels

- Hydrocortisone 5 mg/kg/day IV or PO in two divided doses for 24 to 48 hrs.
- Diazoxide can be given orally 10–25 mg/kg/day in three divided doses. Diazoxide acts by keeping the K_{ATP} channels of the β-cells of the pancreas open, thereby reducing the secretion of insulin. It is therefore useful in states of unregulated insulin secretion like insulinomas.
- Glucagon 100 g/kg subcutaneous or intramuscular (maximum 300 g) up to three doses. Glucagon acts by mobilizing hepatic glycogen stores, enhancing gluconeogenesis and promoting ketogenesis. These effects are not consistently seen in SGA infants. Side effects of glucagon include vomiting, diarrhea and hypokalemia and at high doses, it may stimulate insulin release.
- Octreotide (synthetic somatostatin in dose of 2–10 µg/kg/day) subcutaneously two to three times a day.

Do not use diazoxide and glucagon in small for gestational age infants.

Useful formulae

a. $$\text{GIR (mg/kg/min)} = \frac{\% \text{ of dextrose being infused} \times \text{rate (mL/hr)}}{\text{body weight (in kg)} \times 6}$$

b. $$\text{Infusion rate mg/kg/min)} = \frac{\text{IV rate (mL/kg/day)} \times \% \text{ of dextrose} \times}{144}$$

c. $$\text{Infusion rate (mg/kg/min)} = \text{Fluid rate (mL/kg/day)} \times 0.007 \times \% \text{ of dextrose infused}$$

FOLLOW-UP AND OUTCOME

The outcome of hypoglycemia is determined by factors like, duration, degree of hypoglycemia, rate of cerebral blood flow, cerebral utilization of glucose and also co-morbidities. Special attention should be paid to neurodevelopmental outcome, overall IQ, reading ability, arithmetic proficiency and motor performance.

The infants can be assessed at one month corrected age for vision/eye evaluation. At 3, 6, 9, 12 and 18 months corrected age, the infant is followed-up for growth, neurodevelopment, vision and hearing loss. Vision can be assessed with Teller acuity card and hearing should be assessed by brainstem evoked auditory responses. Neurodevelopment is assessed by the clinical psychologist using DASII 2. MRI at 4–6 weeks provides a good estimate of hypoglycemic injury.[17]

What is the Evidence?

Hypoglycemia and Neurodevelopmental Outcome:

- Systemic review involving 18 studies concluded that there is no good correlation between the two and further well designed good quality studies are needed.[18]
- A recent study involving 35 neonates who had symptomatic hypoglycemia showed that 94% of them had some white abnormalities and on follow-up at 18 months of age, 65% of them had demonstrated some impairment in development.[19]

Table 17.6: Achieving appropriate glucose infusion rate at different daily fluid intakes

Daily fluid volume (mL/kg/d)	Glucose infusion rate (GIR)					
	6 mg/kg/min		8 mg/kg/min		10 mg/kg/min	
	D10	D25	D10	D25	D10	D25
60	42	18	24	36	5	55
75	68	7	49	26	30	45
90	90	–	74	16	55	35
105	85*	–	99	6	80	25
120	100*	–	120	–	97	18

Add 20 mL/kg of normal saline to provide 3 mEq/kg of sodium

REFERENCES

1. Schauberger CW, Pitkin RM, Maternal-perinatal calcium relationships. Obstet Gynecol 1979;53:74–6.

2. Linarelli LG, Bobik J, Bobik C. Newborn urinary cyclic AMP and developmental responsiveness to parathyroid hormone. Pediatrics 1972;50:14–23.

3. Hillman, Rajanasathit S, Slatopolsky E, Haddad JG. Serial measurements of serum calcium, magnesium, parathyroid hormone, calcitonin and 25-hydroxyvitamin D in premature and term infants during the first week of life. Pediatr Res 1977; 11:789–44.

4. Salle BL, Delvin EE, Lapillonne A, Bishop NJ, Glorieux FH. Perinatal metabolism of vitamin D. Am J Clin Nutr 2000;71 (5 suppl):S1317–24.

5. Singh J, Moghal N, Pearce SH, Cheetham T. The investigation of hypocalcaemia and rickets. Arch Dis Child 2003;88:403–7.

6. Oden J, Bourgeois M. Neonatal endocrinology. Indian J Pediatr 2000;67:217–23.

7. Schwartz R, Teramo KA. Effects of diabetic pregnancy on the fetus and newborn. Semin Perinatol 2000;24:120–35.

8. Nekvasil R, Stejskal J, Tuma A. Detection of early onset neonatal hypocalcemia in low birth weight infants by Q-Tc and Q-oTc interval measurement. Acta Paediatr Acad Sci Hung 1980; 21(4):203–10.

9. Marx SJ. Hyperparathyroid and hypoparathyroid disorders. N Engl J Med 2000;343:1863–75.

10. Sharma J, Bajpai A, Kabra M, et al. Hypocalcemia—clinical, biochemical, radiological profile and follow-up in a tertiary hospital in India. Indian Pediatrics 2002;39:276–282.

11. Rigo J, Curtis MD. Disorders of calcium, phosphorus and magnesium metabolism in Richard J Martin, Avory A Fanaroff, Michele C Walsh (Eds). Neonatal Perinatal Medicine-Diseases of the fetus and infant. 8th edition; Elsevier, Pihladelphia, 2006; p. 1508–14.

12. Cowett RM, Damico LB. Capillary (heel stick) *versus* venous blood sampling for determination of glucose concentration in neonate. Biol Neonate 1992;62:32–6.

13. Lucas A, Morley R. Outcome of neonatal hypoglycemia. Br Med J 1999;318:194.

14. Filan PM, Inder TE, Cameron FJ, et al. Neonatal hypoglycemia and occipital cerebral injury. J Pediatr 2006;148:552–5.

15. Singhal PK, Singh M, Paul VK. Prevention of hypoglycemia: a controlled evaluation of sugar fortified milk feeding in small-for-date infants. Indian Pediatr 1992; 29:1365-9.

16. Singhal PK, Singh M, Paul VK, et al. A controlled study of sugar fortified milk feeding in prevention of neonatal hypoglycemia. Indian J Med Res 1991;94:342-5.

17. Duvanel CB, Fawer CL, Cotting J, et al. Long term effects of neonatal hypoglycemia on brain growth and psychomotor development in small-for-gestational age preterm infants. J Pediatr 1999;134:492–8.

18. Boluyt N, van Kempen A, Offringa M. Neurodevelopment after neonatal hypoglycemia: a systematic review and design of an optimal future study. Pediatrics 2006;117:2231–43.

19. Burns CM, Rutherford MA, Boardman JP et al. Patterns of cerebral injury and neurodevelopmental outcomes after symptomatic neonatal hypoglycemia. Pediatrics 2008;122:65–74.

Inborn Errors of Metabolism

Inborn errors of metabolism (IEM) are disorders in which there is a block at some point in the normal metabolic pathway caused by a genetic defect of a specific enzyme. The number of diseases in humans known to be attributable to inherited point defects in metabolism now exceeds 500.[1] While the diseases individually are rare, they collectively account for a significant proportion of neonatal and childhood morbidity and mortality. Diagnosis is important not only for treatment and prognosis but also for genetic counseling and antenatal diagnosis in subsequent pregnancies.

CLINICAL PRESENTATION

Severe illness in the newborn regardless of the underlying cause tends to manifest with non-specific findings, such as poor feeding, drowsiness, lethargy, hypotonia and failure to thrive. IEM should be considered in the differential diagnosis of any sick neonate along with common acquired causes such as sepsis, hypoxic-ischemic encephalopathy, duct-dependant cardiac lesions, congenital adrenal hyperplasia and congenital infections (Table 18.1).

Table 18.1: Clinical pointers towards IEM[2]

- Deterioration after a period of apparent normalcy
- Parental consanguinity
- Family history of neonatal deaths
- Rapidly progressive encephalopathy and seizures of unexplained cause
- Severe metabolic acidosis
- Persistent vomiting
- Peculiar odor
- Acute fatty liver or HELLP (hemolysis, elevated liver enzymes and low platelet counts) syndrome during pregnancy: seen in women carrying fetuses with long-chain-3-hydroxyacyl-coenzyme dehydrogenase deficiency (LCHADD)

Table 18.2: Clinical pointers towards specific IEM

Clinical finding	Disorder
Coarse facies	Lysosomal disorders
Cataract	Galactosemia, Zellweger syndrome
Retinitis pigmentosa	Mitochondrial disorders
Cherry red spot	Lipidosis
Hepatomegaly	Storage disorders, urea cycle defects
Renal enlargement	Zellweger syndrome
Eczema/alopecia	Biotinidase deficiency
Abnormal kinky hair	Menke disease
Decreased pigmentation	Phenylketonuria

A variety of examination findings may provide a clue to the underlying IEM (Table 18.2).[2,3]

PATTERNS OF PRESENTATION

Encephalopathy with or without Metabolic Acidosis

Encephalopathy, seizures and tone abnormalities are predominant presenting features of organic acidemias, urea cycle defects and congenital lactic acidosis. Intractable seizures are prominent in pyridoxine dependency, non-ketotic hyperglycinemia, molybdenum co-factor defect and folinic-acid responsive seizures.

Acute Liver Disease

This could manifest as:

Jaundice alone: Gilbert syndrome, Criggler-Najjar syndrome
Hepatic failure (jaundice, ascites, hypoglycemia, coagulopathy): Tyrosinemia, galactosemia, neonatal hemochromatosis, glycogen storage disease type IV.
Neonatal cholestasis: Alpha-1 antitrypsin deficiency, Niemann-Pick disease type C.
Hypoglycemia: Persistent and severe hypoglycemia may be an indicator of an underlying IEM. Hypoglycemia is a feature of galactosemia, fatty acid oxidation defects, organic acidemias, glycogen storage disorders and disorders of gluconeogenesis.

Dysmorphic Features

Dysmorphic features are seen in peroxisomal disorders, pyruvate dehydrogenase deficiency, congenital disorders of glycosylation (CDG) and lysosomal storage diseases. Some IEMs may present with non-immune hydrops fetalis; these include lysosomal storage disorders and CDG.

Cardiac Disease

Cardiomyopathy is a prominent feature in some IEM including fatty acid oxidation defects, glycogen storage disease type II and mitochondrial electron transport chain defects.

INVESTIGATIONS

Metabolic investigations should be initiated as soon as the possibility is considered. The outcome of treatment of many IEM especially those associated with hyperammonemia is directly related to the rapidity with which problems are detected and appropriate management instituted.

First Line Investigations (Metabolic Screen)

Table 18.3 summarizes the tests to be performed in all babies with suspected IEM.

Table 18.3: List of tests to be performed in all babies with suspected IEM

1. Complete blood count (neutropenia and thrombocytopenia seen in propionic and methylmalonic acidemia)
2. Arterial blood gases and electrolytes
3. Blood glucose
4. Plasma ammonia (normal values in newborn: 90–150 g/dl or 64–107 mol/L)
5. Arterial blood lactate (normal values: 0.5–1.6 mol/L)
6. Liver function tests
7. Urine ketones
8. Urine reducing substances
9. Serum uric acid (low in molybdenum cofactor deficiency)

Figure 18.1 gives the algorithmic approach to a newborn with suspected IEM. Disease category can be diagnosed based on blood ammonia, blood gas analysis and urine ketone testing. Hyperammonemia without acidosis is caused by urea cycle defects.

Metabolic acidosis with or without hyperammonemia is a feature of organic acidemias and fatty acid oxidation defects. Figure 18.2 explains the algorithmic approach to neonate with persistent hypoglycemia and suspected underlying IEM.

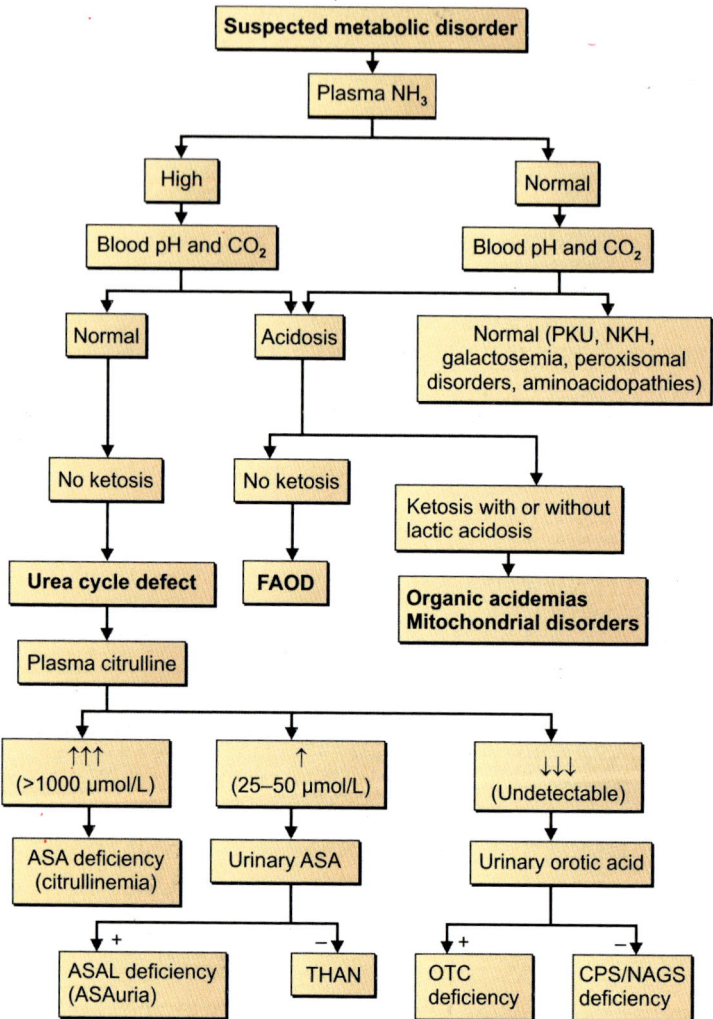

(FAOD: fatty acid oxidation defects, PKU: phenylketonuria, NKH: non-ketotic hyperglycinemia, ASA: argininosuccinic acid, OTC: ornithine transcarbamoylase, CPS: carbamoylphosphate synthetase I, NAGS: N-acetylglutamate synthetase, THAN: transient hyperammonemia of newborn, ASAL: argininosuccinic acid lyase)

Fig 18.1: Approach to newborn with suspected metabolic disorder

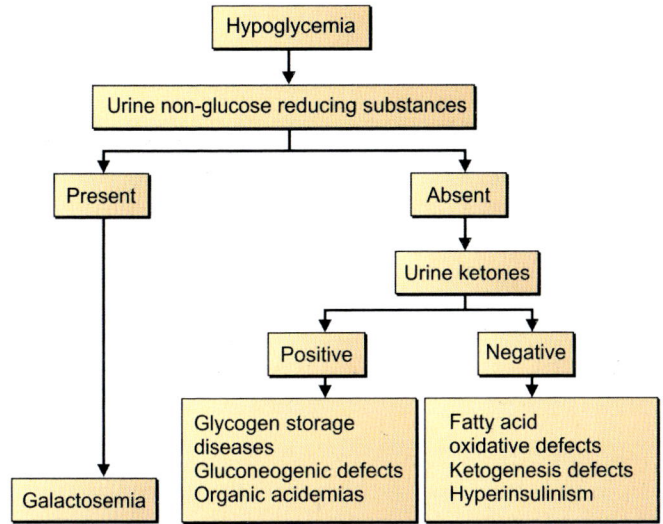

Fig 18.2: Approach to newborn with persistent hypoglycemia and suspected IEM

Table 18.4 explains the categorization of IEM based on simple metabolic screening tests.

Table 18.4: Categorization of neonatal IEM using metabolic screening tests

Acidosis	Ketosis	↑Lactate	↑Ammonia	Diagnosis
−	+	−	−	Maple syrup urine disease
+	+/−	−	+/−	Organic aciduria
+	+/−	+	−	Lactic acidosis
−	−	−	+	Urea cycle
−	−	−	−	Non-ketotic hyperglyceminuria, sulfite oxidase deficiency, peroxisomal, phenylketonuria, galactosemia

Second Line Investigations (Ancillary and Confirmatory Tests)

These tests need to be performed in a targeted manner, based on presumptive diagnosis reached after first line investigations:

1. Gas chromatography mass spectrometry (GCMS) of urine: for diagnosis of organic acidemias.
2. Plasma amino acids and acyl carnitine profile: by tandem mass spectrometry (TMS) for diagnosis of organic acidemias, urea cycle defects, aminoacidopathies and fatty acid oxidation defects.

3. High performance liquid chromatography (HPLC): for quantitative analysis of amino acids in blood and urine; required for diagnosis of organic acidemias and aminoacidopathies.
4. Lactate/pyruvate ratio: In cases with elevated lactate.
5. Urinary orotic acid: In cases with hyperammonemia for classification of urea cycle defect.
6. Enzyme assay: This is required for definitive diagnosis but not available for most IEMs. Available enzyme assays include: Biotinidase assay in cases with suspected biotinidase deficiency (intractable seizures, seborrheic rash, alopecia); and GALT (galactose 1-phosphate uridyl transferase) assay in cases with suspected galactosemia (hypoglycemia, cataracts, reducing sugars in urine).
7. Neuroimaging: MRI may provide helpful pointers towards etiology while results of definitive investigations are pending. Some IEM may be associated with structural malformations, e.g. Zellweger syndrome has diffuse cortical migration and sulcation abnormalities. Agenesis of corpus callosum has been reported in Menke's disease, pyruvate decarboxylase deficiency and non-ketotic hyperglycinemia.[4] Examples of other neuroimaging findings in IEM include:
   • Maple syrup urine disease (MSUD): Brainstem and cerebellar edema
   • Propionic and methylmalonic acidemia: Basal ganglia signal change
   • Glutaric aciduria: Frontotemporal atrophy, subdural hematomas
8. Magnetic resonance spectroscopy (MRS): This test may be helpful in selected disorders, e.g. lactate peak elevated in mitochondrial disorders, leucine peak elevated in MSUD.
9. Electroencephalography (EEG): Some EEG abnormalities may be suggestive of particular IEM, e.g. comb-like rhythm in MSUD, burst suppression in NKH and holocarboxylase synthetase deficiency.[5]
10. Plasma very long chain fatty acid (VLCFA) levels: Elevated in peroxisomal disorders.
11. Mutation analysis when available.
12. CSF amino acid analysis: CSF glycine levels elevated in NKH.

PRECAUTIONS TO BE OBSERVED WHILE COLLECTING SAMPLES

1. Should be collected before specific treatment is started or feeds are stopped, as may be falsely normal if the child is off feeds.
2. Samples for blood ammonia and lactate should be transported in ice and immediately tested. Lactate sample should be arterial and should be collected after 2 hrs fasting in a preheparinized syringe. Ammonia sample is to be collected approximately after 2 hrs of fasting in EDTA vacutainer. Avoid air mixing. Sample should be free flowing.
3. Detailed history including drug details should be provided to the lab (sodium valproate therapy may increase ammonia levels).

Samples to be Obtained in Infant with Suspected IEM when Diagnosis is Uncertain and Death seems Inevitable (Metabolic Autopsy)[6]

1. Blood: 5–10 ml; frozen at $-20°C$; both heparinized (for chromosomal studies) and EDTA (for DNA studies) samples to be taken
2. Urine: Frozen at $-20°C$
3. CSF: Store at $-20°C$
4. Skin biopsy: Including dermis in culture medium or saline with glucose. Store at $4–8°C$. Do not freeze.
5. Liver, muscle, kidney and heart biopsy: As indicated.
6. Clinical photograph (in cases with dysmorphism)
7. Infantogram (in cases with skeletal abnormalities)

TREATMENT OF IEM

In most cases, treatment needs to be instituted empirically without a specific diagnosis. The metabolic screen helps to broadly categorize the patient's IEM (e.g. urea cycle defect, organic acidemia, congenital lactic acidosis, etc.) on the basis of which, empirical treatment can be instituted.

Aims of Treatment

1. To reduce the formation of toxic metabolites by decreasing substrate availability (by stopping feeds and preventing endogenous catabolism).

2. To provide adequate calories.
3. To enhance the excretion of toxic metabolites.
4. To institute co-factor therapy for specific disease and also empirically if diagnosis not established.
5. Supportive care treatment of seizures (avoid sodium valproate as it may increase ammonia levels), maintain euglycemia and normothermia, fluid, electrolyte and acid–base balance, treatment of infection, mechanical ventilation if required.

Management of Hyperammonemia[7, 8]

1. Discontinue all feeds. Provide adequate calories by intravenous glucose and lipids. Maintain glucose infusion rate 8–10 mg/kg/min. Start intravenous lipid 0.5 g/kg/day (up to 3 g/kg/day). After stabilization, gradually add protein 0.25 g/kg till 1.5 g/kg/day.
2. Dialysis is the only means for rapid removal of ammonia, and hemodialysis is more effective and faster than peritoneal dialysis; however, peritoneal dialysis may be more widely available and feasible. Exchange transfusion is not useful.
3. Alternative pathways for nitrogen excretion:
   - · Sodium benzoate (IV or oral)—loading dose 250 mg/kg then 250-400 mg/kg/day in 4 divided doses (intravenous preparation is not available in India).
   - · Sodium phenylbutyrate (not available in India)—loading dose 250 mg/kg followed by 250–500 mg/kg/day.
   - · L-arginine (oral or IV)—300 mg/kg/day (intravenous preparation not available in India).
   - · L-carnitine (oral or IV)—200 mg/kg/day.
4. Supportive care: Treatment of sepsis, seizures, ventilation. Avoid sodium valproate.

Acute Management of Newborn with Suspected Organic Acidemia[9]

1. The patient is kept nil per orally and intravenous glucose is provided.
2. Supportive care: Hydration, treatment of sepsis, seizures, ventilation.
3. Carnitine: 100 mg/kg/day IV or oral.
4. Treat acidosis: Sodium bicarbonate 0.35–0.5 mEq/kg/hr (max 1–2 mEq/kg/hr).

5. Start biotin 10 mg/day orally.
6. Start vitamin B_{12}, 1–2 mg/day I/M (useful in B_{12} responsive forms of methylmalonic acidemias).
7. Start thiamine 300 mg/day (useful in thiamine-responsive variants of MSUD).
8. If hyperammonemia is present, treat as explained above.

Management of Congenital Lactic Acidosis

1. Supportive care: Hydration, treatment of sepsis, seizures, ventilation. Avoid sodium valproate.
2. Treat acidosis: Sodium bicarbonate 0.35–0.5 mEq/kg/hr (max 1–2 mEq/kg/hr).
3. Thiamine: Up to 300 mg/day in 4 divided doses.
4. Riboflavin: 100 mg/day in 4 divided doses.
5. Add co-enzyme Q: 5–15 mg/kg/day.
6. L-carnitine: 50–100 mg/kg orally.

Treatment of Newborn with Refractory Seizures with no Obvious Etiology (Suspected Metabolic Etiology)[10]

1. If patient persists to have seizures despite 2 or 3 anti-epileptic drugs in adequate doses, consider trial of pyridoxine 100 mg intravenously. If intravenous preparation not available, oral pyridoxine can be given (15 mg/kg/day).
2. If seizures persist despite pyridoxine, give trial of biotin 10 mg/day and folinic acid 15 mg/day (folinic acid responsive seizures).
3. Rule out glucose transporter defect: Measure CSF and blood glucose. In glucose transporter defect, CSF glucose level is equal to or less than 1/3rd of the blood glucose level. This disorder responds to the ketogenic diet.

Management of Asymptomatic Newborn with a History of Sibling Death with Suspected IEM

1. After baseline metabolic screen, start oral dextrose feeds (10% dextrose).
2. After 24 hours, repeat screen. If normal, start breast feeds. Monitor sugar, blood gases and urine ketones, blood ammonia 6 hourly.
3. Some authorities recommend starting medium chain triglycerides (MCT oil) before starting breastfeeds,[3] however,

this is not being followed in our center (because of unpalatibility of MCT oil).

4. After 48 hours, repeat metabolic screen. Obtain samples for TMS and urine organic acid tests.

5. The infant will need careful observation and follow-up for the first few months, as IEM may present in different age groups in members of the same family.

LONG-TERM TREATMENT OF IEM

The following modalities are available:

Dietary Treatment

This is the mainstay of treatment in phenylketonuria, maple syrup urine disease, homocystinuria, galactosemia and glycogen storage disease Type I and III. Special diets for PKU and MSUD are commercially available in the west. These are not available in India, but can be imported. These special diets are however, very expensive, and cannot be afforded by most Indian patients. Based on the amino acid content of some common food products available in India, dietary exchanges are calculated and a low phenylalanine diet for PKU and diet low in branched chain amino acids for MSUD are being used in our center. However, there are no studies to document the efficacy of these indigenous diets. Some disorders like urea cycle disorders and organic acidurias require dietary modification (protein restriction) in addition to these modalities.[11]

Enzyme Replacement Therapy (ERT)

ERT is now commercially available for some lysosomal storage disorders.[12] However, these disorders do not manifest in the newborn period, an exception being Pompe's disease (glycogen storage disorder Type II), for which ERT is now available.

Cofactor Replacement Therapy

The catalytic properties of many enzymes depend on the participation of non-protein prosthetic groups, such as vitamins and minerals, as obligatory co-factors. The following co-factors may be beneficial in certain IEM:[13]

- **Thiamine:** Mitochondrial disorders, thiamine responsive variants of MSUD, PDH deficiency and complex I deficiency).

- **Riboflavin:** Glutaric aciduria Type I, Type II, mild variants of ETF, ETF-DH, complex I deficiency.
- **Pyridoxine:** 50% of cases of homocystinuria due to cystathionine β-synthetase deficiency, pyridoxine dependency with seizures, xanthurenic aciduria, primary hyperoxaluria type I, hyperornithenemia with gyrate atrophy.
- **Cobalamin:** Methylmalonic acidemia (*cblA, cblB*), homocystinuria and methylmalonic acidemia (*cblC, cblD, cblF*).
- **Folinic acid:** Hereditary orotic aciduria, methionine synthase deficiency, cerebral folate transporter deficiency, hereditary folate malabsorption, Kearns-Sayre syndrome.
- **Biotin:** Biotinidase deficiency, holocarboxylase synthetase deficiency.

Table 18.5 provides some commercial preparation of commonly used drugs for managing IEM.

Table 18.5: Commercially available formulations used in IEM	
Co-factor	*Trade name, formulation*
Pyridoxine	Tab Benadon (40 mg) (Nicholas Piramal), Inj. Vitneurin (1 ampoule contains 50 mg pyridoxine)
Hydroxycobalamin (Vitamin B$_{12}$)	Inj. Trineurosol (1000 mcg/ml) (Tridoss Laboratories)
Thiamine	Tab Benalgis (75 mg) (Franco India)
Riboflavin	Tab Riboflavin (5 mg) (Shreya)
Biotin	Tab Essvit (5 mg, 10 mg) (Ecopharma)
Carnitine	Syrup L-Carnitor (5 ml = 500 mg), Tab L-Carnitor (500 mg), Inj carnitor (1 g/5 ml) (Elder)
Folinic acid	Tab Leukorin (15 mg) (Samrath)
Sodium benzoate	Satchet 20 g (Hesh Co.)
Arginine	ARG-9 Satchet (3 g) (Noveau Medicament)
Coenzyme Q	Tab CoQ 30 mg, 50 mg (Universal Medicare)

PREVENTION OF IEM

Genetic Counseling and Prenatal Diagnosis

Most of the IEM are single gene defects, inherited in an autosomal recessive manner, with a 25% recurrence risk. Therefore, when the diagnosis is known and confirmed in the index case, prenatal diagnosis can be offered, wherever available for the subsequent pregnancies. The samples required are chorionic villus tissue or amniotic fluid. Modalities available are:[14]

- Substrate or metabolite detection: Useful in phenylketonuria, peroxisomal defects.
- Enzyme assay: Useful in lysosomal storage disorders like Niemann-Pick disease, Gaucher disease.
- DNA based (molecular) diagnosis: Detection of mutation in proband/carrier parents is a prerequisite.

Neonatal Screening

Tandem mass spectrometry is used in some countries for neonatal screening for IEM. Disorders which can be detected by TMS include aminoacidopathies (phenylketonuria, MSUD, homocystinuria, citrullinemia, argininosuccinic aciduria, hepatorenal tyrosinemia), fatty acid oxidation defects, organic acidemias (glutaric aciduria, propionic acidemia, methyl-malonic acidemia, isovaleric acidemia). The cost of this procedure is high. Also, though the test is highly sensitive, the specificity is relatively low; and there are difficulties in inter-pretation of abnormal test results in apparently healthy infants.

REFERENCES

1. Childs B, Valle D, Jimenez-Sanchez. The inborn error and biochemical variability. In: Scriver CR, Beaudet AL, Sly WS and Valle D (Eds). The metabolic and molecular basis of inherited disease, 8th edn. New York: McGraw-Hill, 2001;155–166.

2. A Clinical guide to inherited metabolic diseases. JTR Clarke. 3rd edn. (2006), Cambridge University Press, Cambridge.

3. Cataltepe SU, Levy HL. Inborn errors of metabolism. In: Cloherty JP, Eichenwald EC, Stark AR (Eds). Manual of neonatal care. 6th edn. Lippincott Williams & Wilkins, Philadelphia, 2008; 558–73.

4. Blaser S, Feigenbaum A. A neuroimaging approach to inborn errors of metabolism. Neuroimag Clin N Am 2004;14:307–329.

5. Nordli DR, De Vivo DC. Classification of infantile seizures: Implications for identification and treatment of inborn errors of metabolism. J Child Neurol 2002;17(Suppl 3):S33–38.

6. Leonard JV, Morris AAM. Diagnosis and early management of inborn errors of metabolism presenting around the time of birth. Acta Pediatrica 2006;95:6–14.

7. Summar M. Current strategies for the management of neonatal urea cycle disorders. J Pediatr 2001;38:S30–39.

8. Leonard JV, Morris AAM. Urea cycle disorders. Semin Neonatol 2002;7:27–35.

9. De Baulny HO, Saudubray JM. Branched-chain organic acidurias. Semin Neonatol 2002;7:65–74.

10. Wolf NI, Bast T, Surtees S. Epilepsy in inborn errors of metabolism. Epileptic Disord 2005;7(2):67–81.

11. Kabra M. Dietary management of inborn errors of metabolism. Indian J Pediatr 2002;69:421–26.

12. Brady RO, Schiffmann R. Enzyme-replacement therapy for metabolic storage disorders. Lancet Neurol 2004;3:752–56.

13. Saudubray JM, Sedel F, Walter JH. Clinical approach to treatable inborn metabolic diseases: An introduction. J Inherit Metab Dis 2006;29:261–74.

14. Elias S, Simpson JL, Shulman LP. Techniques for prenatal diagnosis. In: Rimoin DL, Connor JH, Pyeritz RE, Korf BR (Eds). Emery and Rimoin's Principles and practice of medical genetics. Churchill-Livingstone, London 2002;802–25.

19 Congenital Hypothyroidism

Congenital Hypothyroidism (CH) is a preventable cause of mental retardation. The worldwide incidence is 1:3000–4000 live births and the estimated incidence in India is 1:2500–2800 live births.[1] Thyroid dysgenesis is the commonest cause accounting for 75–80% of all cases of CH.

EMBRYOLOGY AND PHYSIOLOGY OF THE THYROID IN THE FETUS

Thyroid gland originates as a proliferation of endodermal epithelial cells at 3 to 4 weeks of gestation. Synthesis and secretion of thyroxine (T4) and triiodothyronine (T3) starts from 12 weeks of gestation. Thyrotropin releasing hormone (TRH) and thyroid stimulating hormone (TSH) are detectable by the end of first trimester, but the activity of the hypothalamic-pituitary thyroid (HPT) axis is low with insufficient production of thyroid hormones until 18 to 20 weeks of gestation. Therefore, the fetus depends on transplacental passage of thyroid hormones during this period. In the second half of gestation, fetal T4 and TSH levels increase progressively.

In the hypothyroid fetus, transplacental passage of maternal thyroid hormones and increased conversion of T4 to T3 in fetal brain by type 2 deiodinase confer neuroprotection, and near normal cognitive outcomes are possible if maternal thyroid function is normal and postnatal therapy is initiated early. In contrast, when both maternal and fetal hypothyroidism are present as in severe iodine deficiency, there is significant neuro-intellectual impairment.[2] Subtle or overt hypothyroidism in the mother during pregnancy also adversely affects the cognitive outcome of the offspring.[3]

NEONATAL PHYSIOLOGY

As a response to the cold ex utero environment, there is an early postnatal surge of TSH, rising to 60–80 mU/L within 30–60 minutes after delivery, with a rapid fall to about 20 mU/L in first 24 hours and further decrease to below 10 mU/L by the end of first week. T4 levels also increase to peak levels of approximately 17 µg/dL at 24–36 hours, with a gradual decline over 4 to 5 weeks. Preterm infants demonstrate a similar but blunted response.

ETIOLOGY OF CONGENITAL HYPOTHYROIDISM

CH can be permanent or transient (Table 19.1).

Table 19.1: Etiology of CH

1. **Permanent hypothyroidism**
   a. Thyroid dysgenesis (aplasia, hypoplasia or ectopia)
   b. Thyroid hormone biosynthetic defects
   c. Iodine deficiency (endemic cretinism)
   d. Hypothalamic-pituitary hypothyroidism
2. **Transient hypothyroidism**
   a. TSH binding inhibitory immunoglobulins
   b. Exposure to goitrogens (iodides or antithyroid drugs)
   c. Transient hypothyroxinemia of prematurity
   d. Sick euthyroid syndrome

Thyroid dysgenesis is the commonest cause of permanent CH affecting 1 in 4000 live births. It is usually sporadic with a 2 : 1 female to male preponderance. Some of the genes proposed as operative in dysgenesis have recently been identified as TITF1, TITF2, PAX8 and TSHR.[4]

Thyroid hormone synthetic defects account for 10–15% of all cases. These are inherited as autosomal recessive disorders. The defect can lie in iodide trapping or organification, iodotyrosine coupling or deiodination and thyroglobulin synthesis or secretion. The commonest of these is a defect in the thyroid peroxidase (TPO) activity leading to impaired oxidation and organification of iodide to iodine. These disorders usually result in goitrous hypothyroidism. *Iodine deficiency* is responsible for endemic cretinism and hypothyroidism in some regions of India.

Hypothalamic pituitary hypothyroidism is rare and has an estimated incidence of 1 in 50,000. It may be isolated or associated with deficiency of other pituitary hormones and present with hypoglycemia and microphallus.

Transient hypothyroidism due to *transplacental transfer of TSH binding inhibitory immunoglobulins (TBII)* from mothers with autoimmune thyroid disease is seen in 1:50,000 births. Their effect wanes off by 3 to 6 months in the majority, but may last up to 9 months.

Exposure to iodine in sick preterm infants, e.g. application of povidone iodine for skin disinfection (Wolff-Chaikoff effect) or intake of iodine containing expectorants by pregnant mothers can also induce transient hypothyroidism.

Transient hypothyroxinemia of prematurity refers to low serum concentration of thyroid hormones in up to 85% of preterm infants in early postnatal life as compared to term infants. This reflects the underdevelopment of the HPT axis. The normal levels of fT4 and TSH in preterm infants are presented in Table 19.2.[5] There has been a concern that transient hypothyroxinemia is associated with adverse neurodevelopmental outcomes and decreased survival in affected infants.[6] However, currently there is no recommendation with respect to routine supplementation of these infants.

Table 19.2: Reference ranges for serum free T4 (fT4) and TSH in preterm infants

Age in weeks	Free T4 (ng/dL)	TSH (mu/L)
25–27	06–2.2	0.2–30.3
28–30	0.6–3.4	0.2–20.6
31–33	1.0–3.8	0.7–20.9
34–36	1.2–4.4	1.2–21.6

Sick euthyroid syndrome reflects suppression of the pituitary's response to TRH, with inappropriately low TSH concentration in the context of low T3 and in the more severe cases, low T4 concentrations.

DIAGNOSIS

Newborn screening: Ideally universal newborn screening at 3 to 4 days of age should be done for detecting CH (coupled with screening of other inborn errors of metabolism, wherever it is undertaken). If screening is being done only for CH, cord blood may also be used. Universal newborn screening is currently being done in many parts of the world. Three approaches are being used for screening:

1. Primary TSH, back up T4
2. Primary T4, back up TSH
3. Concomitant T4 and TSH

The advantages and disadvantages of these approaches are presented in Panel 1.

Panel 1: Approaches to Screen for Congenital Hypothyroidism: Advantages and Disadvantages

1. Primary TSH, back up T4: TSH is measured first and T4 is measured only if TSH is >20 mu/L. This approach is most widely used and cost-effective, but likely to miss central hypothyroidism, thyroid binding globulin (TBG) deficiency and hypothyroxinemia with delayed elevation of TSH.

2. Primary T4, back up TSH: T4 is checked first and if low, TSH is also checked. This is likely to miss milder/subclinical cases of CH in which T4 is initially normal with elevated TSH.

3. Concomitant T4 and TSH: Most sensitive approach but incurs a higher cost.[7]

Screening programs use either percentile based cut-offs (e.g. T4 below 10th centile or TSH above 90th centile)[7] or absolute cut-offs such as T4 <6.5 ug/dL and TSH >20 mu/L. Among infants with proven CH, TSH is >50 mu/L in 90% and T4 is <6.5 ug/dL in greater than 75% of cases.

Abnormal values on screening should always be confirmed by a venous sample (using age appropriate cut-offs given in Table 19.3[8–10]). Most centers initiate treatment after drawing the infants' sample if TSH >30 mu/L or T4 is low, and the decision to continue or withhold treatment is taken after

Table 19.3: Reference ranges for T4, fT4 and TSH in term infants according to postnatal age[6,7]

Age	T4 (g/dL) mean (range)	mean (range) mean (SD)/ range	fT4 (pg/mL) TSH (iU/mL)
Cord blood	10.8 (6.6–15)	13.8 (3.5)	10.0 (1–20)
1–3 days	16.5 (11–21.5)	*	5.6 (1–10)
4–7 days	*	22.3 (3.9)	*
1–2 weeks	12.7 (8.2–17.2)	*	2.3 (0.5–6.5)
2–6 weeks	6.5–16.3**	0.9–2.2	1.7–9.1**
6 weeks to 12 months	11.1 (5.9–13)	*	2.3 (0.5–6.5)

*No data available ** data for median/mean not available

obtaining the venous blood report. For intermediate screening values of TSH, with normal T4 (if available), the treatment is initiated only after confirmation of diagnosis based on the blood report.

In the absence of universal screening, newborns with the following indications should be screened:

1. Family history of CH.
2. History of thyroid disease or anti-thyroid medicine intake in mother.
3. Presence of other conditions like Down syndrome, trisomy 18, neural tube defects, congenital heart disease, metabolic disorders, familial autoimmune disorders and Pierre Robin syndrome, which are associated with higher prevalence of CH.

Thyroid function should be tested in any infant with signs and symptoms of hypothyroidism such as postmaturity, macrosomia or wide open posterior fontanel at birth or prolonged jaundice, constipation, poor feeding, hypotonia, hoarse cry, umbilical hernia, macroglossia or dry edematous skin in infancy. The tests should be performed even in infants who have had a normal newborn screening report.

Once the diagnosis is established, further investigations to determine the etiology should be done. A nuclear scan using sodium pertechnetate (^{99m}Tc) is especially useful in diagnosing true athyrosis or ectopy as well as goitrous hypothyroidism due to dyshormonogenesis. However, since the scan can be done only before initiating treatment, one should not withhold therapy if it is not possible to get it performed immediately.[11,12] A list of diagnostic studies useful in infants with congenital hypothyroidism is presented in Table 19.4 and an algorithmic approach to investigation in Fig. 19.1.

When Should we Ask for Free T4 Levels?

In most situations, T4 (total) levels are sufficient for diagnosis of hypothyroidism and monitoring treatment, but free T4 can be obtained as a more robust marker of the bioavailable T4, when readily accessible. When availability or cost is a constraint, free T4 should be definitely estimated in the following situations:[8,13]

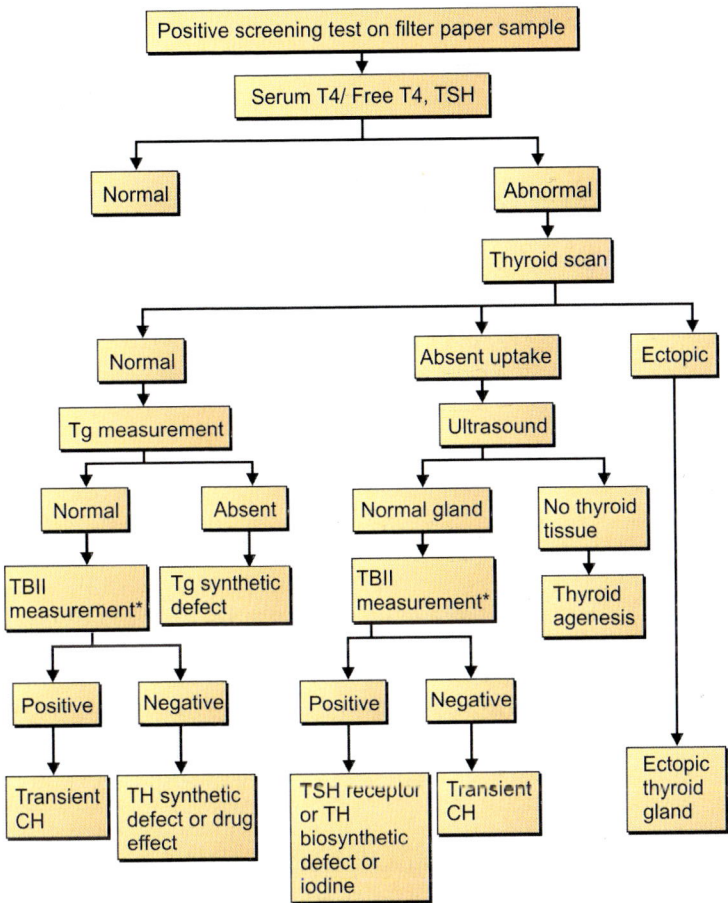

TBII: TSH binding inhibitory immunoglobulin (*not routinely available)
Tg: thymoglobulin, TH: thyroid hormone
Adopted from Fisher DA. Management of congenital hypothyroidism. J Clin
Endocrinol Metab 1991;72:585–8

Fig. 19.1: Approach to a newborn infant with positive screening test for CH

1. In premature or sick newborns, T4 (total) values may be low
   because of abnormal protein binding or low levels of
   thyroxine binding globulin (TBG) due to immaturity of liver
   function, proteinuria or undernutrition. Therefore, free T4
   values provide a better estimate of true thyroid function.

Table 19.4: Diagnostic studies for evaluation of CH

1. Imaging studies will determine location and size of thyroid gland
   a. Scintigraphy (^{99m}Tc or ^{123}I)
   b. Sonography
2. Function studies
   a. ^{123}I uptake
   b. Serum thyroglobulin
3. Suspected inborn error of T4 synthesis
   • ^{123}I uptake and perchlorate discharge
4. Suspected autoimmune thyroid disease
   • Maternal and neonatal serum TBII measurement (not routinely available)
5. Suspected iodine exposure or deficiency
   • Urinary iodine measurement
6. Ancillary test to determine severity of fetal hypothyroidism
   • Radiograph of knee for skeletal maturation

2. A case of low T4 with normal TSH. If free T4 is normal, it can be a case of congenital partial (prevalence 1:4000 to 12000 newborns) or complete (prevalence 1:15000 newborns) TBG deficiency. TBG levels should be evaluated to confirm this but this test is not available routinely. If free T4 is also low along with low T4 with normal TSH, central hypothyroidism should be suspected.
3. During monitoring for adequacy of treatment, we usually monitor T4 (total) level. This assumes a normal TBG level. This can be confirmed by measuring free T4 or TBG levels once at the time of the first post-treatment T4 measurement.

TREATMENT OF CONGENITAL HYPOTHYROIDISM

Term as well as preterm infants with low T4 and elevated TSH should be started on L-thyroxine as soon as the diagnosis is made. The initial dose of L-thyroxine should be 10–15 μg/kg/day with the aim to normalize the T4 level at the earliest.

Those infants with severe hypothyroidism (very low T4, very high TSH and absence of distal femoral and proximal tibial epiphyses on radiograph of knee) should be started with the highest dose of 15 μg/kg/day.[14]

Monitoring of Therapy

• T4 should be kept in the upper half of normal range (10 to 16 μg/dL) or free T4 in the 1.4 to 2.3 ng/dL range with the TSH suppressed in the normal range.

- Check T4 and TSH levels according to the following schedule:
  - 0 to 6 months: Every 6 weeks
  - 6 months to 3 years: Every 3 months
  - Beyond 3 years: Every 6 monthly
  - 6 to 8 weeks after any dosage change.
- Monitor growth and development of the infant.
- Avoid over treatment as it can lead to premature fusion of cranial sutures, acceleration of skeletal maturation and problems with temperament and behavior.

SPECIAL SITUATIONS

1. **Asymptomatic hyperthyrotropinemia (Elevated TSH, normal T4)**
   - Can be transient or permanent.
   - Perinatal iodine exposure is an important cause of transient elevation of TSH in neonatal period.
   - Other causes include defects in biological activity of TSH or TSH receptor, mild thyroid hormone biosynthesis defect, subtle developmental defects or disturbance in the negative feedback control of TSH.
   - There is a controversy regarding need for treatment.
   - Persistently elevated TSH > 10 μU/ml is generally treated. However, in the presence of free T4 levels in upper half of normal range, expectant management can be followed with repetition of tests after 2 weeks.
   - When treatment is started, it should be continued till 3 years of age, with monitoring of thyroid function as detailed above. If TSH and T4 have always been within normal limits with no need for escalation of dose during the first 3 years, thyroid function should be re-evaluated after withholding thyroxine for a period of 6 weeks.[14]
2. **Isolated hypothyroxinemia (Low T4 and normal TSH levels)**
   - This clinical situation is commonly seen in preterm infants due to immaturity of HPT axis and is labeled as 'Transient hypothyroxinemia of prematurity'. As of now, there is insufficient evidence that early treatment with thyroid hormone leads to improved outcomes.
   - Central (hypothalamic/pituitary) hypothyroidism (incidence 1 in 1,00,000) is also characterized by low T4.

TSH may be low or normal. In term infants, with low total as well as free T4, this diagnosis should be considered, especially in presence of midline facial abnormalities, hypoglycemia, microphallus or visual abnormalities. The infant should undergo testing for other pituitary hormones and MR imaging of hypothalamus and pituitary.

- TBG deficiency (rare) can also present with low T4 and normal TSH. Free T4 is normal and no treatment is required

3. **Transient hypothyroidism[15]**

- The causes are listed in Table 19.1.
- Infants with transient hypothyroidism due to maternal goitrogenic drugs need not be treated unless low T4 and elevated TSH values persist beyond 2 weeks. Therapy can be discontinued after 8–12 weeks. Intake of anti-thyroid drugs can be continued by the hyperthyroid mothers during breastfeeding because concentration of these drugs is very low in breast milk.
- In infants born to mothers with autoimmune thyroiditis, treatment should be started if T4 is low. If presence of TBII is documented in the infant, treatment can be discontinued at 3–6 months.[8] However, when TBII estimation is not available, treatment should be continued till the age of 3 years, when T4 and TSH can be tested after withholding thyroxine for 6 weeks.

OUTCOME

The best outcome occurs with L-thyroxine therapy started by 2 weeks of age at 9.5 µg/kg or more per day as compared with lower doses or later start of therapy. Residual defects can include impaired visuospatial processing and selective memory and sensorimotor defects. More than 80% of infants given replacement therapy before three months of age have an IQ greater than 85 but may show signs of minimal brain damage, including impairment of arithmetic ability, speech or fine motor coordination in later life.[7] When treatment is started between 3–6 months, the mean IQ is 71 and when delayed to beyond 6 months, the mean IQ drops to 54.[16]

REFERENCES

1. Desai MP, Upadhye P, Colaco MP, Mehre M, Naik SP, Vaz FE, Nair N, Thomas M. Neonatal screening for congenital hypo-thyroidism using the filter paper thyroxine technique. Indian J Med Res 1994;100:36–42.

2. Fisher DA, Klein AH. Thyroid development and disorders of thyroid function in the newborn. N Engl J Med 1981;304: 702–12.

3. Haddow JE, Palomaki GE, Allan WC, Williams JR, Knight GJ, Gagnon J, O'Heir CE, Mitchell ML, Hermos RJ, Waisbren SE, Faix JD, Klein RZ. Maternal thyroid deficiency during pregnancy and subsequent neuro-psychological development of the child. N Engl J Med 1999;19;341:549–55.

4. Macchia P. Recent advances in understanding the molecular basis of primary congenital hypothyroidism. Mol Med Today 2000;6: 36–42.

5. Adams LM, Emery JR, Clark SJ, Carlton EI, Nelson JC. Reference ranges for newer thyroid function tests in premature infants. J Pediatr 1995;126:122–7.

6. Fisher DA. Thyroid function and dysfunction in premature infants. Pediatr Endocrinol Rev 2007 Jun;4(4):317–28.

7. American Academy of Pediatrics, Rose SR; Section on Endo-crinology and Committee on Genetics, American Thyroid Association, Brown RS, Public Health Committee, Lawson Wilkins Pediatric Endocrine Society, Foley T, Kaplowitz PB, Kaye CI, Sundararajan S, Varma SK. Update of newborn screening and therapy for congenital hypothyroidism. Pediatrics 2006;117: 2290–303.

8. Fisher DA. Disorders of the thyroid in newborns and infants. In Sperling MA, Ed. Pediatric Endocrinology, 2nd edn. Philadelphia: Saunders, 2002;161–86.

9. Soldin OP, Jang M, Guo T, Soldin SJ. Pediatric reference intervals for free thyroxine and free triiodothyronine. Thyroid 2009;19: 699–702.

10. Fisher DA. Disorders of the thyroid in childhood and adolescence. In Sperling MA (Ed). Pediatric Endocrinology, 2nd edn. Philadelphia: Saunders, 2002;187–210.

11. LaFranchi S. Congenital hypothyroidism: etiologies, diagnosis and management. Thyroid 1999;9:735–40.

12. Fisher DA. Management of congenital hypothyroidism. J Clin Endocrinol Metab 1991;72:525–8.

13. Brown RS. The thyroid gland. In Brook CGD, Hindmarsh PC eds. Clinical Pediatric Endocrinology, 4th edn. London: Blackwell Science 2001;288–320.

14. LaFranchi SH, Austin J. How should we be treating children with congenital hypothyroidism? J Pediatr Endocrinol Metab 2007;20: 559–78.

15. Postnatal thyroid hormones for preterm infants with transient hypothyroxinaemia. Cochrane Database Syst Rev 2007;CD005945.

16. Klien AH, Meltzer S, Kenny FM. Improved prognosis in congenital hypothyroidism treated before age three months. J Pediatr 1972;81: 912–5.

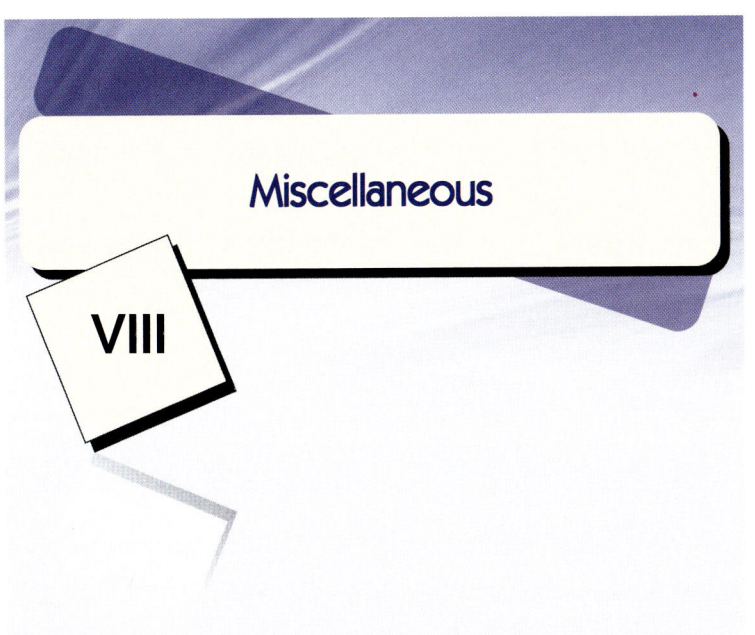

Miscellaneous

VIII

20 | Follow-up of High-risk Neonates

Improving perinatal-neonatal care has led to increased survival of newborns[1] who are at high-risk of post discharge morbidities including growth failure, ongoing medical illnesses, neurosensory impairment and developmental deficits.[2–4]

What is Evidence?

A recent systematic review in Lancet[2] has reported a high prevalence of long term neurodevelopmental sequelae after different intrauterine and neonatal insults, which is as follows: sepsis–40.0%, meningitis–42.0%, HIE–31.0%, preterm birth–31.0%, jaundice–18.0%, tetanus–26.0%, CMV infection–41.0%.

Most common sequelae: Learning difficulties, cognition or developmental delay; cerebral palsy; hearing impairment and visual impairment.

An appropriate and comprehensive follow-up program for high-risk infants will help in early detection and management of any morbidity associated with perinatal events, and shall ensure not only intact survival and optimum growth but also an optimal quality of life for these infants.

SETTING UP OF FOLLOW-UP CARE SERVICES

High-risk clinic: Follow-up of high-risk infants should be done in a dedicated high-risk clinic (HRC). A detailed description is provided under the heading "Procedures".

High-risk follow-up team: High-risk infants' follow-up requires a multi-disciplinary approach and an experienced and dedicated team including personnel from various specialties. We describe here important members of such a team and their respective roles (Table 20.1).

It might not be possible in all set ups to have a complete team of specialists as outlined above. It is, therefore, important that simple tools be available and the nodal person of the team

Table 20.1: Personnel required for follow-up program and their respective roles

Team member	Role(s)
Neonatologist/ pediatrician	• Nodal person of the team
	• To assess growth and nutrition, manage intercurrent illness/chronic morbidities
	• To screen for neurological abnormality and developmental delay
	• Regular assessment of child's progress, care-coordination and counseling
Medical social worker	• Interface between the follow-up care team and family
	• To address parental expectations, social and socio-economic issues
	• To provide emotional support and motivation to family to adjust and cope up with child's condition, and to help in rehabilitation and integration of infants with impairment/disability
Psychologist(s)	• To perform formal neurodevelopment assessment
	• To screen and manage behavioral and other domain specific problems
Early interventionist	• To enhance and facilitate the development of milestones in all domains of development and to promote developmental potential
Occupational therapist	• To improve neuro-motor coordination and perceptual skills, fine motor functions and oro-motor coordination
	• Training in activities of daily living like feeding, bathing and dressing of children with special needs
Physiotherapist	• Assessment and grading of muscle tone and power
	• To plan appropriate training for an infant with tone abnormalities, prescription of appliances/casts and rehabilitation of infants with impairment/disability
Ophthalmologist	• Follow-up and treatment for ROP
	• Visual assessment and management of refractory errors, strabismus, etc.
Neurophysiologist/ speech therapist	• Hearing screening and evaluation, management of hearing impairment, if any
	• To evaluate and manage speech delay and speech therapy
Nutritionist	• Dietary advice regarding complementary feeding
	• Management of infants with failure to thrive and those with special needs (e.g. galactosemia)
Pediatric neurologist*	• Drug therapy, long-term management of neurological illnesses such as refractory seizures

Other specialists from pediatric genetics, pediatric surgery, pediatric cardiology or pediatric gastroenterology, hematology, etc. should be available for consultation and referral as and when required.

have working knowledge of all the domains. It is desirable that all the services ideally be provided under one roof as far as possible and appropriate referrals sought as required. The days and timings of the different clinics and the appointment schedule should be clearly marked on patient's records and multiple visits should be avoided.

WHO NEEDS FOLLOW-UP CARE

A rigorous follow-up of all the neonates discharged from a health facility would neither be practical nor feasible. Therefore, it is important to select a cohort of neonates who are at a higher risk of developing adverse outcomes—'at-risk' or 'high-risk' infants. Selection of high-risk infants should be based on the gestational age, birth weight, occurrence and severity of perinatal/neonatal illnesses, interventions received in the neonatal intensive care unit (NICU), presence of malformations, etc.

There are no standardized criteria for defining high-risk infants even in tertiary care centers. Commonly used criteria have been outlined here (Panel 1). These may be modified depending upon the level of neonatal care provided by the unit and the mix of neonatal population the unit caters to.

Panel 1: High-risk Neonates who need Follow-up Care in a Tertiary Care Setting

1. Birth weight < 1500 g
2. Gestation < 32 weeks
3. Infants with BW of 1500 g or more OR gestation 32 weeks or more
   a. Intrauterine growth centile < 3rd centile
   b. Meningitis
   c. Received mechanical ventilation for 48 hours or more
   d. Hypoxic ischemic encephalopathy stage 2 or higher
   e. Major malformation
   f. Inborn error of metabolism/chromosomal or genetic disorders/intrauterine infections
   g. Symptomatic hypoglycemia
   h. Retrovirus positive mother
   i. Hyperbilirubinemia requiring exchange transfusion OR Rh isoimmunization/cholestasis
   j. Abnormal neurological examination at discharge/seizure
   k. Major morbidities such as chronic lung disease, IVH grade III or more (Papile's classification) and periventricular leucomalacia

PREREQUISITES

Discharge planning: Discharge planning should ideally begin many days before discharge. This gives adequate time to the caretakers to ask questions and practice skills. The following criteria should be fulfilled before discharging a high-risk infant:

• Free of any significant medical/surgical illness
• Should not be on injectable drugs (antibiotics/other)
• Should be on full enteral feeds (either direct breastfeeding or by paladai/spoon)
• For very low birth weight infants, **in addition to above**, the infants should:
  – Have sufficiently mature respiratory control (should ideally be off caffeine/theophylline and apnea free for at least 5 days prior to discharge)
  – Be able to maintain body temperature in an open crib
  – Have had stable weight gain for three consecutive days; and
  – The minimum discharge weight should be 1400–1600 g

It is also important to ensure that any multivitamin/micronutrient supplementation has been started as required, and the vaccination has been done as per schedule based on postnatal age, and that the parents are confident to take care of the baby at home.

It might be necessary in some resource limited settings to individualize some of the above criteria. In such cases, it would be important to call such infants at 3–7 days post-discharge to ensure successful transition of the infant to home care.

Counseling prior to discharge: Counseling plays an important role in the care of these high-risk babies at home; regular counseling sessions should be done before discharge. Parents should be given advice regarding:

• Temperature regulation—proper clothing, cap, socks, kangaroo mother care, etc.
• Feeding—focus should be on exclusive breastfeeding. If required, other type and amount of milk, method of administration and nutritional supplementation, if any, should be advised as per the need of the child.
• Prevention of infections—hand washing, avoidance of visitors, etc.

- Follow-up visits—where and when (Panel 2).
- Danger signs—recognition and where to report if signs are present.
- Vaccination—schedule, next visit, etc.

Panel 2: Follow-up Schedule for High-risk Infants

Very preterm infants (<32 weeks OR <1500 g)
- After 3–7 days of discharge to check if the baby has adjusted well in the home environment
- Every 2 weeks until a body weight of 3 kg (6, 10 and 14 week immunization visits to be covered during these visits)
- At 3, 6, 9,12, 15 and 18 months of corrected age and then every 6 months until 8 years of age
- More visits if required

Infants with other conditions
- Two weeks after discharge
- At 6, 10, 14 weeks of age
- At 6, 9, 12, 15 and 18 months of corrected/postnatal age, as applicable and then every 6 months until 8 years of age
- More visits if required

- Special needs—e.g. next visits for ROP screening, USG/MRI brain, etc.

The family should be provided with the telephone number of the nursery/health care provider, e.g. on-duty doctor in case the family needs to consult for infant's illness in emergency or otherwise.

PROCEDURES

It is important that the family be provided with a structured discharge summary including the details of important events during hospital stay, investigations and treatment received and schedule of follow-up visits. The venue and dates of follow-up should be clearly indicated on the discharge summary.

High-risk clinic: A specified site should be earmarked for follow-up services. The venue, days and timings of the clinic should be fixed. Prior appointments should be given and ad hoc visits discouraged. Registration procedure at the clinic should be simplified to avoid any undue delays.

Venue: Dedicated room(s) in the OPD premises should be designated for high-risk follow-up.

Days and timing: One or more fixed days and time of the week should be allocated for the clinic.

Registration: The high-risk infant should be registered at the clinic on the first visit following hospital discharge. An OPD card for the same should be made.

Record maintenance: A separate file for each high-risk infant should be made on the day of registration of the baby in the HRC. The HRC case file should have a uniform format and include the following information for each infant:
• Demographic and contact details of infants' family
• Detailed diagnosis at discharge
• Details of any intermittent morbidities/any important investigations, e.g. cranial USG/MRI brain
• Reports of hearing and vision (ROP) screening, as applicable
• Nutritional details
• Anthropometry (weight, head circumference at each visit and length)
• Developmental screening chart
• Neurological assessment proforma
• Immunization details
• Doctor's assessment and note

A copy of discharge summary should be maintained in all these files for ready referral. A note of important details and advice should be made in the OPD card also.

Appointments: At the first visit and subsequently, the infant should be given the date for the next visit.

Practical Tips
Corrected age: Age of the child since the expected date of delivery. The correction for gestational immaturity at birth should be done until 24 months age. All developmental milestones, anthropometric parameters are assessed according to corrected age to compensate for the prematurity. The initiation of complementary feeds is also according to corrected age.
Postnatal age: Age of the child since birth. Immunization is done according to postnatal age.

When to Follow-up

The follow-up schedule should be explained to the parents at discharge, and should also be mentioned on the discharge summary.

For the purpose of follow-up visits, at-risk infants can be grouped under two major categories:

- Very preterm or VLBW infants, and
- Infants with other conditions

The follow-up schedule for both these categories has been summarized in Panel 2. This schedule represents minimum number of visits for high-risk neonates. If the baby has ongoing issues or illness, more frequent visits are recommended. Note that first contact of the infant with the health providers after discharge is important and helps in identification of adjustment problems at home. Ideally this contact should be achieved by the home visit, preferably within the first week of discharge.

Very low birth weight babies or those born at less than 32 weeks gestation (or bigger and sick babies) should be followed up for eye check up for retinopathy of prematurity till the postnatal age of 44 weeks (see ROP protocol).

Some neurological abnormalities that are identified in the first year of life are transient or improve whereas findings in other children may worsen over time.[5] By 12 months corrected age, the cognitive and language assessment can be done. By 18–24 months corrected age, there is improved prediction to early school age performance.[6-8] The importance of long-term follow-up lies in the fact that minor neurological disabilities may not be detected early and become apparent only with increasing age. Standard follow-up for many multi-center networks is currently at 18–24 months corrected age.

WHAT SHOULD BE DONE

Table 20.2 summarizes the plan for follow-up.

1. **Assessment of feeding and dietary counseling:** Parents should be asked about the infants' diet and offered dietary counseling at each visit. Breastfeeding frequency and adequacy should be assessed. The amount, dilution and mode of feeding should be noted if supplemental feeding is given. It is a good idea to enquire about source of milk as milk supplied by local vendors is often diluted (dilution has the same impact on the infant whether done by the family or the vendor). It is also important to record the duration of exclusive breastfeeding. If a baby is not gaining adequate weight on exclusive breastfeeding, take care of any illness,

Assessment	Age in months								
	1	2	3	6	9	12	15	18	24........8 yrs
Assessment of feeding and dietary counseling	All visits								
Growth monitoring	All visits								
Immunization	As per schedule (based on postnatal age)								
Ongoing morbidities	All visits and as and when required								
Neurological examination			*	*	*	*	–	*	*
Developmental screening	All visits								
Formal developmental assessment			*	¶	¶	*	–	*	*
Hearing (BERA)			*	¶	¶	¶	–	¶	¶
Ophthalmic evaluation	ROP screening				*	¶	–	¶	¶
USG/MRI brain	As indicated								

Table 20.2: Follow-up plan for high-risk neonates

¶ *if previous test abnormal*

maternal problems which may interfere with feeding and milk output. If poor weight gain persists despite all measures to improve breast milk output, supplementation can be considered.

Complementary feeding should be started at 6 months corrected age. Initially, semisolids should be advised in accordance with the local cultural practices. Spend adequate time on explaining what and how to give. The common practice of giving too little or too dilute complementary food such as rice-water, dal-water, too much of juice, etc. should be discouraged (Table 20.3).[9]

Complementary foods should be varied and include adequate quantities of meat, poultry, fish or eggs as well as vitamin A-rich fruits and vegetables everyday. Where this is not possible, the use of fortified complementary foods and vitamin mineral supplements may be necessary to ensure adequacy of particular nutrient intakes. As infants grow, the consistency of complementary foods should change from semisolid to solid foods and the variety of foods offered should increase. By eight months, infants can eat 'finger foods' and by 12 months, most children can eat the same types of food as the rest of the family. The major problem with the family food is that it is not nutrient-rich.

Table 20.3: Amount and frequency of complementary foods

Age	Foods	Frequency
6–8 months	Thick, soft porridge (khichri/dalia); add sugar and oil mixed with either milk or pounded ground nuts. Mixtures of mashed foods made of potatoes or millet or rice; mix with fish or beans or pounded ground-nuts; add green vegetables.	Breastfeeding plus 2–3 meals per day.
9–11 months	–Do– Give nutritious snacks between meals like egg, banana or bread.	Breastfeeding plus 3–4 meals/day plus one snack between meals.
12–24 months	–Do– Family foods, chopped or mashed if necessary.	3–4 meals/day plus two snacks between meals.

Recommended micro-nutrient supplementation should be provided.

2. **Growth monitoring:** Growth (including weight, head circumference, mid-arm circumference and length) should be monitored and plotted on an appropriate growth chart at each visit. We use Wright's/Ehrenkranz charts (till 40 weeks post menstrual age; PMA) and WHO MGRS growth charts (for preterm infants after 40 weeks PMA and for term infants) for growth monitoring. The infant's growth pattern (slope of the curve) is compared with the standard curve; any deviation should be noted and appropriate remedial action taken.

Anthropometry should be taken for all high-risk infants during follow-up visits.[10] Weight and head circumference should be monitored at each visit and length 3 monthly. These should be marked on the gender specific WHO-MGRS growth charts. The **Corrected age** of the child should be used while using these charts for preterm infants.

3. **Immunization:** Immunization should be ensured according to chronological age. Parents should be offered the option of additional vaccines such as hepatitis B, *Haemophilus influenzae* b and MMR (where not in routine immunization schedule), if they can afford.

4. **Ongoing morbidities surveillance and management:** Ongoing morbidities and their management is one of the most important services a follow-up clinic is meant to

provide. These may relate to prolonged jaundice due to any cause, recurrent exacerbations of respiratory distress in a child with chronic lung disease, gastroesophageal reflux or other feeding difficulties or inadequate weight gain in a preterm infant, anemia in a baby with Rh immunization, cardiac failure in a baby with congenital heart disease, diagnostic evaluation and intermittent illnesses in a baby born to HIV positive mother, etc. The details of any such intermittent morbidity should be systematically recorded in the high-risk file as well as the OPD card of the infant. Details of any intermittent hospitalization and investigations or treatment received should also be recorded for future reference.

5. **Developmental follow-up:** There are three stages of developmental evaluation of a child:[11]
   a. **Surveillance**: It is the process of recognizing children who may be at risk of developmental delays. It incorporates:
      - Eliciting and attending to the parents' concerns about their child's development
      - Documenting and maintaining a developmental history
      - Making accurate observations of the child
      - Identifying risk and protective factors; and
      - Maintaining an accurate record of findings
   b. **Screening:** It is the use of standardized tools to identify and refine the risk recognized on developmental surveillance. Developmental screening does not result in either a diagnosis or treatment plan but rather identifies areas in which a child's development differs from same-age norms. Because development is dynamic in nature and surveillance and screening have limits, periodic screening with a validated instrument should occur so that a problem not detected by surveillance or a single screening can be detected by subsequent screening. Repeated and regular screening is more likely than a single screening to identify problems, especially in later-developing skills such as language. Waiting until a young child misses a major milestone such as walking or talking may result in late rather than early recognition, increasing parental dissatisfaction and anxiety and depriving the child and family of the benefits of early identification and intervention.

c. **Evaluation:** It is a process aimed at identifying specific developmental disorders in children through formal developmental evaluation by a trained developmental pediatrician/child psychologist.

It is recommended that developmental surveillance and screening be incorporated at every visit and any concerns raised be promptly addressed with standardized developmental screening tests. The early identification of developmental problems should lead to further developmental and medical evaluation, diagnosis and treatment including early developmental intervention. It is important that a pediatrician/neonatologist be well versed with the normal developmental milestones, and be able to use the available screening tools effectively so that a formal developmental evaluation be required only for the most deserving cases.

Table 20.4 lists the commonly available and used screening tests in India. There is paucity of evidence for relative benefit of one over the other.

A formal developmental assessment is done using DASII, which is the Indian adaptation of BSID-II, and is considered to be the gold standard to date in Indian

Table 20.4: Developmental screening tests commonly available in India

Test	Domains assessed	Age range	No. of items	Psychometric properties
Trivandrum Development Screening Test (TDSC)[12]	Gross motor, fine motor, vision/hearing and personal/social/language	0–2 years		Sensitivity 66.7%; Specificity 78.8%; Validated against DDST
Denver Developmental Screening Test-II (DDST-II) or Denver-II[13]	Gross motor, language, fine motor, adaptive and personal-social. Also a behavior rating scale	0–6 years	123	Sensitivity 83%; Specificity 43%[13]
Baroda Development Screening Test (BDST)[14]	Motor and mental	0–30 months	54	Sensitivity and specificity of 65–95%

settings. It measures motor and mental domains using 230 items in children between 0 and 30 months of age. However, it is considered ideal that such tools be periodically revalidated to account for the secular trends. Also, since the arrival of BSID-III, which helps assess neurodevelopment in different domains (cognitive, language—receptive and expressive, motor—fine and gross, socio-emotional and adaptive behavior) till 42 months of age, it is desirable that it should be adapted and validated for use in India. Additional tools like VSMS, CBCL and M-CHAT may be used beyond infancy (beginning at 18 months of age) for social-emotional, behavioral and autism evaluation, respectively (Table 20.5).

Also, an objective assessment of the home environment, if feasible, shall be a good adjunct to any developmental evaluation of such children.

Table 20.5: Other tools relevant to developmental evaluation early in life

Test	Brief description	Age
Modified checklist of autism for toddlers (M-CHAT)	To identify children who may benefit from a more thorough developmental and autism evaluation	16–30 months
Vineland social maturity scale (VSMS), Indian adaptation-Malins	Self-help general, self-help eating, self-help dressing, self direction, occupation, communication, locomotion and socialization	0–15 years
Child behavior checklist-language development survey (CBCL-LDS 1½)	Assesses different domains of behavior like emotionally reactive, anxious depressed, somatic complaints, withdrawn, sleep problems, attention problems and aggressive behavior, along with language	1.6–5 years
Also, an objective assessment of the home environment, if feasible, shall be a good adjunct to any developmental evaluation of such children.		

6. **Neurologic examination**: Amiel-Tison neurological assessment is currently the most widely used neurological examination tool during early follow-up of infants. The main focus of neurological examination during the high-risk

follow-up visits is usually evaluation of muscle tone besides vision and hearing, though a complete neurological examination should be performed if indicated in a particular child.

Evaluation of muscle tone is an integral part of the neurological examination. A waxing and waning pattern of neuromotor development from 28 weeks of gestation to the end of first year of life was reported by Amiel-Tison. From 28 to 40 weeks gestation, the acquisition of muscle tone and motor function spreads from lower extremities towards the head (caudo-cephalic progression). After full term, the process is reversed so that relaxation and the motor control proceed downwards for the next 12 to 18 months (cephalo-caudal). So the upper limbs begin to relax and acquire skills before the lower limbs. The axial tone follows a similar pattern. Head control appears first followed by the ability to sit, stand and walk. Hypertonia or hypotonia should be looked for by measuring the following angles: adductor angle, popliteal angle, ankle dorsiflexion and scarf sign; any asymmetry between the extremities should also be recorded. Any history of seizures or involuntary movements should also be recorded.

The following angles should be measured to assess tone as shown in Table 20.6 and Fig. 20.1.

Hypertonia in lower limbs is defined as when either adductor angle is restricted to less than the age specific norms as per Amiel-Tison or if there is scissoring or tight tendo Achilles or restriction of ankle dorsiflexion on extension of knee. Hypertonia in upper limbs is defined as when scarf sign does not cross midline at one year corrected age. Hypertonia of the neck extensors can be inferred by an increased gap between the nape of the neck and examination

Table 20.6: Muscle tone norms (Amiel-Tison)

Age (mo)	Adductor angle	Popliteal angle	Dorsiflexion angle	Scarf sign
0–3	40°–80°	80°–100°	60°–70°	Elbow does not cross midline
4–6	70°–110°	90°–120°	60°–70°	Elbow crosses midline
7–9	110°–140°	110°–160°	60°–70°	Elbow goes beyond axillary line
10–12	140°–160°	150°–170°	60°–70°	—

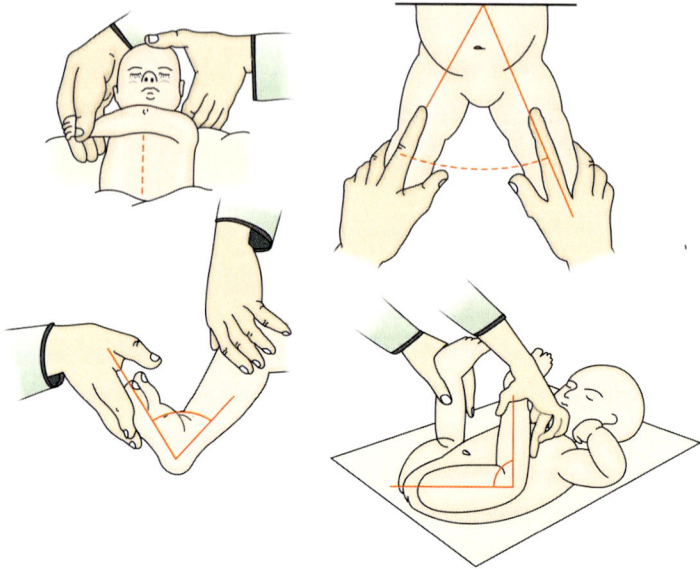

Fig. 20.1: Amiel-Tison method of tone assessment

table with the infant lying in supine position. Truncal extensor hypertonia is present when there is a tendency of body to go into hyperextension or opisthotonus. Cerebral palsy usually presents with definitely abnormal neurological examination with upper motor neuron signs with motor developmental delay.

Any tone abnormality requires a detailed evaluation and management by a trained physiotherapist.

7. **Hearing evaluation:** High-risk infants have higher incidence of moderate to profound hearing loss (2.5–5% *versus* 1% in normal babies). Since clinical screening is often unreliable, brainstem auditory evoked responses (BAER/BERA) should be performed on these infants prior to 3 months of postnatal age.

We do a screening BERA (*A*utomated *A*uditory *B*rainstem *R*esponse-AABR) initially in all cases prior to discharge (but not before 34 weeks PMA for very preterm infants).[15] Those who fail on the first screen are re-screened prior to discharge to minimize the false positivity rates.[16] Those failing on second screen are referred for a diagnostic BERA in the Department of ENT.

For units using otoacoustic emissions (OAE) for the initial hearing screening, it is recommended that a two stage screening be done for high-risk infants, using TEOAE and/ or DPOAE first, followed by AABR for those who fail the first screen by OAE. This approach has been shown to minimize the false positive results.[17]

However, even after a two-stage screening with OAE pass followed by AABR pass, incidence of permanent hearing loss has been shown to be significant.[18] Therefore, it is important to evaluate for hearing and language-communication skill at each follow-up visit.[19]

8. **Vision assessment**: Besides the check-up for retinopathy of prematurity which should start in the NICU and continue till 40 to 44 weeks post-conceptional age or till the retinal vessels have matured (refer protocol on retinopathy of prematurity), the children should have an assessment for eye problems in the newborn period and then at all subsequent routine health supervision visits.

The eye evaluation during follow-up should include the following:[20]

Ocular history: Parents observations are valuable and should be sought. Relevant questions are:

1. Does your child see well?
2. Does your child hold objects close to his or her face when trying to focus?
3. Do your child's eyes appear straight or do they seem to cross or drift or seem hazy?
4. Do your child's eyes appear unusual?

How to assess visual impairment: In children younger than 3 years or in any non-verbal child, vision assessment is accomplished by evaluating the child's ability to fix and follow objects. A standard assessment strategy is to determine whether each eye can fixate on an object, maintain fixation and then follow the object in different gaze positions. Failure to perform these maneuvers indicates significant visual impairment. The assessment should be performed binocularly and then mono-ocularly. If poor fix and following is noted binocularly after 3 months of age, a significant bilateral eye or brain abnormality is suspected, and referral for more formal assessment is advisable. It is important to ensure that the child is awake and alert, because disinterest or poor co-operation can mimic a poor vision response.

In addition, an external penlight evaluation of the lids, conjunctiva, sclera, cornea and iris should be done along with assessment of ocular alignment, as development of strabismus in children may occur at any age, and can represent serious orbital, intraocular or intracranial disease. Pupils should also be examined and a red reflex test performed to detect opacities in the visual axis, such as cataract or corneal abnormality and abnormalities of the back of the eye, such as retinoblastoma or retinal detachment. When both eyes are examined simultaneously, potentially amblyopic conditions such as asymmetric refractive errors and strabismus may also be identified.

Visual acuity should be assessed at 9 months of age using the Teller Acuity Cards (TAC)/Cardiff Acuity Cards (CAC).

Rehabilitation for visual impairment should be early so that the child gets appropriate stimulation. The child should be provided with glasses or corrective surgery as appropriate.

9. Role of neuroimaging[21]

For preterm neonates: Routine screening cranial ultrasound (CUS) is recommended for all preterm infants < 32 weeks gestation once between 7 and 14 days of age. It should optimally be repeated between 36 and 40 weeks PMA. Though MRI brain in preterm neonates detects more abnormalities as compared to CUS performed on same day, there is insufficient data from follow-up studies to indicate whether these additional findings provide more information about the neurodevelopmental prognosis. *Therefore, a routine MRI of all very low birth weight preterm infants with abnormal results of CUS is not currently recommended.*

For term infants: Non contrast CT should be performed to detect hemorrhagic lesions in the encephalopathic term infant with a history of birth trauma, low hematocrit or coagulopathy. If CT findings are inconclusive, MRI should be performed between day 2 and 8 to assess location and extent (pattern) of injury and predict neurodevelopmental outcome.

EARLY ENRICHMENT

The evidence with regard to the usefulness of early stimulation and intervention for high-risk neonates is limited to preterm and low birth weight infants, mostly from developed countries.[21]

What is Evidence?

1. The Newborn Individualized Developmental Care and Assessment Program (NIDCAP) developed to stimulate preterm infants at levels adapted to the child's degree of neurological maturity shows promising findings, primarily on cognitive and motor development, though the scientific evidence on the effects is limited.[22]
2. Early intervention programs (beginning in NICU and post hospital discharge) suggest positive influence on cognitive and motor development.[23,24]
3. Early intervention programs from birth to nine years for children with physical disabilities result in positive outcomes for both children and families.[25]

A few measures that may help have been outlined below:

Birth to 2 months	Tactile and kinesthetic	Place your baby's head and neck on the crook of your elbow and forearm while lifting or carrying her.
2 to 4 months	Tactile and kinesthetic	Help your baby to roll by placing her on either side and calling her name or making a sound with the rattle from behind encouraging her to turn.
4 to 6 months	Auditory	– Play different types of music for her to listen. – Make her sit in front of the mirror and imitate the sounds that she makes.
	Visual	– Roll a medium size ball gently in front of her for her to follow.
	Tactile	– Give her small light rattles to hold in each hand.
	Tactile and kinesthetic	– Encourage her sit by herself leaning on her arms and taking their support.
	Communication	– Start an activity that she enjoys and then stop to see if she moves her body in the same manner to indicate her desire to continue the play.
6 to 8 months	General	– Give her a spoon to bang on a steel plate, small drum to bang her hand on, rattle to shake, paper to crumble and tear (please be there when she is playing with paper). – Cover your face with a plain cloth, slowly remove it and say jha or thuki and hug her. Repeat the activities couple of times on yourself and then take her hand to pull of the cloth. Once she is familiar with the game, cover her face and you pull of the cloth, clap and show excitement.

Contd...

Contd...

- Call the child by one name only and encourage her to respond by smiling at her if she looks.
- Make her sit independently for 5 to 10 mins by putting her brightly colored and musical toys in front of her. If she loses balance, after some time help her to sit again by holding her from the hips lightly.
- Encourage crawling when she is on her tummy by placing her favorite toy in front of her just a little out of her reach so that she has to stretch her hands and push herself forward.
- Repeat the sounds of da da, ma ma, ga ga, ba ba that she makes. Pretend you understand them and answer back in your mother tongue with different intonations.
- Keep talking to her and naming all the family members as come to her, hold or play with her.

8 to 10 months

- Put two blocks in each hand and encourage her to bang them together while looking at them. Encourage her to clap her hands.
- Hold her hand and help her to take out toys one by one from a tub filled with toys. Once she has learnt to take out the toys, hold her hand and encourage her to drop the toys back into the tub one by one.
- When a family member leaves, ask her to wave bye bye.
- Take her in your lap and show her picture books with single, large, colorful pictures of everyday objects and animals. You name and point at the pictures.
- Object permanence.

10 to 12 months

- Show her the functions of objects used in daily life, like glass for drinking, mobile for talking, comb for the hair.
- Encourage her to hold furniture and take some step around it.

12 to 15 months

- Take her hand and help her to point to a toy or any food item she wants. You say the name of the toy and encourage her to take out a sound resembling the name.
- Hold her lightly from the back and give her the confidence to take few steps on her own.

HOW TO ENSURE A GOOD FOLLOW-UP RATE

A good follow-up rate may be ensured through the following:

The importance of follow-up should be routinely empha-sized to the parents during the hospital stay. Elder members of the family, especially grandmothers should be involved in the process.

The permanent and present addresses of the families should be maintained along with phone numbers. It shall be ideal if a person of follow-up team like the medical social worker can make an early visit to the baby's home, either at discharge or within 48–72 hours of discharge.

1. It is highly desirable that a permanent 24 × 7 helpline no. be provided to the family at discharge to contact in case of any problem. Regular contact with the parents with inquiry about the status of the child during follow-up shall be helpful.
2. An easily accessible, less time consuming and hassle free organizational flow of follow-up services including provision of comprehensive assessments under one roof shall encourage parents to come for regular follow-ups.
3. A person who serves as care coordinator and handles all appointments and services shall add to the quality of care experience of the families coming for follow-up.

Practical Tip

The most important determinant if the family would come for follow-up is the availability of comprehensive and reliable clinical services that family can access easily and with dignity.

REFERENCES

1. National neonatology forum of India, National neonatal perinatal database 2002–2003.
2. Mwaniki MK, Atieno M, Lawn JE, Newton CR. Long-term neurodevelopmental outcomes after intrauterine and neonatal insults: A systematic review. Lancet 2012 Feb 4;379(9814):445–52. Epub 2012 Jan 13.
3. Nair MKC, Chacko DS, Paul MK, Nair L, George B, Kumar GS. Low birth weight babies–outcome at 13 years. Indian Pediatrics, vol 46 supplement, Jan 2009;S71–74.

4. Chaudhari S, Otiv M, Chitale A, Pandit A, Hoge m. Pune low birth weight study–cognitive abilities and educational performance at twelve years. Indian Pediatr 2004 Feb;41:121–8.

5. Drillien C. Abnormal neurological signs in the first year of life in low birth weight infants: possible prognostic significance. Dev Med Child Neurol 1997;14:575–84.

6. Weisglas-Kuperus N, Baerts W, Smrkovsky M, Sauer PJ. Effects of biological and social factors on the cognitive development of very low birth weight children. Pediatrics 1993;92:658–665.

7. Dezoete JA, MacArthur BA, Tuck B. Prediction of Bayley and Stanford-Binet scores with a group of very low birth weight children. Child Care Health Dev 2003;29:367–372.

8. Lee H, Barratt MS. Cognitive development of preterm low birth weight children at 5–8 years old. J Dev Behav Pediatr 1993;14:242–49.

9. Guiding principles for complementary feeding of the breastfed child. Freely downloadable from WHO website (*http://whqlibdoc.who.int/paho/2003/a85622.pdf*).

10. Bhandari N, Taneja S, Rongsen T, Chetia J, Sharma P, Bahl R, Kashyap DK, Bhan MK for the WHO Multicenter Growth Reference Study Group. Implementation of the WHO Multicenter Growth Reference Study in India.

11. Council on Children with Disabilities, Section on Developmental Behavioral Pediatrics, Bright Futures Steering Committee and Medical Home Initiatives for Children with Special Needs Project Advisory Committee. Identifying infants and young children with developmental disorders in the medical home: an algorithm for developmental surveillance and screening. Pediatrics 2006;118:405–20.

12. Trivandrum Development Screening Chart.

13. Glascoe FP, Byrne KE, Ashford LG, Johnson KL, Chang B, Strickland B. Accuracy of the Denver-II in developmental screening. Pediatrics 1992 Jun;89:1221–5.

14. Baroda Development Screening Test for Children.

15. Coenraad S, Toll MS, Hoeve HL, Goedegebure A. Auditory brainstem response morphology and analysis in very preterm neonatal intensive care unit infants. Laryngoscope 2011;121:2245–9. doi: 10.1002/lary.22140. Epub 2011 Sep 6.

16. Clemens CJ, Davis SA. Minimizing false-positives in universal newborn hearing screening: a simple solution. Pediatrics 2001 Mar;107:E29.

17. Lin HC, Shu MT, Lee KS, Ho GM, Fu TY, Bruna S, Lin G. Comparison of hearing screening programs between one step with

transient evoked otoacoustic emissions (TEOAE) and two steps with TEOAE and automated auditory brainstem response. Laryngoscope 2005 Nov;115:1957–62.

18. Johnson JL, White KR, Widen JE, Gravel JS, James M, Kennalley T, Maxon AB, Spivak L, Sullivan-Mahoney M, Vohr BR, Weirather Y, Holstrum J. A multicenter evaluation of how many infants with permanent hearing loss pass a two-stage otoacoustic emissions/automated auditory brainstem response newborn hearing screening protocol. Pediatrics 2005 Sep;116:663–72.

19. Harlor AD Jr, Bower C; Committee on Practice and Ambulatory Medicine; Section on Otolaryngology-Head and Neck Surgery. Hearing assessment in infants and children: recommendations beyond neonatal screening. Pediatrics 2009 Oct;124:1252–63.

20. Committee on Practice and Ambulatory Medicine, Section on Ophthalmology. American Association of Certified Orthoptists; American Association for Pediatric Ophthalmology and Strabismus; American Academy of Ophthalmology. Eye examination in infants, children and young adults by pediatricians. Pediatrics 2003 Apr;111:902–7.

21. McCormick MC, Brooks-Gunn J, Buka SL, Goldman J, Yu J, Salganik M, Scott DT, Bennett FC, Kay LL, Bernbaum JC, Bauer CR, Martin C, Woods ER, Martin A, Casey PH. Early intervention in low birth weight premature infants: results at 18 years of age for the Infant Health and Development Program. Pediatrics 2006 Mar;117(3):771 80.

22. Wallin L, Eriksson M. Newborn Individual Development Care and Assessment Program (NIDCAP): a systematic review of the literature. Worldviews Evid Based Nurs 2009;6:54–69. Epub 2009 Apr 29.

23. Spittle AJ, Orton J, Doyle LW, Boyd R. Early developmental intervention programs post hospital discharge to prevent motor and cognitive impairments in preterm infants. Cochrane Database Syst Rev 2007 Apr 18;(2):CD005495.

24. Blauw-Hospers CH, Hadders-Algra M. A systematic review of the effects of early intervention on motor development. Dev Med Child Neurol 2005 Jun;47:421–32.

25. Ziviani J, Feeney R, Rodger S, Watter P. Systematic review of early intervention programmes for children from birth to nine years who have a physical disability. Aust Occup Ther J 2010 Aug;57: 210–23.

21 Retinopathy of Prematurity (ROP)

Retinopathy of prematurity (ROP) is a vaso-proliferative disorder of the retina among preterm infants. Neonates born before 32 weeks of gestation are at risk of developing ROP. However, preterm infants born at 32 weeks or later can also develop severe ROP if they have been sick or required prolonged oxygen therapy. Nearly one-fourth of neonates undergoing screening may show some degree of ROP which fortunately regresses on its own in majority of affected infants. In a few, it progresses to the stage of retinal detachment and blindness. Timely screening and treatment of ROP can prevent blindness and minimize visual handicaps.

What is Evidence?

Studies from India have reported ROP in 20–52% of screened neonates.[1–9] More recent studies have reported lower rates of ROP ranging from 20 to 30%.[1,2]

CLASSIFICATION OF ROP

International classification of ROP (ICROP) is used for classifying ROP.[15] ICROP describes vascularization of the retina and characterizes ROP by its position (zone), severity (stage) and extent (clock hours) (Fig. 21.1 and Table 21.1).

Aggressive posterior ROP (AP-ROP): A rapidly progressing, severe form of ROP, which if untreated, usually progresses rapidly to stage 5 ROP. The characteristic features of this type of ROP include its posterior location, prominence of plus disease and the ill-defined nature of the retinopathy. It may not have classical ridge or extraretinal fibrovascular proliferation, but rather have innocuous looking retina and tortuous vessels forming arcades. This type of ROP is likely to get missed by inexperienced examiners. Observed most commonly in Zone I, it may also occur in posterior Zone II.

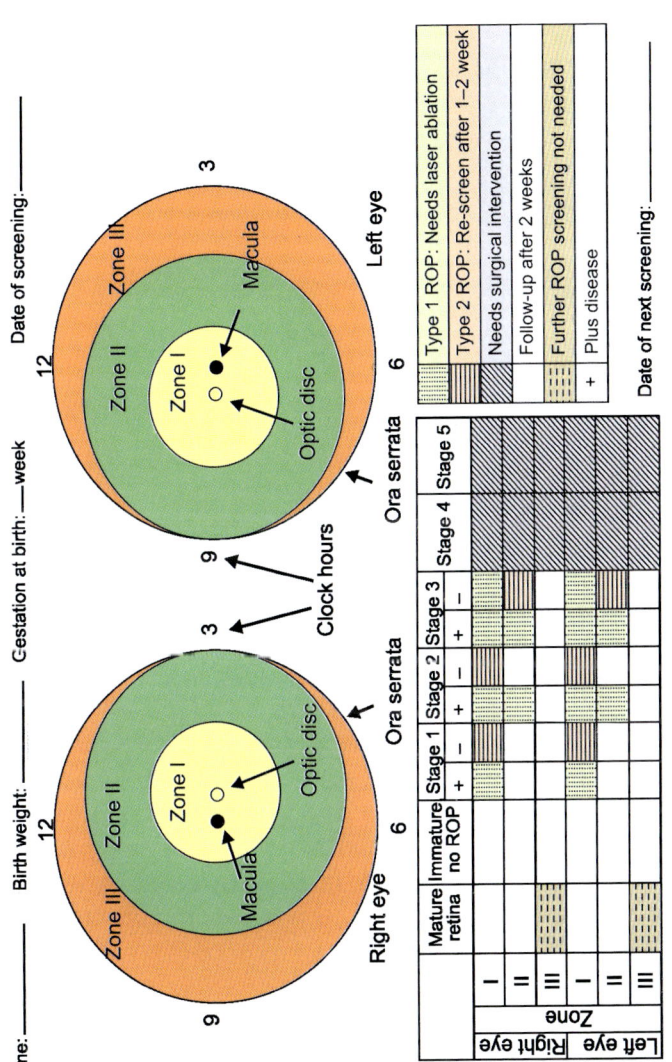

Fig. 21.1: Classification of retinopathy of prematurity

Table 21.1: Classification of ROP (ICROP)[15]

Location	Zone I	Circle with optic nerve at its centre and a radius of twice the distance from optic nerve to macula
	Zone II	Concentric circle from edge of zone I to ora serrata nasally and equator temporally
	Zone III	Lateral crescent from zone II to ora serrata temporally
Severity	Stage 1	Presence of thin white **demarcation line** separating vascular from avascular retina
	Stage 2	Addition of depth and width to the demarcation line of stage 1, so as the line becomes **ridge**
	Stage 3	Presence of **extra retinal fibrovascular proliferation** with abnormal vessels and fibrous tissue extending from ridge to vitreous
	Stage 4	**Partial retinal detachment** not involving macula (4A) and involving macula (4B)
	Stage 5	**Complete retinal detachment**
Plus disease		Presence of dilatation and tortuosity of retinal vessels at posterior pole of eye. Also associated with papillary rigidity and vitreous haze.
Extent		Extent of ROP described in 3 clock hours (a total of 12 clock hours of 30° each)

PROTOCOL FOR SCREENING

The aim of the screening program is to detect ROP early, follow it up closely during its evolution and treat if it assumes potentially serious severity level.

Which Infants should be Screened

Selecting neonates for screening depends on risk of ROP at different gestation. *Gestation and birth weight cut-off for screening shifts lower as the quality of care improves.* Based on current incidence and risk factors reported in Indian literature, the following group of neonates should be screened:

1. Babies with birth weight < 1500 g
2. Babies born at < 32 weeks of gestation
3. Selected preterm infants with a birth weight between 1500 and 2000 g or gestation of more than 32 weeks with sickness like cardio-respiratory instability, prolonged oxygen therapy, repeated episodes of apnea of prematurity, anemia needing blood transfusion and neonatal sepsis or believed by their

attending pediatrician or neonatologist to be at high risk. This 'third criterion' is important as it brings in many larger babies into the screening guidelines ambit without raising the screening parameters.[19]

Other risk factors of developing ROP include anemia, blood transfusion, sepsis, apnea, hypotension and poor weight gain. In general, other risk factors are surrogate markers of sickness in the baby. Therefore, sicker the baby, higher is the risk.[3]

When and How often to Screen

First screening examination should be carried out at 32 weeks of post menstrual age (PMA) or 4 weeks of postnatal age, whichever is later.[20]

Practical Tip

A good rule to remember is to perform first screening at 4 weeks of PMA.

What is Evidence?

Progression of ROP follows a distinct timeline as per PMA rather than postnatal age (PNA) of the infant. Hardly any ROP is detected before 32 weeks of PMA. However, ROP usually does not develop before 3 weeks of PNA.

The median age at detection of stage 1 ROP is 34 weeks. Threshold ROP appears at 34 to 38 weeks. Vascularization is complete by 44 weeks of gestation. Therefore, critical phase during screening is 34 to 38 weeks when the infant is likely to reach the threshold stage of disease and may require treatment for prevention of blindness.

Follow-up examinations are normally required every one to two weeks depending upon ROP staging, and should be recommended by the examining ophthalmologist.

ROP screening can be terminated once there is complete vascularization of retina without any ROP or if the ROP has shown regression. This normally happens at around 40 to 44 weeks of PMA.

Where to Examine the Baby

Neonates are best examined in the neonatal unit itself under supervision of attending pediatrician/neonatologist. It is not wise to transport small babies to ophthalmic outpatient or ward for examination.

How to Dilate the Pupils

Pupils are dilated with phenylephrine 2.5% and tropicamide 0.5–1%. One drop of tropicamide is instilled every 10–15 minutes up to 4 times starting 1 hour before the scheduled time for examination. This is followed by phenylephrine, just one drop before examination. Phenylephrine is available in 10% concentration; it should be diluted 4 times before use in neonates. Repeated instillation of phenylephrine is avoided for the fear of hypertension.

Practical Tip

If pupils are not dilating despite administration of adequate mydriatic drops, severe ROP (plus disease) should be suspected.

What does the Examination Entail

Screening of ROP involves indirect ophthalmoscopy (IO) using 20D or 28/30D lens by an experienced ophthalmologist. After instilling a topical anesthetic drop like proparacaine, a wire speculum is inserted to keep the eyelids apart. First, the anterior segment of the eye is examined to look for tunica vasculosa lentis, pupillary dilation and lens/media clarity followed by the posterior pole to look for plus disease, followed by sequential examination of all clock hours of the peripheral retina. A sclera depressor is often used to indent the eye externally to examine areas of interest, rotate and stabilize the eye.

How to Record Findings during Screening

Ophthalmological notes should be made after each ROP examination, detailing zone, stage and extent in terms of clock hours of any ROP and the presence of any pre-plus or plus disease. These notes should include a recommendation for the timing of the next examination (if any) and be kept with the baby's medical record (*see* Fig. 21.1).

What Precautions to take during Examination

ROP screening examination can have short-term effects on blood pressure, heart rate and respiratory function in the premature baby.[14] The examination should be kept as brief as possible and precaution is taken to ensure that emergency situations can be dealt with promptly and effectively.

Discomfort to the baby should be minimized by administering oral sucrose just before examination, pre-treatment of the eyes with a topical proparacaine and swaddling the baby. Baby should not be fed just before examination to avoid vomiting and aspiration. Hand hygiene should be practiced to maintain asepsis.

What is Evidence?

A systematic review and meta-analysis comprising four studies has reported that oral sucrose reduces pain during eye examination.[14] Of two studies reporting the role of topical proparacaine drops, one has reported significant pain reduction.

Use of Wide-field Digital Camera (RetCam) for Screening

A wide-field digital camera (RetCam) capable of retinal imaging in preterm infants has been evaluated as an alternative to IO for screening. Retinal images taken by camera can be stored, transmitted to expert, reviewed, analyzed and sequentially compared over time and are useful for telemedicine purposes. However, due to high cost and limitations in diagnostic accuracy particularly with poor image quality, RetCam cannot replace IO in current scenario. Digital fundus images acquired by RetCam can serve as a useful adjunct to conventional bedside ROP screening by IO.

What is Evidence?

Studies comparing RetCam with indirect ophthalmoscopy (IO) have reported variable sensitivity but good specificity.[13]

TREATMENT OF ROP

The treatment involves ablation of peripheral normal avascular retina and thereby abolishing hypoxic drive of retina (mediated by over-expression of vascular endothelial growth factor, VEGF). This results in regression of established ROP. Care is taken not to touch the retina with ROP as it would result in severe bleeding.

Indication for Peripheral Retinal Ablation

Treatment of ROP is based on differentiation of the following two types of ROP:

Type 1 ROP:
- Zone I, any stage ROP with plus disease
- Zone II, stage 3 ROP without plus disease
- Zone III, stage 2 or 3 ROP with plus disease

Type 2 ROP:
- Zone I, stage 1 or 2 ROP without plus disease
- Zone II, stage 3 ROP without plus disease

Peripheral retinal ablation should be carried out for all cases with type 1 ROP and continued serial examinations are advised for type 2 ROP.

What is Evidence?

Classification of ROP into type 1 and 2 is based on results of Early Treatment for Retinopathy of Prematurity Randomized Trial (ETROP).[12] Before ETROP study, laser ablation was performed in neonates with threshold ROP, a classification based on location and stage of ROP.

ETROP study demonstrated improved visual outcome if laser ablation is performed in eyes with 'high-risk' pre-threshold ROP. Type 1 ROP includes threshold ROP and subset of pre-threshold ROP likely to benefit from early treatment.

Treatment Modalities

Peripheral retinal ablation is carried out either by cryotherapy or by diode laser. Diode laser ablation has largely replaced cryotherapy as it is associated with a lower rate of postoperative ocular and systemic complications and lesser damage to the adjacent tissues. Additionally, 'laser spots' on retina are visible during the procedure minimizing the skip areas requiring retreatment. The procedure can be carried out under general anesthesia or under sedation depending on the feasibility and expertise.

What is Evidence?

In a Cochrane systematic review, peripheral retinal ablation as compared to no treatment was associated with improved structural and functional outcome in treated eyes.[11] Due to ablation of peripheral avascular retina, visual fields were reduced in treated eyes.

Pre-anesthetic Preparation

Oral feeds should be discontinued 3 hours prior to the procedure (Table 21.2). Baby should be started on intravenous

Table 21.2: Preparation for laser ablative therapy

- Take consent
- Ensure good pupillary dilatation
- Nil by mouth 3 hrs prior to procedure
- Start on intravenous fluids
- Put on vital sign monitor/pulse oximeter
- Warmer for maintaining temperature
- Arrange equipment and check functioning thereof
  - Endotracheal tubes No. 2.5, 3, 3.5
  - Resuscitation bag and face masks (appropriate sizes)
  - Oxygen delivery system
  - Syringes, infusion pumps, ventilator

fluids, and put on cardio-respiratory monitor. Dilatation of pupil is ensured (as described earlier).

Anesthesia/Sedation

Topical anesthesia alone provides insufficient analgesia for ROP treatment and should not be solely relied upon. Ideally, babies should be treated under general anesthesia or under opioid sedation. If shifting to operation theatre is not possible, babies may be treated more rapidly in the neonatal unit.

Procedure

Both the eyes can be treated at the same sitting unless contraindicated by instability of the baby. If baby is not tolerating the procedure, consider abandoning the procedure for the time being. Vital signs and oxygen saturation should be monitored very closely.

MONITORING AFTER LASER THERAPY

After laser therapy, first examination should take place 5–7 days after treatment and should be continued at least weekly for signs of decreasing activity and regression. Re-treatment should be performed usually 10–14 days after initial treatment when there has been a failure of the ROP to regress.

Postoperative Care

- The baby should be closely monitored. If condition permits, oral feeds can be started shortly after the procedure.

- Premature babies especially those with chronic lung disease may have increase or re-appearance of apneic episodes or an increased in oxygen requirement. Therefore, they should be carefully monitored for 48–72 hours after the procedure.
- Antibiotic drops (such as chloramphenicol) should be instilled 6–8 hourly for 2–3 days.

Bevacizumab

Intravitreal injection of bevacizumab, a neutralizing anti-VEGF molecule has been demonstrated to diminish the neovascular response significantly in animal models and human studies. As VEGF is an important mediator of lung growth and brain development, and there is significant systemic absorption of anti-VEGF mediation after intravitreal injection, there are concerns regarding toxicity of such therapy. Due to lack of data on potentially serious systemic adverse effects, administration of intravitreal bevacizumab (anti-VEGF monoclonal antibody) is not routinely recommended in neonates with ROP. It may be used only when laser photocoagulation fails and after taking informed consent from the parents.

What is Evidence?

A multi-centre RCT showed that intravitreal injection of bevacizumab is superior to conventional laser therapy in infants with treatable ROP (stage 3+) in zone I but not in zone II.[16] Additional advantage of bevacizumab was that retinal vessels continued to grow as opposed to permanent destruction of the same with laser therapy.[17,18] The trial was not large enough to rule out potential serious side effects of this treatment modality.

PREVENTION

Antenatal Steroids

Use of antenatal steroids (ANS) is a well-known approach to prevent respiratory distress and intraventricular hemorrhage (two important risk factors of ROP). Though antenatal steroids have not reduced occurrence of ROP as it saves smaller babies who are at higher risk of developing ROP. As ANS reduces sickness level in preterm infants, they are likely to reduce severe ROP.

Judicious Oxygen Therapy

Oxygen is a drug and it should be used judiciously. Each neonatal unit should have a written policy regarding when and how to use oxygen with appropriate target saturations.

If a preterm neonate <32 weeks gestation needs resuscitation at birth, inhaled oxygen concentration (FiO_2) should be titrated to prevent hyperoxia and achieve gradual increase in oxygen saturation (70% at 3 minute and 80% at 5 minute after birth).[21] During acute care of a sick preterm neonate, ROP is more likely to develop if partial pressure of oxygen in arterial blood is more than 80 mmHg.

Oxygen level in blood should be continuously monitored using pulse oximetry keeping a saturation target of 90–93%, with limits set at 88% and 95%. It is important that a work culture is inculcated wherein physicians and nurses respond to monitor alarms.

What is Evidence?

A large scale RCT (SUPPORT trial) indicated that maintaining low saturations (85–89%) as compared to high saturations (91–95%) in preterm infants <28 weeks did not reduce composite outcome of death or severe ROP but it resulted in lower severe ROP and higher death rates.[10]

Therefore, it is recommended that saturations in preterm neonates be maintained between 90% and 95%. Saturations should be monitored in preterm infants receiving oxygen therapy to prevent hyperoxia or hypoxia.

Judicious Use of Blood Transfusions

Transfusion of packed RBCs is another risk factor of ROP. Adult RBCs are rich in 2, 3 DPG and adult Hb binds less firmly to oxygen, thus releasing more oxygen to the retinal tissue. Packed cell transfusions should be given as per protocol (Refer to Blood Component Transfusion Protocol).

Other Interventions

Supplementation of high doses of vitamin E or reduced ambient light exposure is not associated with reduced incidence of ROP. In neonates with early stages of ROP, administration of supplementation oxygen to achieve oxygen saturation in supraphysiological range and to reduce retinal hypoxia is not associated with reduction in progression of ROP.

QUALITY IMPROVEMENT

Protocolized Approach

- All units caring for babies at risk of ROP should have a written protocol in relation to the screening and treatment of ROP. This should include responsibilities for follow-up of babies transferred or discharged from the unit before screening is complete.
- If babies are transferred either before ROP screening is initiated or when it has been started but not completed, it is the responsibility of the consultant neonatologist to ensure that the neonatal team in the receiving unit is aware of the need to start or continue ROP screening.
- Whenever possible, ROP screening should be completed prior to discharge. There should be a record of all babies who require review and the arrangements for their follow-up.
- For babies discharged home before screening is complete, the first follow-up outpatient appointment must be made before hospital discharge and the importance of attendance explained to the parents.

Auditing

The following outcomes should be regularly audited in units with ROP screening and treatment program:

- Completeness of screening program: Percentage of eligible babies who receive at least one ROP eye examination.
- Timing of first screen: Percentage of eligible babies receiving first ROP screening exam by 4 weeks of postnatal age.
- Timing of treatment: Percentage of babies needing ROP treatment for their ROP who are treated within 48 hours of the decision to treat being made.

REFERENCES

1. Kumar P, Sankar MJ, Deorari A, et al. Risk factors for severe retinopathy of prematurity in preterm low birth weight neonates. Indian J Pediatr 2011;78:812–6.
2. Aggarwal R, Deorari AK, Azad RV, et al. Changing profile of retinopathy of prematurity. J Trop Pediatr 2002;48:239–42.

3. Maheshwari R, Kumar H, Paul VK, Singh M, Deorari AK, Tiwari HK. Incidence and risk factors of retinopathy of prematurity in a tertiary care newborn unit in New Delhi. Natl Med J India 1996; 9:211–4.

4. Narayan S, Aggarwal R, Upadhyay A, Deorari AK, Singh M, Paul VK. Survival and morbidity in extremely low birth weight (ELBW) infants. Indian Pediatr 2003;40:130–5.

5. Charan R, Dogra MR, Gupta A, Narang A. The incidence of retinopathy of prematurity in a neonatal care unit. Indian J Ophthalmol 1995;43:123–6.

6. Dutta S, Narang S, Narang A, Dogra M, Gupta A. Risk factors of threshold retinopathy of prematurity. Indian Pediatr 2004;41: 665–71.

7. Vinekar A, Dogra MR, Sangtam T, Narang A, Gupta A. Retinopathy of prematurity in Asian Indian babies weighing greater than 1250 grams at birth: Ten year data from a tertiary care center in a developing country. Indian J Ophthalmol 2007; 55:331–6.

8. Rekha S, Battu RR. Retinopathy of prematurity: incidence and risk factors. Indian Pediatr 1996;33:999–1003.

9. Gopal L, Sharma T, Ramachandran S, Shanmugasundaram R, Asha V. Retinopathy of prematurity: A study. Indian J Ophthalmol 1995;43:59–61.

10. Carlo WA, Finer NN, Walsh MC, et al. Target ranges of oxygen saturation in extremely preterm infants. N Engl J Med 2010; 362:1959–69.

11. Andersen CC, Phelps DL. Peripheral retinal ablation for threshold retinopathy of prematurity in preterm infants. Cochrane Database Syst Rev 2000;CD001693.

12. Good WV. Final results of the Early Treatment for Retinopathy of Prematurity (ETROP) randomized trial. Trans Am Ophthalmol Soc 2004;102:233-48; Discussion 48–50.

13. Kemper AR, Wallace DK, Quinn GE. Systematic review of digital imaging screening strategies for retinopathy of prematurity. Pediatrics 2008;122:825–30.

14. Sun X, Lemyre B, Barrowman N, O'Connor M. Pain management during eye examinations for retinopathy of prematurity in preterm infants: a systematic review. Acta Paediatr 2010;99:329–34.

15. The International Classification of Retinopathy of Prematurity revisited. Arch Ophthalmol 2005;123:991–9.

16. Mintz-Hittner HA, Kennedy KA, Chuang AZ. Efficacy of intravitreal bevacizumab for stage 3+ retinopathy of prematurity. N Engl J Med 2011;364:603–15.
17. Good WV, Palmer EA. Bevacizumab for retinopathy of prematurity. N Engl J Med 2011;364:2359; author reply 61–2.
18. Gilbert CE, Zin A, Darlow B. Bevacizumab for retinopathy of prematurity. N Engl J Med 2011;364:2359–60; author reply 61–2.
19. Adhikari S, Badhu BP, Bhatta NK, Rajbhandari RS, Kalakheti BK. Retinopathy of prematurity in a tertiary care hospital in eastern Nepal. JNMA J Nepal Med Assoc 2008;47:24–7.
20. Screening examination of premature infants for retinopathy of prematurity. Pediatrics 2006;117:572–6.
21. York JR, Landers S, Kirby RS, Arbogast PG, Penn JS. Arterial oxygen fluctuation and retinopathy of prematurity in very-low-birth-weight infants. J Perinatol 2004;24:82–7.

Acute Renal Failure

Acute renal failure (ARF) is a common clinical condition in neonatal intensive care unit (NICU). There is a wide variation in the incidence of ARF across studies. It affects approximately 1–24% of newborns in the NICU.[1,2] In a recent report from a tertiary centre of Thailand, the prevalence of ARF among newborns was found to be 6.3%, with more than 65% developing within 7 days of birth.[3] ARF is an acute reduction in glomerular filtration rate (GFR) with both failure to remove solutes and water leading to concurrent net solute and water retention—oligoanuric renal failure.[2]

CLASSIFICATION OF ACUTE RENAL FAILURE

Based on the urine output, ARF can be of two types:
1. Oligoanuric
2. Non-oliguric

Based on the site of origin of insult, ARF can be of three types:[4]
1. Pre-renal (75–80%)
2. Intrinsic renal (10–15%)
3. Post-renal (5%)

Persistence of insult can convert pre-renal or post-renal failure to intrinsic renal failure. However, there is an increasing awareness that even moderate decrease in renal function is important in the critically ill neonates and contributes significantly to morbidity as well as mortality.

DIAGNOSIS OF ARF

Neonatal ARF is defined as:
- Plasma creatinine more than 1.5 mg/dL for at least 24 to 48 hours if mother's renal function is normal.[2]
- Serum creatinine rising more than 0.3 mg/dL over 48 hours.

- Serum creatinine fails to fall below maternal plasma creatinine within 5–7 days.

Plasma Creatinine

Some studies use the doubling criterion, that is, if the neonate's creatinine increases two times between any two measurements, he would be said to have ARF. The above definitions have reasonable accuracy in term neonates. In preterm neonates, there is a transient increase in serum creatinine, peaking on day 4, followed by a progressive decline to normal neonatal levels by a postnatal age of 3 to 4 weeks. This occurs due to re-absorption of creatinine across the permeable tubules.

Urine Output

Oliguria: It has been defined as urine output less than 1 mL/kg/hr after first day of life for both term and preterm neonates. However, some term neonates may void for the first time at around 24 hrs of life. It has been seen that 17% of newborns void in the delivery room, approximately 90% by 24 hours and 99% void by 48 hours.[1]

Practical Tips
ARF can also present with normal urine output in one-third of the cases, especially in asphyxiated neonates. Further, in VLBW infants without ARF, there could be an oliguric phase that resolves spontaneously in the first a few days of life.[1] Anuria can also occur in syndrome of inappropriate ADH secretion in absence of ARF.

CONCEPT OF ACUTE KIDNEY INJURY (AKI)

An attempt has been made to define renal failure bringing uniformity across age, gender and body mass index and reduce the need for a baseline value of serum creatinine. The result of such an attempt is the concept of acute kidney injury (AKI).[5]

DEFINITION OF ACUTE KIDNEY INJURY (AKI)

An abrupt (within 48 hours) reduction in kidney function currently defined as an absolute increase in serum creatinine of more than or equal to 0.3 mg/dL (≥26.4 mol/L), a percentage increase in serum creatinine of more than or equal to 50% (1.5-fold) from the baseline or a reduction in urine output (documented oliguria of less than 0.5 mL/kg per hour for >6 hours). Thus, the concept of AKI creates a new paradigm which encompasses not only established renal failure but also functional impairment relative to the physiological demand.[5]

Pre-renal versus Intrinsic Renal Failure

- The usefulness of differentiating pre-renal from intrinsic renal failure was believed to lie in the fact that in the former, the damage to the kidneys is yet to begin, whereas in the latter it already has. However, with the increasing recognition of AKI as a continuum of volume responsiveness through unresponsiveness, this distinction has blurred out. There is a definite role of appropriate fluid therapy in reversing the renal damage in the former.[5]
- When a baby has not passed urine in the past 12 hrs, the first thing is to look for distended bladder by palpation of the abdomen or by ultrasound (if available at bed side) (Fig. 22.1). *It is better to avoid catheterization of the bladder*

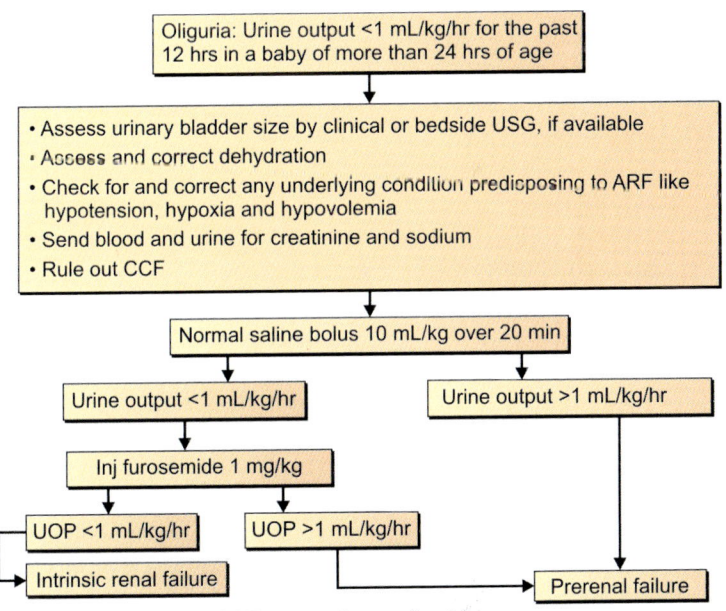

UOP: urine output; CCF: congestive cardiac failure

Fig. 22.1: Approach to a neonate with oliguria

to prevent infection, but it may be necessary in sick babies. If required, it has to be done with a 5 Fr lubricated feeding tube under strict asepsis. *Compression of the bladder (supra pubic pressure) should be avoided especially in preterm infants for the fear of VUR and rarely bladder rupture.* [1]

- After confirming the absence of urine in the bladder, a fluid challenge can be given. The common causes of pre-renal azotemia are hypovolemia, systemic hypotension and hypoxia (in more than 80% of cases).[2] In the absence of obvious signs of fluid overload, a normal saline bolus of 10 mL/kg can be given over 20 min (or 20 mL/kg over 2 hrs). In spite of the fluid challenge, if urine output fails to ensue, furosemide can be given in a single dose of 1 mg/kg (in a non-dehydrated patient).

Approach to a Neonate with Renal Failure

History

a. Pre-natal history:
   - History of maternal drug intake like enalapril or indo-methacin, which decreases glomerular filtration should be sought.
   - Maternal uncontrolled diabetes may be associated with genitourinary malformations.
   - Oligohydramnios may result from fetal oliguria due to bilateral congenital renal disease, bilateral lower urinary tract obstruction or maternal drugs. Likewise, poly-hydramnios may result from a defect in urinary concentration whereas hydrops may be the first sign of congenital nephrotic syndrome.

b. Family history: It may be present in cases of polycystic kidney disease, renal tubular disorders and congenital nephrotic syndrome.

c. Natal history:
   - Perinatal asphyxia, respiratory distress, sepsis and shock may predispose the kidneys to anoxic injury culminating in acute tubular necrosis.
   - Oliguria in asphyxia may result from pre-renal failure mediated by endothelin, intrinsic renal failure (ATN) or SIADH.

- Micturition history: As much as 7% newborns do not void in the first 24 hours. The most common cause of delayed micturition is inadequate perfusion of the kidneys. However, intrinsic renal disorders and urinary tract obstruction need to be ruled out.

Physical Examination

Examination must include assessment of hydration (edema/dehydration), vital signs including blood pressure and a search for dysmorphic features (abnormal ears, pre-auricular pits, ambiguous genitalia, hypospadias, abdominal wall defects, aniridia, Potter facies), which are associated with renal malformations. Spontaneous pneumothorax may be associated with renal abnormalities. Abdominal masses are present in 0.8% newborns, most of which are genitourinary in origin. A suprapubic mass could indicate a palpable bladder. In males, the urine stream should be carefully observed as thin stream, dribbling or post voidal residual bladder suggest posterior urethral valve.

What is Evidence?

Routine renal ultrasound for babies with single umbilical artery:

Studies indicate that 10% of babies with single umbilical artery (SUA) have an associated major congenital renal malformation. However, a recent meta-analysis ascertains that 14 cases of SUA will have to be screened to pick up one major renal malformation, which could also be picked up with a good pediatric follow-up. So the value of routine ultrasound screening of all babies with SUA for renal malformations is not established.[6]

LABORATORY INVESTIGATIONS

Babies with ARF must be investigated not only to look for the cause but also for the complications. Apart from serum creatinine and blood urea, serum electrolytes, arterial blood gas analysis, urine sodium and urine creatinine must be done.

Role of Indices

Differentiation of pre-renal and intrinsic renal failure can be done on the basis of urinary indices (Table 22.1). The important pre-requisite is that the urine sample for measuring indices must be obtained *prior to fluid and diuretic challenge*. Among

Table 22.1: Parameters to differentiate pre-renal from intrinsic renal failure[1]

Parameters	Pre-renal	Intrinsic renal
Urinary Na	<20 mEq/L	>50 mEq/L
Renal failure index*	Low <1	High >4
Fractional excretion of Na$	<1	>3

*Renal failure index (RFI): $\dfrac{\text{Urinary Na} \times \text{Plasma creatinine}}{\text{Plasma Na} \times \text{Urine creatinine}}$

$Fractional excretion of sodium (FENa): $\dfrac{\text{Urinary Na} \times \text{Plasma creatinine}}{\text{Plasma Na} \times \text{Urine creatinine}} \times 100$

the indices available, fractional excretion of Na (FENa) is the most preferred. FENa more than 2.5–3.0% is associated with intrinsic ARF.

Preterm babies lose more sodium in the urine due to the tubular immaturity, hence, a FENa of more than 6% can be used to define intrinsic ARF in babies born between 29 and 32 weeks of gestation.[7] Likewise, renal failure index (RFI) more than 4 in term and more than 8 in preterm babies <32 weeks is suggestive of intrinsic ARF.

Urine microscopic analysis: The presence of granular and hyaline casts, RBC, protein and tubular cells suggests an intrinsic cause. In asphyxia, there is an increase in epithelial cells and transient microscopic hematuria with leucocytes. The excretion of low molecular weight proteins like β_2-glycoprotein is a sensitive indicator of tubular damage as in asphyxia.

Radiological Evaluation

Ultrasonography and Doppler studies: Useful in ruling out congenital anomalies like polycystic kidneys, dysplasia of kidneys and obstructive causes like posterior urethral valves. Renal Doppler studies are useful in diagnosing vascular thrombosis.

Voiding cysto-urethrography can identify lesions of the lower urinary tract that cause obstruction, such as posterior urethral valves.

Etiology of Renal Failure

Having differentiated pre-renal from intrinsic renal failure, look for the exact etiology of renal failure. There are several causes of ARF (Table 22.2).

Table 22.2: Etiology of neonatal renal failure

I. Congenital malformations
    - Renal agenesis
    - Renal hypoplasia/dysplasia
    - Cystic diseases of kidney, e.g. autosomal recessive polycystic kidney

II. Acquired renal disorders
    - Acute tubular necrosis
        - Perinatal asphyxia
        - Perinatal hypoxia due to respiratory distress syndrome, traumatic delivery
        - Sepsis
        - Hypovolemia due to dehydration, severe patent ductus arteriosus, intraventricular hemorrhage, postoperative, increased insensible water loss
    - Vascular
        - Arterial thrombosis or embolism or stenosis
        - Venous thrombosis (infants of diabetic mother, dehydration, polycythemia)
    - Drugs:
        - Maternal use of ACE* inhibitors, indomethacin
        - Neonatal: Indomethacin, aminoglycosides, radiographic contrast media

III. Urinary tract obstruction
    - Posterior urethral valves
    - Pelviureteric obstruction, ureterovesical obstruction

*ACE: Angiotensin converting enzyme.

In one series of newborns with ARF, sepsis was the most common cause of AKI (30.9%) followed by hypovolemia (18.7%), kidney, ureter and bladder (KUB) anomalies (12.2%), congestive heart failure (12.2%) and birth asphyxia (11.5%).[3]

Some Special Considerations

- A neonate with oliguric ARF, hematuria, hypertension with/without loss of femoral pulses suffers from bilateral renal artery thrombosis. Thrombolysis/thrombectomy is indicated in refractory hypertension in such a neonate.
- Renal venous thromboses should be suspected in any newborn who presents with bilateral flank mass, proteinuria, hematuria with/without oliguria and thrombocytopenia in the presence of a setting like polycythemia, severe dehydration and maternal diabetes.

MANAGEMENT OF ACUTE RENAL FAILURE

Fluid Management

- Fluids must be restricted to replenish insensible water loss (IWL) along with urinary loss. The urinary loss must be replaced volume for volume. The insensible water loss in a term neonate is 25 mL/kg/day. In preterm neonates, this can vary between 40 and100 mL/kg/day depending on gestation, postnatal age, use of radiant warmers, photo-therapy, etc.[8]

- Fluids requirement should be revised based on urine output, weight and assessment of extracellular volume status, preferably every 8 hourly.

- The insensible water losses should be replaced with 5–10% dextrose. The urine output should be replaced volume by volume with N/5 saline.[5]

- During the polyuric phase, hourly monitoring of urine output and serial monitoring of serum electrolytes with appropriate replacement of sodium, potassium and water are indicated to prevent dehydration, hyponatremia and hypokalemia.[1]

ELECTROLYTE DISTURBANCES

Hyponatremia

Babies can have hyponatremia in oliguric renal failure.

Hyponatremia is due to dilution secondary to water reten-tion, hence, has to be corrected with fluid restriction. In most of the cases, there is no sodium deficit.

- If serum sodium is between 120 and 135 mEq/L, restriction of fluids will suffice. Serum sodium must be monitored at least 12 hrly.

- If hyponatremia is associated with symptoms like seizures or if serum sodium is less than 120 mEq/L, it requires prompt correction with 3% hypertonic saline over 2 hours, using the formula:

  Na required (mEq) = [Na desired – Na actual] × body weight (kg) × 0.8

- Hyponatremia unresponsive to above therapy is an indication for dialysis.

- Babies with non-oliguric ARF may have urinary sodium losses of up to 10 mEq/kg/day and these must be replaced.

- Care should be taken not to increase the serum sodium by more than 0.5 mEq/L/h.

Hyperkalemia

Hyperkalemia ($K^+ > 6.5$ mEq/L[1]): It is one of the most dangerous complications of ARF. It results from reduction in glomerular filtration rate, acidosis, immature tubular response to aldosterone and cellular breakdown.

Practical Tip

If hyperkalemia is associated with hypoglycemia, hyponatremia and hypotension, consider a diagnosis of adrenal insufficiency.

- The first step in the management of hyperkalemia is to stop all potassium in the fluids as well as drugs which can accentuate hyperkalemia (indomethacin, ACE inhibitors, potassium sparing diuretics).
- ECG will help in diagnosing cardiac effects of hyperkalemia. If ECG changes are evident, IV calcium gluconate 10% is given. This will decrease the myocardial excitability but will not lower the potassium levels.
- This should immediately be followed by methods to decrease the potassium levels (Table 22.3). Hyperkalemia which is unresponsive to medications is one of the most common indications for instituting dialysis.

Practical Tips[1]

- Saturate the plastic tubing with insulin solution before infusing to the baby.
- Oral administration of resins is associated with the risk of concretions, hypernatremia and fluid overload—avoid in VLBW infants and those with poor peristalsis.
- Salbutamol aerosol may not be very effective in neonates.

Hypocalcemia

Hypocalcemia can develop in babies with ARF due to hyperphosphatemia and skeletal resistance to parathyroid hormone. Symptomatic hypocalcemia should be corrected by infusing 10% calcium gluconate at a dose of 0.5–1 mL/kg over 5–10 min under cardiac monitoring. Also, during the oliguric phase, phosphorus/magnesium administration is to be avoided.

ROLE OF DOPAMINE

At doses less than 5 mEq/L, dopamine acts via DA_1 and DA_2 receptors to increase renal blood flow. But preterm infants are hypersensitive to alpha receptors and hence, even low doses

Table 22.3: Management of hyperkalemia[1]

Level of K+	Medication	Dose	Mechanism/degree of effect	Onset of action
ECG changes suggestive of hyperkalemia	Calcium gluconate (10%)	0.5 to 1 mL/kg over 5–10 min	Modifies myocardial excitability, no decrease in K levels	5–10 min
6.5–7.5 mEq/L	1. Glucose and insulin	0.5 g/kg/h of glucose and 0.1 U/kg/hr infusion of insulin	Intracellular uptake of potassium	30 min
	2. Salbutamol IV infusion	4 µg/kg over 20 min	Intracellular uptake of potassium	30–40 min
More than 6.0 mEq/L	Cation exchange resin (Na/Ca polystyrene sulfonate)	1 g/kg intrarectally q 6 h	Exchange of K for Na or Ca 1 g/kg reduces K levels by 1 mEq/kg	1–2 hrs May take up to 6 hours
More than 7.5 mEq/L	1. Exchange transfusion	Washed RBC reconstituted with 5% albumin	Uptake of K by RBC	Minutes
	2. Peritoneal dialysis	Use a dialysate with low K concentration	Dialysis	Minutes

of dopamine can cause vasoconstriction and raise renal vascular resistance.[9] This may explain the difficulty in dosing of dopamine for improving renal function and therefore dopamine for prevention or treatment of ARF is not recommended.[11,12] Dopamine when combined with furosemide causes natriuresis and diuresis in preterm infants with RDS and oliguria.[10]

Nutrition

- The goal is to provide 100 kcal/kg/day as babies with ARF are catabolic. Proteins or amino acids can be provided in a dose of 1–2 g/kg/day.[13]
- If enteral feeding is possible, breast milk can be used, failing which, low phosphate formula can be given. Caloric density can be increased by adding medium chain triglycerides.
- If the baby is on parenteral nutrition, a central venous catheter may be needed to infuse hypertonic glucose.

Acidosis

Mild metabolic acidosis is common in babies with ARF. If pH is <7.2 and bicarbonate <18 mEq/L, sodium bicarbonate is given in a dose of 1–2 mEq/kg over 3–4 hrs. But monitoring for fluid overload, hypernatremia, intracranial hemorrhage and hypocalcemia is needed. Babies with persistent acidosis require dialysis.

Hypertension

Fluid overload in neonatal ARF can result in hypertension, which can be controlled with fluid restriction and anti-hypertensive agents. The development of severe hypertension in the setting of neonatal ARF should raise the suspicion for renal artery or venous thrombosis.

Commonly used anti-hypertensives in newborns are oral amlodipine (0.1–0.3 mg/kg/dose every 12–24 hourly), enalapril (0.1–0.4 mg/kg/day every 6–12 hourly, with careful monitoring of potassium and renal functions) and intravenous diazoxide (2–5 mg/kg/dose over 5 min every 4–24 hourly).[1]

RENAL REPLACEMENT THERAPY

The indications of renal replacement therapy are:
- Hyperkalemia refractory to medication
- Hyponatremia with volume overload (pulmonary edema, severe hypertension)

- Metabolic acidosis (TCO_2 <16–18 mEq/L)
- Hypocalcemia
- Hyperphosphatemia refractory to therapy
- Inability to provide adequate nutrition due to fluid restriction.

The two mechanisms of renal replacement therapy are ultrafiltration (removal of water) and dialysis (removal of solutes). Dialysis is a process of removal of plasma solutes by diffusion down their concentration gradient across a semi-permeable membrane. Filtration involves removal of protein free plasma across a membrane by convection.

Peritoneal dialysis (PD) catheters: Peritoneal access in most institutes is achieved by a stiff catheter and trocar, but when used beyond 48–72 hours, infection rates are high.[14] Risk of infection and visceral injury is less with soft PD catheters made of silicone polymer of methyl-silicate, either in curled or straight configurations.[15,16]

Most of the catheters have side holes that allow for easy ingress and egress of fluid. Permanent catheters have cuffs. Straight Tenckhoff and coiled catheters are available. Coiled Tenckhoff catheters are useful for chronic dialysis.

Detailed description of drug dose modification in ARF is available in literature.[5]

Procedure

- The first step involves creating a fluid filled reservoir by infusing 20–30 mL/kg dialysate into the peritoneum using a cannula.
- After this, the catheter is inserted into the peritoneal cavity and connected to a three-way cannula. The common sites of insertion are in the midline below the umbilicus, right or left lower quadrant of the abdomen. Urinary bladder must be emptied before insertion of the catheter.
- The dialysate fluid is connected to a pediatric burette set and its terminal end is connected to one of the ports of three-way cannula. The remaining port of the three ways is connected to an intravenous (IV) set, the end of which is let into a sterile container (empty IV fluid bottle).

- The abdomen is filled with 20–30 mL/kg of dialysis fluid infused over 10 min. A dwell time of 20 to 30 min is used before draining the fluid over 10 min. The dwell time can be reduced in case of respiratory compromise.
- A total of 20–40 cycles can be used or it can be continued till the desired effect is obtained.
- Blood sugar, serum electrolytes and blood gas should be monitored every 6 hourly and serum creatinine every 24 hourly. At the end of the procedure, the catheter can be removed and the tip and the fluid are sent for culture.

Dialysate Fluids

- The common dialysate fluid contains 1.7% dextrose with lactate. If higher gradient is required as in case of fluid overload, 3% solution can be used. This can be prepared by adding 25 mL of 50% dextrose to one liter of 1.7% PD fluid.
- In case of liver failure as in asphyxia, lactate free bicarbonate containing fluid has to be used as these babies may be unable to metabolize lactate quickly.

  If baby becomes hypokalemic during the procedure, add one mL of KCl to one liter of dialysate fluid.

Composition of Dialysis Solutions[5]

- Osmotic agent: Dextrose 1.4–3.9 g/dL
- Base: Lactate 35–40 mEq/L or bicarbonate 34 mEq/L
- Sodium 132–134 mEq/L, calcium 1.25–1.75 mM/L
- Magnesium 0.25–0.75 mM/L, chloride 95–103.5 mEq/L

COMPLICATIONS OF PERITONEAL DIALYSIS (PD)

PD is an invasive procedure and the following complications/contraindications need to be remembered:

- The chief complication of PD is peritonitis, the common organisms being coagulase negative Staphylococcus, *S. aureus* and gram-negative bacteria.[5]
- Catheter related bleeding, catheter malfunction, perforation of abdominal viscera, adhesion of catheter tip to omentum.
- Hyperglycemia can occur when higher concentrations of dextrose are used.

- PD cannot be done in babies with necrotizing enterocolitis, babies who underwent abdominal surgery and in those with severe respiratory compromise as it may worsen the abdominal distension.
- Hypothermia must be prevented by using pre-warmed dialysis fluid.
- PD will be less effective in poor cardiac output or gut hypoperfusion.

Hemofiltration and hemodiafiltration are effective in neonates with ARF in whom PD is contraindicated. The complication rates are less. Hemofiltration is particularly useful in the presence of fluid overload, but it needs a vascular access with large sized catheters and adequate mean arterial blood pressure. Hemodiafiltration is more useful in the presence of fluid overload and azotemia with electrolyte disturbances.[2]

Outcome

Non-oliguric renal failure has a better prognosis when compared to oliguric renal failure. Mortality ranges from 25 to 78% in oligoanuric renal failure.[17] Long-term abnormalities in GFR and tubular function are common in babies who survive ARF and is secondary to hyperfiltration in the surviving nephrons.

Follow-up

All babies who develop ARF need follow-up. Adequacy of growth and nutrition, blood pressure and renal function status has to be monitored. Newborns who have had ARF are predisposed to the development of chronic renal failure in the future. Long-term follow-up of extremely low birth weight infants who had neonatal ARF has shown that the risk factors for progression of renal disease at 1 year of age included a random urinary protein/creatinine ratio of greater than 0.6, serum creatinine greater than 0.6 mg/dL and a tendency to obesity with a body mass index greater than the 85th percentile.[18]

REFERENCES

1. Suhas M, Nafday, et al. In Renal Disease—Avery's neonatology pathophysiology and management of newborn, 6th edn. MG MacDonald (Ed); Lippincott Williams & Wilkins, 981–1065.

2. Gouyon JB, Guignard JP. Management of acute renal failure in newborns. Pediatr Nephrol 2000;14:1037–1044.

3. Vachvanichsanong P, McNeil E, Dissaneevate S, Dissaneewate P, Chanvitan P, Janjindamai W. Neonatal acute kidney injury in a tertiary centre in a developing country. Nephrol Dial Transplant 2012;27:973–7.

4. Hentschel R, Lodige B, Bulla M. Renal insufficiency in the neonatal period. Clin Nephrol 1996;46:54–8.

5. Bagga A, Sinha A, Gulati A. Protocols in pediatric nephrology, 1st edn. CBS Publishers and Distributors Pvt Ltd.

6. Thummala MR, Raju TN, Langenberg P. Isolated single umbilical artery anomaly and the risk for congenital malformations: a meta-analysis. J Pediatr Surg 1998;33:580–5.

7. Ishizaki Y, etal, Evaluation of diagnostic criteria of acute renal failure in premature infants. Acta Paediatr Jpn 1983,35:311-315.

8. Chawla D, Agarwal R, Deorari AK, Paul VK. Fluid and electrolyte management in term and preterm neonates. AIIMS-NICU protocols 2008, www.newbornwhocc.org.

9. Seri I. Effects of low dose dopamine infusion on cardiovascular and renal functions cerebral blood flow and plasma cathecolamines levels in sick preterm neonates. Pediatric Res 1993; 34:742–749.

10. Tulassy T, Seri I, Acute oliguria in preterm infants with hyaline membrane disease; interaction of dopamine and furosemide. Acta Pediatr Scand 1986;75:420–424.

11. Barrington K, Brion LP. Dopamine *versus* no treatment to prevent renal dysfunction in indomethacin-treated preterm newborn infants. Cochrane Database of Systematic Reviews 2002, Issue 3. Art. No.:CD003213.

12. Friedrich JO, Adhikari N, Herridge MS. Meta-analysis: Low dose dopamine increases urine output but does not prevent renal dysfunction or death. Ann Intern Med 2005;142:510–24.

13. Philippe SF Jacquelyyn RE, Tivadar T, Seri I. In Acute and chronic renal failure, Avery's diseases of newborn, 8th edn. William

Taeusch, Roberta Ballard, and Christine A (Eds). Gleason, Saunders 2005;1298–1306.

14. Gulati A, Bagga A. Management of acute renal failure in the pediatric intensive care unit. Indian J Pediatr 2011;78:718–25.

15. Coulthard MG, Brayan V, Managing acute renal failure in very low birth weight infants. Arch dis child 1995;73:F187–92.

16. Marsha ML, Annabelle NC, Peter DY. Neonatal peritoneal dialysis. Neo Reviews 2005;.6:e384–91.

17. Chevalier R. Prognostic factors in neonatal acute renal failure. Pediatrics 1984;74:165–272.

18. Annabelle NC, Minnie MS. Acute renal failure management in the neonate. Neo Reviews 2005;6:e369–76.

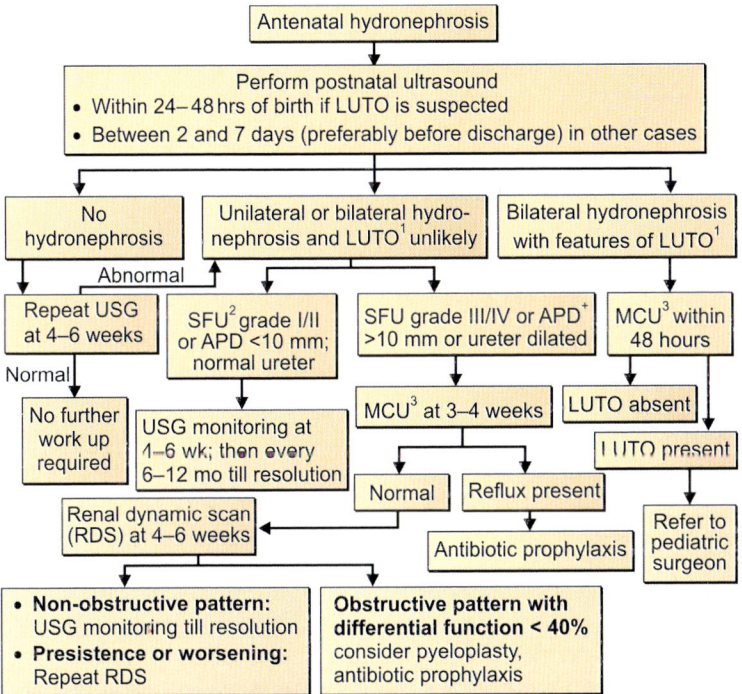

ADP: anterior posterior diameter of renal pelvis; LUTO: lower urinary tract obstruction; MCU: micturating cystourethrogram

[1]LUTO is suggested by bilateral hydroureteronephrosis associated with oligohydramnios and/or bladder wall thickness or dilatation

[2]Society of Fetal Urology (SFU) grading for hydronephrosis: • Grade 0: No splitting of renal pelvis; • Grade I: Urine in pelvis barely splits pelvis; • Grade II: Urine fills intra-renal pelvis $\pm$ urine fills extra-renal major calyces dilated; • Grade III: SFU Gr II and minor calyces uniformly dilated and normal parenchyma; • Grade IV: SFU Gr III and thin parenchyma

[3]All patients planned for MCU should receive antibiotic prophylaxis.

Improving Quality of Care in NICU

INTRODUCTION

A broad based definition of quality is "the degree to which health services for individuals and populations increase the likelihood of desired health outcomes and are consistent with current professional knowledge".[1,2] This has assumed importance as there has been a renewed interest in neonatology and resulted in mushrooming of NICUs across the country. Though there are various perspectives of improving quality of care, the present document aims at focusing on more practical aspects.

MINIMIZING ERRORS

Errors occur at various levels in the unit. They can be broadly classified as follows:

Asepsis Routine

- Not performing optimum hand hygiene in lieu of wearing sterile gloves. Gloves contain many minute pores and hence, it is important that the hand is made sterile before putting on gloves, which is only an additional safety measure.
- Disinfectant solution for hand cleansing should not be used at the first time entry in the NICU or if the hands are obviously soiled, when hand washing needs to be done.
- A check on rate of use of soap/sterile papers/disinfectant solutions, a clock in front of washing area, a CCTV camera, etc. can be adopted to ensure compliance of hand hygiene.

Medication Errors[3–5]

- The common drugs wherein medication errors occur are: narcotics, electrolytes and parenteral nutrition, vasopressors antibiotics, caffeine, albuterol, heparin, furosemide, pheno-barbital.

• Counterchecks on the dose, final concentration of solution and rate of infusion needs to be done at various levels during use of these drugs.

• Improvement of patient identification policies, habit of reading back aloud the orders for medication, writing legible prescriptions, encouraging patients' active participation, identification of all look-alikes, sound-alike medications go a long way in minimizing medication errors.

Equipment Related Errors

• Maintenance of detailed inventory with a regular time table of checks and balances ensure the upkeep of equipment.[6]

• Counter-checking the functionality of equipment with standards is needed to be done regularly. Some of the examples are:
  – Checks on functionality of pop-off valve of an ambu bag.
  – Usage of standardized weights for checking accuracy of weighing machines.
  – Use of oxygen analyzer for checking the FiO_2 delivered.
  – Counter-checks with lab for measures of bilirubin from micro-bilirubinometer, glucose from glucometer and electrolytes from ABG reports.
  – Use of flux meter at different positions under a photo-therapy machine.
  – Maintenance of log time on the use of phototherapy tube lights for its timely replacement.
  – Generation of adequate good quality waveforms on pulse oxymeter.

Pre-analytical Lab Errors

There is an exhaustive list. Some of the commonly encountered scenarios are mentioned in Table 24.1.

OPTIMAL USE OF INVESTIGATIONS

The use of lab/radiological investigations needs to be optimized to avert unnecessary costs and harm to babies. Though its use varies, some of the common areas of improvement are as follows:

Table 24.1: Common sampling errors and pre-analytical variables affecting lab reports

Analysis	Anticipated errors	Effects of error	Corrective measures
Arterial blood sampling for ABG	Excess heparin Less volume Presence of air bubbles Sample not cooled	↓ $PaCO_2$ Wrong reading ↓ $PaCO_2$, ↑ PaO_2 ↑ $PaCO_2$, ↓pH,	Flush heparin in syringe At least 0.6 mL Remove air bubbles Collect in a slush of ice
Serum potassium	Squeezed sample	↑	Free flowing sample
Serum sodium	Small sample volume Lipemic serum (Secondary to TPN)	→ →	Adequate sample Collect fresh sample
Glucose by strip	Use of betadine swab	↑ (Betadine is an oxidizing agent)	Use spirit swab to clean skin and sample after dry
Glucose by lab	Prolonged waiting time, wrong vial for sample collection	→	Avoid delay in transport
CSF Study	Prolonged waiting time Traumatic tap	↓ CSF glucose Degeneration of cells CSF culture sterility ↑ Cell count and protein levels	Avoid delay in transport Bedside direct culture on plate Proper technique Use appropriate diluents for sufficient time for RBC lysis
Bilirubin estimation	Prolonged exposure to ambient light/waiting time	→	Avoid delay in estimation/transport

Contd...

Table 24.1: Common sampling errors and pre-analytical variables affecting lab reports *(Contd....)*

Analysis	Anticipated errors	Effects of error	Corrective measures
PCV by capillary	Inadequate centrifuge time	↑	10,000 rpm for 3 minutes
Urine electrolyte analysis by ABG machine	Improper dilution	↑	Dilute specimen as recommended
FeNa estimation	Prior furosemide administration	↑	Avoid prior diuretic administration
Micro ESR	Coexisting anemia	↑	To be reported with PCV
Blood culture	Less volume	False negative report	At least 1 ml of blood
	Improper technique	Contaminant/commensal growth	Sterile technique for sample collection
Serum creatinine	High maternal levels	↑	To be reported
Thyroid hormone assay	Samples taken postnatally till day 3rd of life	↑	Either cord blood samples or after 72 hrs of life
Blood sample karyotyping/ chromosomal studies	Presence of sepsis/unsterile technique	Poor yield	Sterile technique for sample collection

- Routine use of X-rays to check position of endotracheal tubes after intubation is unnecessary and increases costs of care.
- Micro-sampling needs to be practiced and multiple tests such as micro-ESR, serum bilirubin estimation, CRP, PCV, VBG and blood sugar can be done in a single setting.

STANDARD OPERATING PROCEDURES

Standard operating procedures (SOPs) incorporate the best clinical practices.[7] Such SOPs need to be laid down for commonly done practices such as neonatal transport, use of CPAP, surfactant administration, long lines insertion, peripheral IV line insertion, parenteral nutrition, preparation for receipt of a high risk neonate in the NICU, etc.

Such SOPs should have predictable use of bundles of consumables and personnel, so that all the members of the team are on same grid of working.

POLICIES

Having NICU protocols and policies based on current best evidence should be in place. They can include various aspects such as various protocols mentioned in the book, besides policies such as breastfeeding, pain control, developmentally supportive care, kangaroo mother care, discharge of high risk babies, antibiotic use, antibiotic cycling, surveillance cultures of units, golden first minute management.

DOCUMENTATION/ACCOUNTING

Prompt and timely documentation of census, patient parameters, equipment use, iatrogenic complications, medication errors, sepsis rates, perinatal statistics, indents, log book maintenance of residents working, log books of the equipment in use, etc. would go in a long way in maintaining continuum of research, calculating costs of care and self improvement.

A paperless approach based on tailor-made software would be of immense help.

REFERENCES

1. Lohr K. Medicare: A Strategy for Quality Assurance. Washington, DC: National Academy Press; 1990.

2. Kohn L, Corrigan J, Donaldson M. To err is human: building a safer health system. Institute of Medicine. Washington, DC: National Academy Press; 2000.

3. National Coordinating Council for Medication Error Reporting and Prevention Taxonomy of Medication Errors, Copyright 1998. Available at: http://www.nccmerp.org/pdf/taxo 2001;07–31.pdf. Accessed September 18, 2007.

4. Walsh KE, Kaushal R, Chessare JB. How to avoid paediatric medication errors: a user's guide to the literature. Arch Dis Child 2005;90(7):698–702.

5. Stavroudis TA, Miller MR, Lehmann CU. Medication Errors in Neonates. Clin Perinatol 2008;35:141–161.

6. Deorari AK, Paul VK. Neonatal equipment: everything you would like to know. 4th edn. Sagar Publications 2010.

7. Deorari AK, Paul VK, Scotland J, Singhal N, McMillan D. Practical Procedures for the newborn nursery: a manual for physicians and nurses. 3rd edn. Sagar Publications 2010.

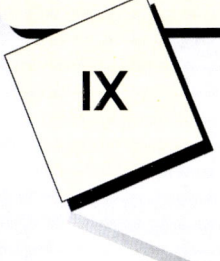

Therapies and Diagnostic Modalities

IX

Continuous positive airway pressure (CPAP), often thought to be the 'missing link' between supplemental oxygen and mechanical ventilation, is gaining immense popularity in neonatal intensive care units (NICU). Being technically simple, inexpensive and effective, it has become the primary mode of respiratory support in very preterm infants admitted in NICUs. The evidence, clinical studies and the controversies regarding its use have been extensively reviewed and are not discussed here.[1,2] This protocol deals mainly with the practical aspects of CPAP administration in neonates.

DEFINITION AND BACKGROUND

CPAP refers to the application of positive pressure to the airway of a spontaneously breathing infant throughout the respiratory cycle.

The first clinical use of CPAP was reported by Gregory et al in a landmark report in 1971. They described the use of CPAP via endotracheal tube or a head box in preterm infants with respiratory distress syndrome (RDS).[3] Shortly after this, Kattwinkel reported successful use of nasal prongs to provide CPAP in these infants.[4] After the initial enthusiasm, it gradually fell out of favor in 1980s because of the advent of newer modes of ventilation (such as high frequency ventilation) and the perceived complications of CPAP (such as air leak). However, reports of significantly lower incidence of chronic lung disease (CLD) from a neonatal unit in Columbia University, that used more CPAP (Hudson prongs) as compared to other North American Centers have led to a resurgence of interest in CPAP over the past 15 years.[5]

CPAP: How does it Work

CPAP predominantly helps by preventing collapse of the alveoli with marginal stability. Preterm infants have difficulty in establishing and maintaining lung volumes due to surfactant deficiency, muscle hypotonia, slow clearance of lung fluid and a compliant chest wall. CPAP results in recruitment of alveoli, thus increasing the functional residual capacity (FRC) and hence prevents alveolar collapse.

Components of CPAP System

The components of a CPAP system are:
1. Gas source: To provide continuous supply of warm humidified and blended gases, i.e. air and oxygen.
2. Pressure generator: To create the positive pressure in the circuit.
3. Patient interface/delivery system: To connect the CPAP circuit to the infant's airway.

DEVICES USED FOR PRESSURE GENERATION

The pressure sources of CPAP can be broadly grouped into:[6]
1. Continuous flow devices
2. Variable flow devices (Fig. 25.1)

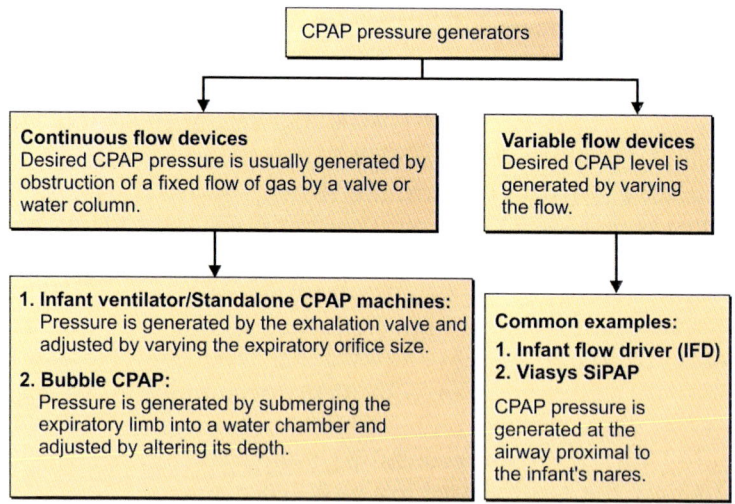

Fig. 25.1: Types of CPAP devices

Continuous Flow (Bubble) CPAP: A typical bubble CPAP setup is shown in Panel 2. One has to remember that though classified as a continuous flow device, flow may still need to be adjusted to maintain continuous bubbling in the water chamber and thus the required level of CPAP.

Variable Flow CPAP: A typical example is the *Infant flow driver (IFD)*. It uses the *Bernoulli effect* via dual injector jets directed towards each nasal prong to maintain a constant pressure. If the infant requires more inspiratory flow, the venturi action of the injector jets entrains additional flow. When the infant makes a spontaneous expiratory effort, there is a 'fluidic flip' that causes the flow from the injector limb to flip around and to leave the generator chamber via the expiratory limb (*Coanda effect*). So, unlike the other methods of CPAP where the infant has to exhale against the incoming gas flow, the 'fluidic flip' of the variable flow devices assists in exhalation thereby reducing the work of breathing.

The advantages and disadvantages of each of these methods are given in Table 25.1.

DEVICES USED FOR CPAP DELIVERY (PATIENT INTERFACE)

Various devices used for CPAP delivery include:
1. Nasal prongs (single/double or bi-nasal)
2. Long (or) nasopharyngeal prongs
3. Nasal cannula
4. Nasal masks (Fig. 25.2).

⎫ Commonly
⎬ used
⎭

Face mask, endotracheal tube and head box are no longer used for CPAP delivery in neonates. Endotracheal CPAP is not recommended because it has been found to increase the work of breathing (as the infant has to breathe 'through a straw').

The advantages and disadvantages of each of these methods have been summarized in Table 25.2.

INDICATIONS FOR CPAP

The common clinical indications of CPAP have been listed in Panel 1.

Table 25.1: A comparison of CPAP devices used for pressure generation[7]

Devices	Examples	Advantages	Disadvantages	Remarks
Conventional ventilator derived CPAP	Bear Cub, Bird-VIP, Draeger Baby log, Newport, Sechrist, Siemens, SLE, etc.	• No need of a separate equipment • Can be easily switched over to mechanical ventilation, if CPAP fails	• Expensive • Standard flow of 5–8L/min may be insufficient in the presence of high leak • Difficult to know if the set flow is sufficient or not (insufficient flow can lead to increased WOB)	Of practical utility in units having ventilators but not so in a small hospital/nursing home without a neonatal ventilator.
Standalone CPAP machines (Indigenous CPAP)	Lectromedik, Meditrin, Phoenix, Shreeyash, Zeal	• Economical • Useful for small hospitals • Can have bubble CPAP option	• Most of them do not have proper blenders and/or pressure manometer • Flow has to be altered to ensure proper bubbling • It is difficult to detect high flow which can lead to over distension of the lungs	Though inexpensive, they have not been tested adequately; niggling issues observed during daily use
Bubble CPAP	Indian: Mediserve, Meditrin Imported: Fisher and Paykel	• Simple and inexpensive • Oscillations produced by continuous bubbling might contribute to gas exchange (akin to HFV) • Can identify large leaks at the nares (bubbling stops)		oscillations delivered at the nares are transmitted up to the alveoli. Still, the standalone option makes it an easy and cost effective proposition in developing countries.
Variable flow devices	Arabella, IFD, Viasys SiPAP	• Maintains more uniform pressure • Might decrease the WOB • Recruits lung volume more effectively	• Expensive • Requires more technical expertise	On theoretical grounds, this device scores more than the other two. However, the prohibitive cost and the lack of evidence regarding its superiority preclude its widespread use.

(WOB: work of breathing; HFV: high frequency ventilation; IFD: infant flow driver)

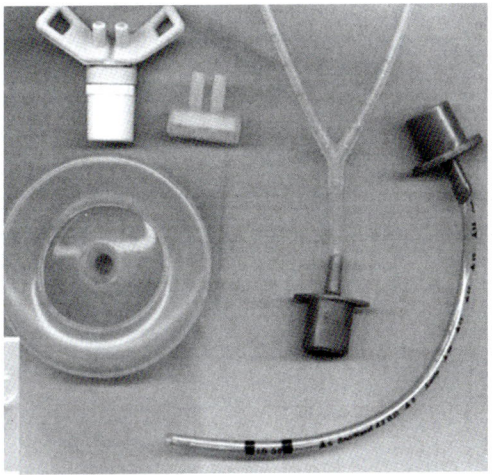

Fig. 25.2: CPAP delivery systems

Panel 1: Common Indications

1. Respiratory distress syndrome (RDS)
2. Apnea of prematurity (especially obstructive apnea)
3. Post-extubation in preterm VLBW infants
4. Transient tachypnea of newborn (TTNB)/delayed adaptation

Other indications

1. Pneumonia
2. Meconium aspiration/other aspiration syndromes
3. Pulmonary edema/pulmonary hemorrhage
4. Laryngomalacia/tracheomalacia/bronchomalacia

Practically, CPAP is very useful in preterm (<35 weeks) infants with respiratory distress of any etiology. Some of these indications have been briefly described below:

1. *RDS:* The most common indication for CPAP is mild to moderate RDS where it helps by preventing collapse of alveoli with marginal stability. The recruitment of more alveoli helps to increase the FRC, thus helping in better oxygenation (Fig. 25.1). Numerous studies have proved its efficacy in reducing the need for mechanical ventilation and probably the incidence of chronic lung disease in infants with RDS.[10,11] Recently, a multi-centric study on CPAP versus intubation and ventilation at 5 minutes of age in infants born at 25–28 weeks' gestation found significant reduction in the

Table 25.2: Advantages and disadvantages of common CPAP delivery systems

Devices	Advantages	Disadvantages	Remarks
Nasal prongs (single-/bi-nasal) Example: • Argyle • Hudson • IFD prongs	• Simple device • Lower resistance leads to greater transmission of pressure • Mouth leak acts like a 'pop-off' mechanism	• Relatively difficult to fix • Risk of trauma to nasal septum and turbinates • Leak through mouth means end expiration pressure is variable	Studies have shown that they are more effective than naso-pharyngeal prongs in post-extubation settings[8]
Nasopharyngeal prongs (e.g. using a cut endotracheal tube) Length is estimated by measuring the distance from the earlobe to the tip of the chin or nose; Tube placement is confirmed by direct visualization of the tip behind the uvula	• Easy availability • Economical • More secure fixation	• More easily blocked by secretions • Likely to get kinked	Though economical and are easily available, they are found to be inferior to short bi-nasal prongs[8]
Nasal cannulae (with an outer diameter of 3 mm and flows up to 2 L/min)	Ease of application	• Unreliable pressure delivery • FiO_2 delivered may be high • Large leaks around the cannula	• Mainly tried in apnea of prematurity—paucity of data in other conditions[9] • Still experimental
Nasal masks	Minimal nasal trauma	Difficulty in obtaining an adequate seal	New generation masks are yet to be studied in detail

(IFD, infant flow driver)
In our unit, we use short bi-nasal prongs for delivering CPAP (both ventilator and bubble CPAP).

need for oxygen at 28 days of life although this benefit did not extend to the need for oxygen at 36 weeks PMA.[12]

The beneficial effect of CPAP in preterm infants could be enhanced by administering early surfactant. In this approach, if respiratory distress progresses even after initiating CPAP, the baby is intubated, given surfactant *and* then extubated and put back on CPAP again. Known as INSURE (**In**tubation-**Sur**factant-**Ex**tubation), this approach might further reduce the need for subsequent ventilation and improve the outcome in extreme preterm infants.[13] *We routinely employ INSURE technique for babies born after 27 weeks' gestation and requiring surfactant therapy.*

2. *Apnea of prematurity:* CPAP is typically used when clinically significant episodes of apnea occur despite optimal methylxanthine therapy.

3. *Post-extubation in VLBW infants:* CPAP reduces the incidence of apnea, respiratory acidosis and increased oxygen requirement in VLBW infants extubated after a period of mechanical ventilation.

4. *Delayed adaptation/TTNB:* In this condition associated with excess lung fluid, CPAP helps by maintaining the lung expansion. Though useful in premature infants, it is not tolerated by most term and near-term neonates with TTNB

5. *Pneumonia:* CPAP can be tried in stable infants with mild to moderate respiratory distress due to pneumonia. It helps in this condition by maintaining the lung expansion preventing any collapse due to fluids and secretions.

6. *Meconium aspiration syndrome:* Use of CPAP is contro-versial in this condition as most of these infants would already have hyper-expanded lung fields. Moreover, they are unlikely to tolerate CPAP well. CPAP is only indicated in a rare infant with predominant collapse/atelectasis in the chest X-ray.

We use CPAP predominantly in preterm infants (<35 weeks and birth weight <1800 g) with respiratory distress, apnea of prematurity, delayed adaptation and pneumonia; also, we extubate VLBW infants to CPAP routinely. We occasionally use CPAP in near-term and term infants with TTNB and pneumonia.

CONTRAINDICATIONS OF CPAP

The important contraindications for CPAP include:

1. Progressive respiratory failure with $PaCO_2$ levels >60 mmHg and/or inability to maintain oxygenation (PaO_2 <50 mmHg)
2. Congenital malformations of the airway (choanal atresia, cleft palate, tracheo-esophageal fistula, congenital diaphragmatic hernia, etc.)
3. Severe cardiovascular instability (hypotension)
4. Poor respiratory drive that is not improved by CPAP.

GUIDELINES FOR CPAP THERAPY

When to Initiate CPAP

Early CPAP: It is important to note that CPAP helps mainly by *preventing* the alveolar collapse in infants with surfactant deficiency. Once atelectasis and collapse have occurred, CPAP might not help much. Therefore, all preterm infants (< 35 weeks' gestation) with any sign of respiratory distress (tachypnea/chest indrawing/grunting) should be started immediately on CPAP.

Prophylactic CPAP: Extending the logic behind early CPAP, some have advocated the use of prophylactic CPAP (before the onset of respiratory distress) in preterm VLBW infants as majority of them would eventually develop respiratory distress. However, there is no evidence for any additional benefit with this approach; indeed, there are concerns regarding increased adverse effects such as intraventricular hemorrhage. Hence, prophylactic CPAP is NOT recommended at present.[14]

How to Set-up a CPAP Apparatus

The steps in setting-up a bubble CPAP are summarized in Panel 2.

How to Fix the CPAP Delivery System (Nasal Cannula)

The most difficult aspect of using nasal CPAP is the positioning and fixation of the patient interface. The optimal technique of fixation depends on the type of delivery system used; the exact technique used does not matter as long as the device is secure and not traumatizing.

Short bi-nasal prongs: It is important to choose the appropriate sized prong that snugly fits in the nasal cavity to avoid a

Panel 2: Steps of Initiation and Nursing Care during CPAP[7]

A. How to Set-up a Bubble CPAP

1. Connect the air and oxygen tubing (pressurized gases from either central manifold or from compressor and oxygen cylinder, respectively).
2. Attach both to the air-oxygen blender.
3. Set the flow using flow meter (usually at 5–8 L/min).
4. Set-up the inspiratory limb:
   a. From the flow meter to the humidifier, and
   b. From the humidifier to the patient end (e.g. nasal cannula); fill water in the humidifier and humidify the gases to 34–37°C.
5. Set-up the expiratory limb from the patient end to a chamber filled with sterile water. Immerse it under the water up to the required depth (which is determined by the intended pressure—e.g. to deliver 5 cm H_2O, immerse up to 5 cm mark in the tube).
6. Attach a pressure manometer at the patient end.
7. Set required pressure and FiO_2, low pressure alarm and apnea alarm.

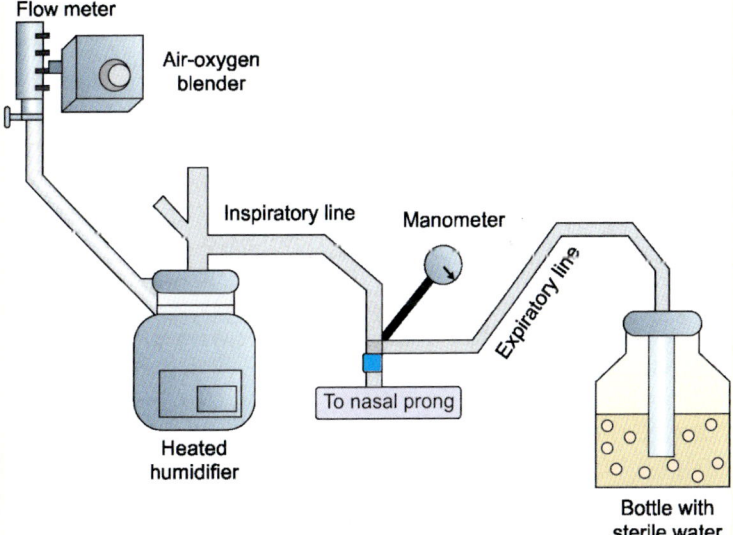

Flow meter

Air-oxygen blender

Inspiratory line

Manometer

Expiratory line

To nasal prong

Heated humidifier

Bottle with sterile water

8. Occlude the patient end of the ventilator circuit with your palm and observe if:
   a. Bubbling occurs in the water chamber—If there are no bubbles, look for any leak in the circuit. If no leak is found, increase the flow by 1 L/min and recheck.
   b. The set pressure is delivered (see the manometer reading)—If it is less than the set pressure, look for any leaks in the circuit/around the cannula. If no leak is found, increase the flow and recheck.

B. **Initiation of CPAP**
 1. Place a roll under infants' shoulder to slightly extend the neck.
 2. Application of prongs:
    a. Choose the correct size prong (the prongs should fill the nasal opening without stretching the skin).
    b. Apply a thin strip of *Tegaderm* on overlying skin of septum.
    c. Place the prongs with the curve downwards and fix as shown in Fig. 25.3.
 3. Attach the patient end of the ventilator circuit to the cannula.
 4. Attach a pulse-oximeter to the infant.

C. **Nursing Care**
 1. Monitor the infant frequently (*see text*); observe if the baby is comfortable.
 2. Pass an orogastric tube. Keep the proximal end of tube open. If the infant is being fed while on CPAP, close the tube for half an hour after giving feeds and keep it open for the next 90 minutes (if fed 2 hourly).
 3. Do regular but gentle nasal suction to clear the mucus 4 hourly or as and when required.
 4. Clean the nasal cannula and check its patency once per shift.
 5. Change the infant's position regularly every 2–4 hours and check the skin condition frequently for redness and sores.

significant leak. However, to avoid causing any injury, it should be fixed straight and not pressed hard against the nasal septum.

We use a modified cap (made from adult cotton socks) and tapes to secure the bi-nasal prongs (Fig. 25.3).

Steps of Initiation and Nursing Care before and during CPAP

The steps of initiation and nursing care during CPAP therapy are given in Panel 2.

Protocol for CPAP Therapy

Table 25.3 outlines the protocol for CPAP therapy in the three most common neonatal conditions.

MONITORING WHILE ON CPAP

The following parameters need to be monitored while the infant is on CPAP:
1. Continuous monitoring of respiratory rate, heart rate, SpO_2
2. Serial monitoring of
    a. Severity of respiratory distress by using Downe's or Silverman score

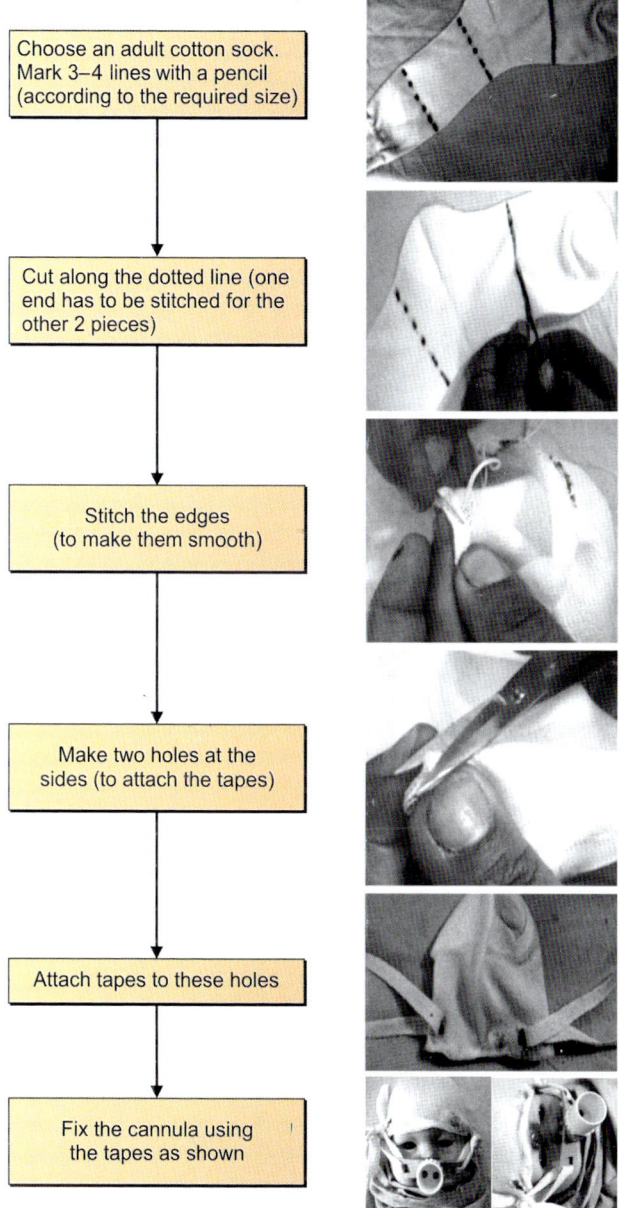

Choose an adult cotton sock. Mark 3–4 lines with a pencil (according to the required size)

Cut along the dotted line (one end has to be stitched for the other 2 pieces)

Stitch the edges (to make them smooth)

Make two holes at the sides (to attach the tapes)

Attach tapes to these holes

Fix the cannula using the tapes as shown

Fig. 25.3: Steps in fixation of CPAP nasal cannula

Table 25.3: Protocol for CPAP therapy in the three common neonatal conditions

	Indications		
	RDS	Apnea of prematurity	Post extubation
How to initiate CPAP?			
Pressure	• Start at 5 cm H_2O	• Start at 4 cm H_2O	• Start at 4–5 cm H_2O
FiO_2	• 0.4 to 0.5 (titrate based on SpO_2)	• 0.21–0.4 (as decided)	• 0.05 to 0.1 above the pre-extubation FiO_2
What to do if there is no improvement?			
Pressure	• Increase in steps of 1–2 cm H_2O to reach a maximum of 7–8 cm H_2O	• Increase up to 5 cm H_2O (further increase is not warranted usually in this condition—may lead to hyperinflation)	• Increased in steps of 1–2 cm H_2O to reach a maximum of 7–8 cm H_2O
FiO_2	• Increase in steps of 0.05 (if oxygenation is still compromised) up to a maximum of 0.8	• FiO_2 increase does not help much	• Increase in steps of 0.05 to a maximum of 0.8
Failure of CPAP	Worsening respiratory distress, as indicated by Silverman scoring and/or hypoxemia (PaO_2 <50 mm Hg)/hypercarbia ($PaCO_2$ >60 mmHg) despite CPAP pressure of 7–8 cm H_2O and FiO_2 of 0.8 (*Likely to occur in infants with severe RDS, associated sepsis and in ELBW infants who have not received ANS*)[18]	Recurrent episodes of apnea requiring PPV (*Likely to occur in infants with central apnea and apnea secondary to sepsis/pneumonia*)	Same as for RDS (*Likely to occur in ELBW infants in sepsis/pneumonia, PDA, metabolic acidosis and collapse*)
Weaning from CPAP			
• When to wean	• When there is no respiratory distress and SpO_2/blood gases are normal	• No episodes of apnea/desaturation/bradycardia for at least 12–24 hrs	• Same as RDS
• How to wean	• Reduce FiO_2 in steps of 0.05 to 0.4, then decrease pressure in steps of 1–2 cm H_2O until 3–4 cm H_2O (infants clinical condition will guide the speed of weaning)	• Same as for RDS	

b. Arterial blood gases (ABGs)

c. Perfusion—CFT, BP, peripheral pulses, urine output

d. Abdominal girth

The **target** saturation and blood gases during CPAP therapy are: **SpO_2—90–95%; PaO_2—50 to 70 mmHg; $PaCO_2$—45 to 50 mmHg.**

HAZARDS/COMPLICATIONS OF CPAP

CPAP though less invasive and generally safer than IMV, is not free of side effects.

1. Pulmonary air leaks are probably the most important clinically significant adverse effect of CPAP.[15] It occurs following over distension of the lungs caused by inappropriately high pressures. They tend to occur when the lung compliance starts improving and the oxygen requirements also show a reduction. One has to note that the two recent trials on CPAP for RDS have shown either a trend or a definite increase in the incidence of pneumothorax.[12,16] Therefore, extra vigilance is required during CPAP therapy.

2. Decreased cardiac output due to reduction in the venous return decreased right ventricular stroke volume and altered dispensability of left ventricle.[17] This effect can be minimized by using optimal CPAP and achieving adequate intravascular volume.

3. Impedance of pulmonary blood flow with increased pulmonary vascular resistance (with inappropriately high CPAP pressure).

4. Gastric distension and 'CPAP belly syndrome'. These complications are rarely seen nowadays. The risk is further minimized by routine use of orogastric tube.

5. Nasal irritation, damage to the septal mucosa or skin damage and necrosis from the fixing devices.

REFERENCES

1. Sankar MJ, Deorari AK. CPAP—A gentler mode of ventilation. J Neonatol 2007;21:160–5.

2. Upadhyay A, Deorari AK. Continuous positive airway pressure-a gentler approach to ventilation. Indian Pediatr 2004;41:459–69.

3. Gregory GA, Kitterman JA, Phibbs RH, et al. Treatment of idiopathic respiratory distress syndrome with continuous positive airway pressure. N Engl J Med 1971;284:333–40.

4. Kattwinkel J, Nearman HS, Fanaroff AA, Katona PG, Klaus MH. Apnea of prematurity. Comparative therapeutic effects of cutaneous stimulation and nasal continuous positive airway pressure. J Pediatr 1975;86:588–92.

5. Avery ME, Tooley WH, Keller JP, et al. Is chronic lung disease in low birth weight infants preventable? A survey of eight centers. Pediatrics 1987;79:26–30.

6. Courtney SE, Barrington KJ. Continuous positive airway pressure and non-invasive ventilation. Clin Perinatol. 2007;34:73–92.

7. Continuous positive airway pressure machines. In: Deorari AK, Paul VK (Eds). Neonatal Equipment. 3rd edn. New Delhi: Sagar Publications 2006;p. 129–37.

8. De Paoli AG, Davis PG, Faber B, Morley CJ. Devices and pressure sources for administration of nasal continuous positive airway pressure (NCPAP) in preterm neonates. Cochrane Database of Syst Rev 2002;CD002977.

9. Sreenan C, Lemke RP, Hudson-Mason A, et al. High-flow nasal cannulae in the management of apnea of prematurity: a comparison with conventional nasal continuous positive airway pressure. Pediatrics 2001;107:1081–3.

10. Gittermann MK, Fusch C, Gittermann AR, Regazzoni BM, Moessinger AC. Early nasal continuous positive airway pressure treatment reduces need for intubation in very low birth infants. Eur J Pediatr 1997;156:384–8.

11. Poets CF, Sens B. Changes in intubation rates and outcome of VLBW—population based study. Pediatrics 1996;98:24–7.

12. Morley CJ, Davis PG, Doyle LW, Brion LP, Hascoet JM, Carlin JB. COIN Trial Investigators. Nasal CPAP or intubation at birth for very preterm infants. N Engl J Med 2008;358:700–8.

13. Verder H, Robertson B, Greisen G, Ebbesen F, Albertsen P, Lundstron JT. Surfactant therapy and nasal continuous positive airway pressure for newborns with respiratory distress syndrome. Danish-Swedish Multicentre Study Group. N Engl J Med 1994; 331:1051–5.

14. Subramaniam P, Henderson-Smart DJ, Davis PG. Prophylactic nasal continuous positive airways pressure for preventing morbidity and mortality in very preterm infants. Cochrane Database of Syst Rev 2005;CD001243.

15. Hall RT, Rhodes PG: Pneumothorax and pneumomediastinum in infants with idiopathic respiratory distress syndrome receiving CPAP. Pediatrics 1975;55:493.

16. Buckmaster AG, Arnolda G, Wright IM, Foster JP, Henderson-Smart DJ. Continuous positive airway pressure therapy for infants with respiratory distress in non tertiary care centers: a randomized, controlled trial. Pediatrics 2007;120:509–18.

17. Tittley JG, Fremes SE, Weisel RD, Christakis GT, Evans PJ, Madonik MM, et al. Hemodynamic and myocardial metabolic consequences of PEEP. Chest 1985;88:496–502.

18. Pillai MS, Sankar MJ, Mani K, Agarwal R, Paul VK, Deorari AK. Clinical prediction score for nasal CPAP failure in pre-term VLBW neonates with early onset respiratory distress. J Trop Pediatr 2011;57:274–9.

26   Kangaroo Mother Care

Kangaroo mother care (KMC) is a method of care of preterm or low birth weight (LBW) infants by placing them in skin-to-skin (STS) contact with mother or other caregiver in order to ensure optimum growth and development of the infant.[1-4] Initially devised as an alternative to conventional technology-based care, KMC is now considered as a standard of care for LBW infants for all settings as an adjunct or alternative to conventional technology-based care.

Benefits of KMC: What is Evidence?[5]

A Cochrane review on benefits of KMC demonstrated that:
- Improved exclusive breastfeeding rates at discharge (RR 1.21; 95% CI, 1.08–1.36), at 1–3 months of (RR 1.20; 95% CI: 1.01–1.43) and a trend towards improved rates at 6–12 months (RR 1.29; 95% CI 0.95–1.76)
- Reduction in the risk of mortality (seven trials, 1614 infants; RR 0.60; 95% CI 0.39–0.93;)
- Reduction in nosocomial infection/sepsis (RR 0.42, 95% CI 0.24 to 0.73)
- Reduction in hypothermia (RR 0.23, 95% CI 0.10 to 0.55)
- Reduction in length of hospital stay (mean difference 2.4 days, 95% CI 0.7 to 4.1)

COMPONENTS OF KMC[6-8]

Kangaroo Position

The kangaroo position consists of skin-to-skin contact (SSC) between the mother and the infant in a vertical position, between the mother's breasts. The provider must keep herself in a semi-reclining position to avoid the gastric reflux in the infant. The kangaroo position is maintained until the infant no longer tolerates it—as indicated by sweating in the baby or baby refusing to stay in KMC position. When continuous care is not possible, the kangaroo position can be used intermittently, providing the proven emotional and breastfeeding promotion benefits. The kangaroo position must be offered for as long as possible (but at least 1–2 hr/sitting).

Kangaroo Nutrition

Kangaroo nutrition is to provide exclusive breastfeeding or breast milk feeding.

Kangaroo Discharge and Follow-up

Early home discharge in the kangaroo position from the neonatal unit is one of the original components of the KMC intervention. Mothers at home require adequate support and follow-up, hence, a follow-up program and access to emergency services must be ensured.

KMC IN DIFFERENT SETTINGS

KMC may be used in three different scenarios:

No Specialized Care for LBW Neonates

LBW infants born at home or at first level health facility with no specialized care and no possibility of being transferred to a proper healthcare unit can be provided KMC as the sole modality of care. In such cases, KMC including skin-to-skin contact, breastfeeding and the best possible health care follow-up represent the best available means for survival of non-sick preterm infants.

Specialized Care but Limited Resources

Here, KMC represents an effective alternative to technology-based care, which allows better utilization of available resources.

Specialized Care and Adequate Resources

KMC is used as an adjunct to technology-based care to establish healthy bonding between mother and infant and to increase the breastfeeding rates. The intermittent kangaroo position in hospital is the most widely used component in such a setting.

REQUIREMENTS FOR KMC IMPLEMENTATION[6–8]

KMC is feasible everywhere as it does not require any equipment. The requirements of KMC are as follows:

Appropriate Health Facility

a. The health facility (the hospital or the neonatal ward) should allow entry of the parents in the neonatal unit at all times.
b. A room near to or at the neonatal unit, furnished with comfortable seats for the mothers, is needed for KMC practice and for education of mothers and families.
c. Reclining chairs in the nursery and postnatal wards, and beds with adjustable back rest should be arranged.
d. Mother can also provide KMC sitting on an ordinary chair or in a semi-reclining posture on a bed with the help of pillows. Make sure mother is not lying flat in the bed.

Appropriate Supporting Staff and Professionals

a. The presence of a nurse available full time, trained in assisting mothers in KMC is indispensable.
b. Staff should receive adequate training on KMC including nutrition of LBW infants. Additional training is needed in expression and storage of breast milk, using alternate methods of feeding and monitoring of growth of LBW infants. The training may best be done by exposing them to units already practicing KMC.
c. Educational material such as information sheets, posters and video films on KMC in local language should be available to the mothers, families and the community.

Good Quality Follow-up

a. Early discharge in kangaroo position should not be attempted if adequate and appropriate follow-up cannot be ensured.
b. KMC should be provided as an in-hospital activity, allowing mothers and infants to stay together for as long as needed.

Institutional, Social and Community Support

a. The requirement for a successful KMC program can be summarized in three words: communication, sensitivity and education.
b. Apart from supporting the mother, family members should also be encouraged to provide KMC when mother takes rest.
c. Mother would need her family's cooperation to deal with her conventional responsibilities of household chores.
d. Community awareness about the benefits should be created.

ELIGIBILITY OF KMC [6-8]

Baby

All stable LBW babies are eligible for KMC. However, sick and very small babies (<1200 g) needing special care should be cared under radiant warmer initially. KMC should be started after the baby is hemodynamically stable. Short KMC sessions can be initiated during recovery with ongoing medical treatment (IV fluids, oxygen therapy). KMC can be provided while the baby is being fed via orogastric tube or on oxygen therapy. Figure 26.1 shows the timing of KMC initiation for different birth weight categories.

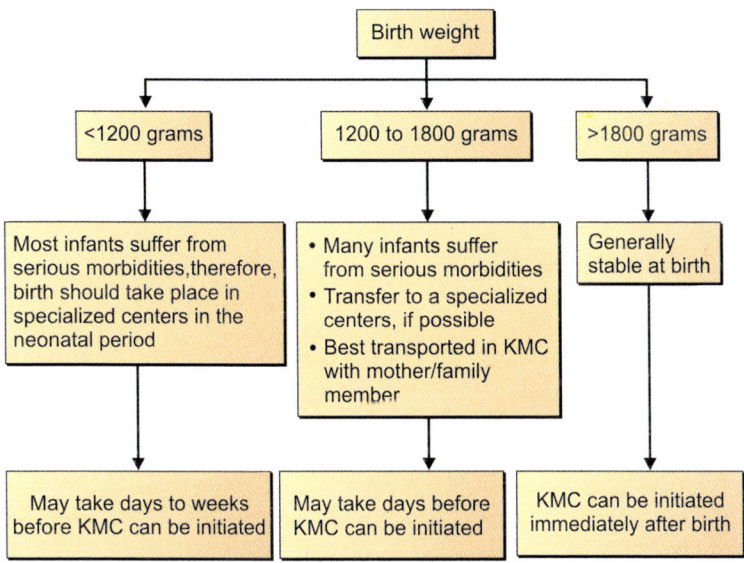

Fig. 26.1: Timing of KMC initiation for different birth-weight categories

Mother

All mothers can provide KMC, irrespective of age, parity, education, culture and religion.[6]

The following points must be taken into consideration when counseling on KMC:

1. **Willingness:** The mother must be willing to provide KMC. Healthcare providers should counsel and motivate her.

2. **General health and nutrition:** The mother should be free from serious illness to be able to provide KMC. She should receive adequate diet and supplements.

3. **Hygiene:** The mother should maintain good hygiene: Daily bath/sponging, change of clothes, hand washing, short and clean finger nails.

INITIATION OF KMC

Counseling

a. When baby is ready for KMC, arrange a time that is convenient to the mother and her baby.

b. Demonstrate to her the KMC procedure in a caring way. Answer her queries and allay her anxieties.

c. Encourage her to bring her mother/mother-in-law, husband or any other member of the family.

d. It helps in building positive attitude of the family and ensuring family support to the mother which is particularly crucial for post-discharge home-based KMC.[8]

e. It is helpful if the mother starting KMC interacts with other families practicing KMC.

Mother's Clothing

a. Mother can wear any front-open dresses as per local culture. This may include a sari, a blouse, a front-open gown, a suit or a simple shirt (Fig. 26.2).

b. KMC can be done with special apparel (such as KEM bag or AIIMS KMC jacket) designed to suit the needs of mothers.

c. Any other suitable apparel that can retain the baby for extended period of time can be adapted locally.

Baby's Clothing

Baby is dressed with cap, socks, nappy and front-open sleeveless shirt.

KMC PROCEDURE[6-8]

Kangaroo Positioning (Fig. 26.3)

a. The baby should be placed between the mother's breasts in an upright position.

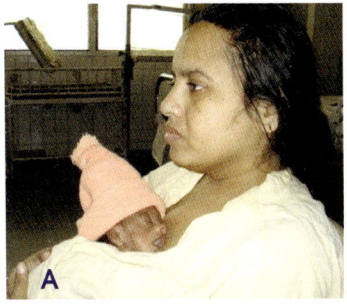 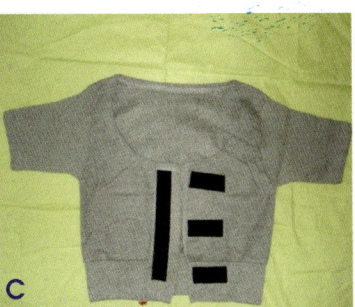

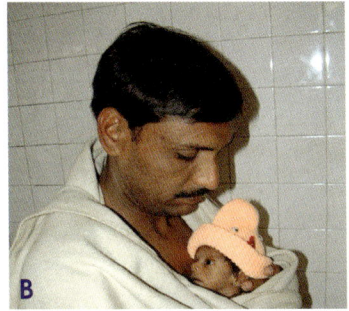 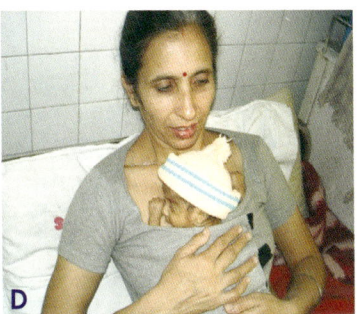

Fig. 26.2: Mother (A) and father (B) practicing KMC in front-open gown and shawl. AIIMS KMC jacket (C) and mother performing KMC using AIIMS KMC jacket (D)

b. The head should be turned to one side and in a slightly exten-ded position. This slightly extended head position keeps the airway open and allows eye-to-eye contact between the mother and her baby.

c. The hips should be flexed and abducted in a "frog" position; the arms should also be flexed. Baby's abdomen should be at the level of the mother's epigastrium. Mother's breathing stimulates the baby, thus reducing the occurrence of apnea.

d. Support the baby's bottom with a sling/binder.

Monitoring

a. Babies receiving KMC should be monitored carefully especially during the initial stages.

b. Make sure that baby's neck position is neither too flexed nor too extended, airway is clear, breathing is regular, color is pink and baby is maintaining temperature.

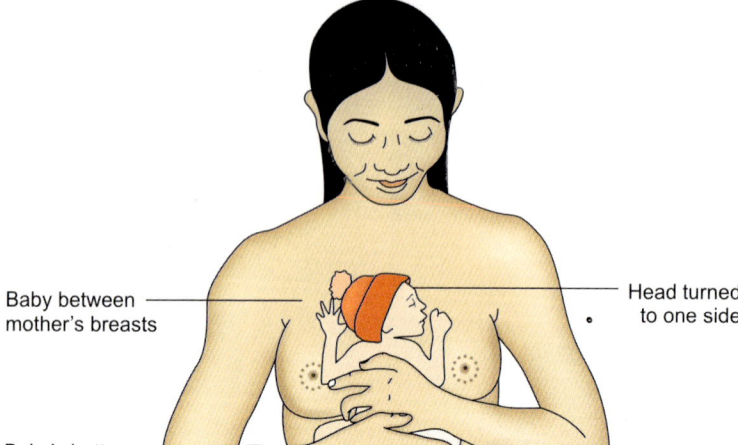

Baby between mother's breasts

Head turned to one side

Baby's bottom supported

Frog-leg position

Fig. 26.3: Positioning in KMC

c. Mother should be involved in observing the baby during KMC so that she herself can continue monitoring at home.

Feeding

a. The mother should be explained how to breastfeed while the baby is in KMC position.

b. Holding the baby near the breast stimulates milk production.[5,6]

c. She may express milk while the baby is still in KMC position. The baby could be fed with paladai, spoon or gastric tube, depending on the condition of the baby.

Duration

a. Skin-to-skin contact should start gradually in the nursery, with a smooth transition from conventional care to continuous KMC.

b. Sessions that last less than one hour should be avoided because frequent handling may be stressful for the baby.

c. The length of skin-to-skin contacts should be gradually increased up to 24 hours a day, interrupted only for changing diapers.

d. When the baby does not require intensive care, she should be transferred to the KMC ward where KMC should be continued.

KMC DURING SLEEP AND RESTING[7]

The mother can sleep with baby in kangaroo position in reclined or semi-recumbent position about 30 degrees from horizontal (Fig. 26.4A). This can be done with an adjustable bed or with pillows on an ordinary bed. A comfortable chair with an adjustable back may be used for resting during the day (Fig. 26.4B).

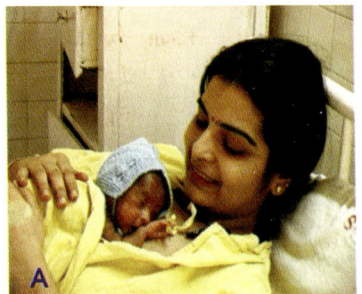 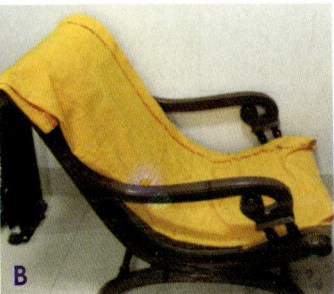

Fig. 26.4: Mother practicing KMC in reclining posture (A) and AIIMS KMC chair (B)

Discharge Criteria

The standard policy of the unit for discharge from the hospital should be followed (refer to AIIMS protocol on LBW feeding).[7]

When to Discontinue KMC

When the mother and baby are comfortable, KMC is continued for as long as possible, in the hospital and then at home. Often this is desirable until the baby's gestation reaches term or the weight is around 2500 g. The baby starts wriggling to show that she is uncomfortable, pulls her limbs out, cries and fusses every time the mother tries to put her back in skin-to-skin position. This is the time to wean the baby from KMC. Mothers can provide skin-to-skin contact occasionally after giving the baby a bath and during cold nights.

Post-discharge Follow-up

Close follow-up is a fundamental pre-requisite of KMC practice. Baby is followed once or twice a week till 37–40 weeks of gestation or till the baby reaches 2.5 to 3 kg of weight. (Refer to AIIMS protocol on follow-up of high risk neonates).

REFERENCES

1. Ludington-Hoe SM, Hadeed AJ, Anderson GC. Physiological response to skin-to-skin contact in hospitalized premature infants. J Perinatol 1991;11:19–24.

2. Whitelaw A, Heisterkamp G, Sleath K, Acolet D, Richards M. Skin-to-skin contact for very low birth weight infants and their mothers. Arch Dis Child 1988;63:1377–81.

3. Sloan NL, Camacho LW, Rojas EP, Stern C. Kangaroo mother method: randomized controlled trial of an alternative method of care for stabilized low birth weight infants. Maternidad Isidro Ayora Study Team. Lancet 1994;344:782–5.

4. Charpak N, Ruiz-Pelaez JG, Charpak Y. Rey-Martinez Kangaroo Mother Program: an alternative way of caring for low birth weight infants. One year mortality in a two cohort study. Pediatrics 1994; 94:804–10.

5. Conde-Agudelo A, Belizán JM, Diaz-Rossello J. Kangaroo mother care to reduce morbidity and mortality in low birth weight infants. Cochrane Database Syst Rev 2011 Mar 16;(3):CD002771.

6. Udani RH, Nanavati RN. Training manual on kangaroo mother care. Published by the Department of Neonatology. KEM Hospital and Seth GS Medical College Mumbai, September 2004.

7. Website of KMC India Network. Guidelines for parents and health providers are available online at *www.kmcindia.org.*

8. World Health Organization. Kangaroo mother care: a practical guide. Department of Reproductive Health and Research, WHO, Geneva. 2003.

Surfactant Replacement Therapy

Surfactant replacement therapy (SRT) has been a major stepping stone in the history of neonatology that has saved innumerable lives all over the world.

TYPES OF SURFACTANTS

The types of surfactants can be classified into two groups as follows (Fig. 27.1):

Natural	Minced lung extracts	1. Surfactant TA (Surfacten) 2. Beractant (Survanta) 3. Poractant alfa (Curosurf)
	Lung lavage extracts	1. CLSE (bLES) 2. Calfactant (Infasurf) 3. SF-RI1 (Alveofact)
	Amniotic fluid extract	1. Human surfactant
Synthetic	Old synthetic (protein-free)	1. Pumactant (ALEC) 2. Colfosceril palmitate 3. Exosurf 4. Turfsurf (Belfast surfactant)
	New synthetic (protein analogues)	1. Lucinactant (Surfaxin) 2. rSP-C surfactant (Venticute)

Fig. 27.1: Types of surfactants

INDICATIONS FOR SURFACTANT THERAPY

Surfactant replacement is done mainly for respiratory distress syndrome (RDS), but it can be used in other conditions where surfactant is inactivated such as meconium aspiration syndrome, pneumonia, pulmonary hemorrhage, congenital diaphragmatic hernia and acute respiratory distress syndrome (ARDS). In RDS, surfactant can be administered either prophylactically or as rescue therapy (Fig. 27.2).

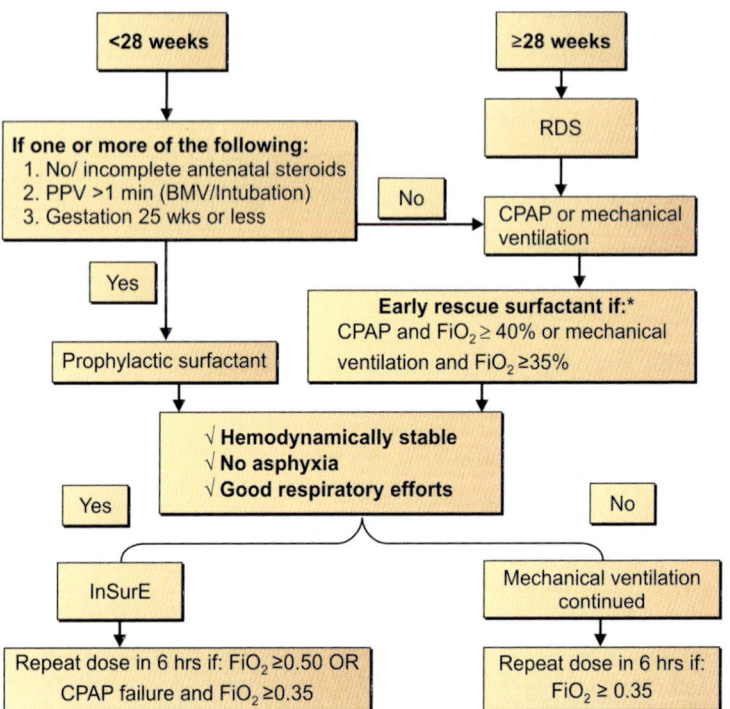

*Chest X-ray findings of RDS, if available can be considered. However, surfactant administration should not be delayed for the want of X-ray.

Fig. 27.2: Protocol for surfactant administration in neonates

1. **Prophylactic:** Surfactant is administered in the delivery room within 15 min of birth, irrespective of the presence of symptoms of RDS. Prophylactic SRT should be given to infnats <25 wk gestation or infants of 26–27 wk gestation. If they have not received complete antenatal steroids or required PPV >1 min (Fig. 27.2).[1–3]

2. **Early rescue:** Surfactant is administered in an infant with features of RDS within 2 hours. Early administration of surfactant is advantageous as the presence of lung fluid helps in uniform distribution of the surfactant. It also ensures that surfactant is administered before widespread atelectasis develops in the lungs.

3. **Late rescue:** Surfactant is administered in an infant with features of RDS after 2 hours. It is done usually in outborn neonates who are transported late to the referral centres.

There are at least three preparations of natural surfactants available in India (Table 27.1). All the preparations are safe and effective notwithstanding minor variations reported in the literature.[4]

We choose the cheapest available preparation.

Table 27.1: Common brands available in India

Surfactant preparations	Survanta (Abbott)	Curosurf (Nicholas)	Neosurf (Cipla)
Dose phospholipids	4 mL/kg (100 mg/kg)	2.5 mL/kg (200 mg/kg)	5 mL/kg (135 mg/kg)
Available formulation	4 and 8 mL	2.5 and 1.5 mL	5 and 3 mL
Cost (₹)	8,200 to 13,500	11,780 to 20,900	4,900 to 79,500

PROCEDURE FOR SURFACTANT ADMINISTRATION

Standard method of surfactant administration is through the endotracheal tube after intubation of the infant (Table 27.2).

Table 27.2: Procedure for surfactant administration*

1. A physician experienced in surfactant administration should administer the surfactant.
2. Warm the surfactant prior to administration (for 8 minutes if the vial is held between the palms of the hands or for 20 minutes at room temperature). The vial should not be heated.
3. Do not shake the surfactant.
4. Intubate the baby with appropriate size endotracheal tube.
5. Assess breath sounds for equality.
6. Infant should be connected to a pulse oximeter and oxygen saturation and heart rate monitored throughout the procedure.
7. Insert a feeding tube through the ET tube such that its tip project just beyond the ET tube.
8. Administer the surfactant through the feeding tube or through the side port of the ET tube (if available).
9. Surfactant is given as bolus dose in four aliquots.
10. Connect the infant to ventilator, resuscitation bag or a T piece and ventilate carefully till saturation and heart rate stabilizes before administering next aliquot.
11. No position change is required between the aliquots.
12. Avoid suctioning for at least 2 hours after administration.

*Strict asepsis should be observed throughout the procedure.

Natural surfactant works best if given as a rapid bolus into the lungs as it leads to homogeneous distribution and results in rapid improvement in oxygenation.

InSurE stands for Intubate – Surfactant – Extubate to CPAP. In infants with signs and symptoms of RDS, intubation and early surfactant therapy followed by extubation to nasal CPAP (nCPAP) when compared with later surfactant administration was associated with a lower incidence of mechanical ventilation [typical RR 0.67, 95% CI 0.57, 0.79], air leak syndromes [typical RR 0.52, 95% CI 0.28, 0.96] and BPD [typical RR 0.51, 95% CI 0.26, 0.99]. InSurE technique may not be successful in the presence of severe birth asphyxia, lack of complete course of antenatal steroids, extreme prematurity, delayed administration of surfactant and shock.

REPEAT DOSE OF SURFACTANT

Repeat doses of surfactant may be required in an infant with severe disease or if the administered surfactant is inhibited by edema fluid, proteins and inflammatory mediators, which are present in the alveoli after lung injury due to mechanical ventilation, delayed surfactant administration or sepsis. Infants may require repeat doses of surfactant if they require $FiO_2 \geq 0.35$ and mean airway pressure (MAP) >7 cm H_2O to maintain a PaO_2 50–70 mmHg and $PaCO_2$ <50 mmHg.[5] The use of repetitive dosing has decreased in clinical practice, probably because more attention is being paid to avoiding lung injury prior to the first dose.

ADVERSE REACTIONS OF SURFACTANT ADMINISTRATION

Transient hypoxia and bradycardia can occur because of acute airway obstruction immediately following surfactant instillation. There is an increase in the risk of pulmonary hemorrhage following surfactant therapy. Trials in which natural surfactants were used reported a higher incidence (5–6%) of pulmonary hemorrhage as compared with trials of synthetic surfactant (1–3%). Pulmonary hemorrhage is due to pulmonary vasodilatation resulting in increased pulmonary blood flow.

POOR RESPONSE TO SURFACTANT

Some infants may not show expected response to surfactant administered. These non-responders either have lung injury prior to birth (such as infection), treatment, pulmonary hypoplasia or a cardiovascular explanation for the lack of response (low blood pressure, congenital heart disease), etc.

REFERENCES

1. Rojas-Reyes MX, Morley CJ, Soll R. Prophylactic versus selective use of surfactant in preventing morbidity and mortality in preterm infants. Cochrane Database of Systematic Reviews 2012, Issue 3. Art. No.: CD000510. DOI:10.1002/14651858.CD000510.pub2.
2. SUPPORT Study Group of the Eunice Kennedy Shriver NICHD Neonatal Research Network, Finer NN, Carlo WA, Walsh MC, Rich W, Gantz MG, Laptook AR, Yoder BA, Faix RG, Das A, Poole WK, Donovan EF, Newman NS, Ambalavanan N, Frantz ID 3rd, Buchter S, Sánchez PJ, Kennedy KA, Laroia N, Poindexter BB, Cotten CM, Van Meurs KP, Duara S, Narendran V, Sood BG, O'Shea TM, Bell EF, Bhandari V, Watterberg KL, Higgins RD. Early CPAP versus Surfactant in Extremely Preterm Infants. N Engl J Med 2010 May 27;362(21):1970–9.
3. Sandri F, Plavka R, Ancora G, Simeoni U, Stranak Z, Martinelli S, Mosca F, Nona J, Thomson M, Verder H, Fabbri L, Halliday H; CURPAP Study Group. Prophylactic or early selective surfactant combined with nCPAP in very preterm infants. Pediatrics 2010 Jun;125(6):e1402–9.
4. Soll R, Blanco F. Natural surfactant extract versus synthetic surfactant for neonatal respiratory distress syndrome. Cochrane Database of Systematic Reviews 2001, Issue 2. Art. No.: CD000144. DOI: 10.1002/14651858.CD000144.
5. Katz LA, Klein JM. Repeat surfactant therapy for postsurfactant slump. J Perinatol 2006 Jul;26(7):414–22. Epub 2006 May 18. PubMed PMID:16724122.

28 | Parenteral Nutrition

The goal of nutrition management in neonates, especially very low birth weight (VLBW) infants is the achievement of postnatal growth at a rate that approximates the intrauterine growth of a normal fetus at the same postmenstrual age. Although, this is best achieved with optimal enteral nutrition, early enteral feeding is commonly limited by immaturity of gastrointestinal motor function, manifested principally as delayed stomach emptying, gastroesophageal reflux, abdominal distension and infrequent stooling. Likewise, establishing an alternative source of nutrition becomes a life-sustaining intervention in surgical neonates with congenital or acquired disease causing gastrointestinal failure.

Importance of Nutrition: What is Evidence?

Suboptimal nutrient intake during neonatal period has been associated with increased vulnerability to infections, greater need of ventilatory support, poor growth and neurodevelopment outcome, susceptibility to cardiovascular diseases and reduced cell growth in specific organ systems (heart, kidney and pancreas).[1,2]

INDICATIONS FOR PARENTERAL NUTRITION

Parenteral nutrition (PN) should be considered in neonates who are not on significant enteral feeds for more than 3–5 days or are anticipated to be receiving less than 50% of total energy requirement by day 7 of life (Table 28.1).

Energy

A daily energy intake of 110–120 kcal/kg is needed to meet the metabolic demands of a healthy preterm neonate and to allow for growth rate comparable to intrauterine growth rate.[3,4]

Table 28.1: Indications of parenteral nutrition

- Birth weight less than 1000 g
- Birth weight 1000–1500 g and anticipated to be not on significant feeds for 3 or more days
- Birth weight more than 1500 g and anticipated to be not on significant feeds for 5 or more days
- Surgical conditions in neonates precluding enteral intake for significant period: necrotizing enterocolitis, gastroschisis, omphalocele, tracheo-esophageal fistula, intestinal atresia, malrotation, short bowel syndrome and meconium ileus, CDH

Energy requirement of term neonate is 90–100 kcal/kg/day. Energy intake of sick neonates (e.g. acute respiratory illness, chronic lung disease, necrotizing enterocolitis) is not exactly known but is likely to be near upper limits of the energy requirement of preterm infant.

10% dextrose solution provides 0.34 kcal/mL. 10% lipid solution provides 0.9 kcal/mL and 20% lipid solution provides 1.1 kcal/mL. If sufficient amount of non-protein energy is not provided, amino acids are catabolized for energy production. Adequate balance between nitrogen and non-protein energy sources (protein/energy ratio: 3–4 g/100 kcal) is needed to promote protein accretion.[5] Balance between carbohydrates and fat is needed to prevent excessive fat deposition and excessive production of CO_2. The ideal distribution of calories should be 50–55% carbohydrate, 10–15% proteins and 30–35% fats.

Amino Acids

PN should provide 3.0–3.5 g/kg/day of amino acid (AA). An optimal AA solution should contain essential (valine, leucine, isoleucine, methionine, phenylalanine, threonine, lysine and histidine) and conditionally essential (cysteine, tyrosine, glutamine, arginine, proline, glycine and taurine). Amino acids should not have excess of glycine and methionine and should not contain sorbitol. AA infusion should be started on the first day of birth preferably soon after birth. To avoid negative protein balance, one should start with at least 1.5 g/kg/d and then increase by 1 g/kg/d to maximum of 3.5 g/kg/d.

AA solutions are available as 10% and 20% preparations.

Proteins in PN: What is Evidence?

The amount started on day 1 of PN has varied from 0.5 to 3.0 g/kg/d in different studies.[6] Although, intake of about 1.5 g/kg/d is needed to prevent negative nitrogen balance, higher intake of 3–3.5 g/kg/d can be safely administered starting from first day of birth.[2] Early provision of protein is critical to attain positive nitrogen balance and accretion, as preterm babies lose about 1% of their protein stores daily.[7]

CARBOHYDRATES

Carbohydrates are the main energy substrate for the neonates receiving PN. The amount of carbohydrate delivered in form of dextrose is commonly initiated at the endogenous hepatic glucose production and utilization rate of 4 to 6 mg/kg/min. This provides energy intake of 40–50 kcal/kg/d and preserves carbohydrate stores. Once the GIR supports acceptable serum glucose values, it is advanced in a gradual, stepwise fashion (2 mg/kg/min/day) to a suggested maximum glucose oxidative rate for neonates of 12–13 mg/kg/min to support growth and maintained there unless serum glucose values change significantly. Insulin infusion should not be used to increase the GIR. However, if infant is developing high glucose levels despite glucose infusion rate of 4–6 mg/kg/minute, insulin infusion can be started.

Glucose is available as 5%, 10%, 25% and 50% solutions.

Carbohydrates in PN: What is Evidence?

Excessive carbohydrate delivery above the amount that can be oxidized for energy and glycogen storage can lead to an increase in basal metabolic rate, fat deposition, cholestasis or hepatic steatosis.[8–10] Use of insulin to achieve higher glucose infusion rate and promote growth has been associated with lactic acidosis.[11]

LIPIDS

Intravenous lipid (IVL) can be started on the first day at dose of 1.0 g/kg/d and then increased gradually in stepwise fashion to 3.0 g/kg/d.[4] In preterm neonates with hyperbilirubinemia in range of exchange transfusion threshold, lipids may be restricted to minimum amounts (1 g/kg/d) that will provide only the essential fatty acids.[12]

IVL emulsions are available in two strengths: 10% and 20%. Use of 20% lipid emulsion is preferable to a 10% solution to decrease the risk of hypertriglyceridemia, hypercholesterolemia and hyperphospholipidemia.[13] When lipids are exposed to light, they form potentially toxic lipid hydroperoxides. Hence, lipid syringes and tubing should be covered by aluminum foil.

Lipids in PN: What is Evidence?

Even a short delay of 3 to 7 days in supplying lipids to parenterally fed preterm infants leads to biochemical EFA deficiency.[14]

MINERALS

Sodium, potassium, chloride, calcium, magnesium and phosphorus need to be provided in PN solution as per their daily needs (Table 28.2). Except phosphate, all these minerals are easily available in India. Sodium, potassium and chloride are essential to life and requirements are dependent on obligatory losses, abnormal losses and amounts necessary for growth. Calcium, phosphorus and magnesium are the most abundant minerals in the body. They are closely interrelated to each other in metabolism, the formation of tissue structure and function. Estimated and advisable intakes (Table 28.2) are based on accretion studies and urinary and fecal losses from balance studies.[15]

Table 28.2: Daily requirement of minerals

Mineral	Requirement
Sodium	0–3 mEq/kg/d (1st week of life), 2–3 mEq/kg/d (beyond 1st week in term neonates), 3–5 mEq/kg/d (beyond 1st week in preterm neonates)
Potassium	0–2 mEq/kg/d (1st week of life), 1–3 mEq/kg/d (beyond 1st week)
Chloride	2–3 mEq/kg/d
Calcium	150–200 mg/kg/day
Magnesium	15–25 mg/d
Phosphate	20–40 mg/kg/d

VITAMINS

Vitamins are added in PN solution to meet the daily requirement (Table 28.3). Separate preparations of fat-soluble and water-soluble vitamins suitable for neonates are not available in India. Multivitamin injection (MVI), when added in a dose of 1.5 mL/kg to lipid solution meets the need of vitamin A and most other vitamin. Furthermore, intravenous vitamin delivery may be less due to photo-degradation of vitamins A, D, E, K, B_2, B_6, B_{12}, C and folic acid, and adsorption of vitamins A, D and E into the vinyl delivery bags and tubing. Vitamin K needs to be given separately as weekly intramuscular injections. Although vitamin B_{12} is not present in MVI, its deficiency is not manifested unless the neonate is on long-term PN.

Table 28.3: Recommended vitamin intake

Vitamin	Term (daily dose)	Preterm (dose/kg/day)
Vitamin A (IU)	2300	1640
Vitamin D (IU)	400	160
Vitamin E (IU)	7	2.8
Vitamin K (µg)	200	80
Vitamin B_6 (µg)	1000	180
Vitamin B_{12} (µg)	1	0.3
Vitamin C (mg)	80	25
Biotin (µg)	20	6
Folic acid (µg)	140	56
Niacin (mg)	17	6.8
Pantothenic acid (mg)	5	2
Riboflavin (µg)	1400	150
Thiamine (µg)	1200	350

TRACE ELEMENTS

Trace elements like zinc, copper, manganese, selenium, fluorine and iodine should be provided in PN solutions.[4] Zinc is universally recommended from day one of TPN, whereas the other trace minerals are generally provided after 2 weeks of TPN without any appreciable enteral feeding. Copper, selenium, molybdenum and iron can be delivered separately also. Dosage of zinc to be provided is 150–400 micrograms/ kg/d even with short-term PN, but a suitable preparation is difficult to find in Indian market.

EVIDENCE-BASED RECOMMENDATIONS

Evidence-based recommendations for use of PN constituents are summarized in Table 28.4.

Table 28.4: Recommendations for parenteral nutrition

Component	Recommendations
Fluids	Day 1: 60–80 mL/kg/d. Postnatal weight loss up to 3% per day to a maximum of 10 to 15% is acceptable. This is achieved by progressively increasing the fluid intake to 120–150 mL/kg/d by one week of age.
Energy	An intake of 50 kcal/kg/d is sufficient to match ongoing expenditure, but it does not meet additional requirements of growth. The goal energy intake is 100–120 kcal/kg/d (higher in infants with chronic lung disease).
Protein	Optimal parenteral amino acid intake is 3.5 g/kg/d. Parenteral amino acids can begin from day 1 at 1–1.5 gm/kg/d.
Carbo-hydrates	From day one, 6 mg/kg/min can be infused, increased by 2 mg/ kg/min/d to 12–14 mg/kg/min and adjusted to maintain euglycemia. Insulin is only used in infants who continue to have hyperglycemia associated with glycosuria and osmotic dieresis even after the glucose intake has been reduced to 4 to 6 mg/kg/ min. Insulin is given as a continuous infusion commencing at a rate of 0.05 units/kg/h, increasing as required for persistent hyperglycemia. Infants on insulin therapy require close monitoring for development of hypoglycemia.
Fat	Intravenous fat, 1 g/kg/d can be started from day 1. This is increased to 2 g/kg/d and 3 g/kg/d over the next two days. It is delivered as a continuous infusion of 20% intravenous fat via a syringe pump, separate from the infusate containing the amino acids and glucose. The syringe and infusion line should be shielded from ambient light.
Minerals and trace elements	Minerals should include: sodium, chloride, potassium, calcium, phosphorus, magnesium. Trace elements should include: zinc, copper, selenium, manganese, iodine, chromium and molybdenum.
Vitamins	Vitamins must be added to the fat emulsion to minimize loss during administration due to adherence to tubing and photodegradation.

DISPENSING PN SOLUTION

Steps for calculation and preparing PN are as follows:
1. Determine total fluid requirement for the day.
2. Subtract amount of fluid to be used for medications (e.g. diluting and infusing antibiotics) and enteral feeds.
3. Plan AA, IVL and glucose to be given over 24 hrs.
4. Take IVL suspension in one syringe and add MVI into it.
5. In second syringe, mix AA, dextrose, electrolytes and trace elements.
6. IVL + MVI suspension is infused separately from AA-glucose-minerals solution, although they can be mixed at the site of infusion using a three-way adapter.
7. Amount of each PN component.

Amount of a PN component =

$$\frac{(\text{Amount to be given per body weight} \times \text{Body weight})}{(\text{Strength of solution})}$$

For example, for a baby weighing 1.5 kg to be given 3 mEq/kg of sodium, amount of 3% NaCl to be used is:

$$\text{Amount of 3\% NaCl} = \frac{(3\ \text{mEq/kg} \times 1.5\ \text{kg})}{(0.5\ \text{mEq/mL})} = 9\ \text{mL}$$

Computer assisted prescribing of PN should be encouraged as this can save time, improve the quality of nutritional care and reduce errors.[16] All PN solutions should be administered with accurate flow control. The infusion system should undergo regular visual inspection. Peripheral infusions should be checked frequently for signs of extravasation.

ROUTE OF ADMINISTRATION

PN can be delivered through peripheral or central venous lines. Short-term PN can be given through peripheral venous line. Peripheral access offers the advantage of a lower risk of infection.

However, nutrition delivery is limited with peripheral lines due to constraints created by a solution's osmolarity. The limiting factor in deciding route of delivery is osmolarity of the AA-glucose solution which is dependent on dextrose concentration. A dextrose concentration greater than 12.5% has an acidic pH and can be irritating to the peripheral veins. In addition to dextrose, electrolytes and minerals added to the solution increase the osmolarity of the solution. Hypertonic solution need to be administered through central venous line.

Increasing use of peripherally inserted central catheters (PICC) has facilitated administration of PN while avoiding many potential complications of surgically inserted central lines. Another attractive option in neonates is central line inserted through umbilical vein. Umbilical venous catheter can be used for up to 14 days after which risk of complications increases.[17,18]

Position of central line should be confirmed by X-ray before starting infusion through it. To avoid risk of pericardial tamponade, tip of the central catheter should lie outside the pericardial sac (on the chest X-ray is at least 0.5 cm outside the cardiac outline). In comparison to catheters made of stiffer material (polyvinylchloride, polypropylene, polyethylene), softer catheters (silicone and polyurethane) are less thrombogenic and less traumatic and are therefore, preferable for long-term use. The venous access used for PN should not be interrupted for giving antibiotics or other medications. For this, a separate intravenous line should be established.

MONITORING AND COMPLICATIONS

Meticulous monitoring is needed in a neonate receiving PN (Table 28.5). Monitoring should be more frequent in the initial stages. Once a steady metabolic stage has been achieved, monitoring can be reduced to once a week.

Complications of PN can be nutrient-related or venous access-related. Nutrient related complications include hypoglycemia and hyperglycemia (glucose-related), azotemia and metabolic acidosis (protein-related), hypertriglyceridemia (triglyceride >200 mg/dL) (lipid-related), cholestasis and trace element deficiency. Most of these complications can be avoided by proper monitoring and provision of nutrients. PN-related cholestasis is usually a complication of long-term PN and can be avoided by provision of minimal-enteral nutrition. Catheter-related complications include occlusion, dislodgement and infection.

Table 28.5: Monitoring schedule for a neonate on parenteral nutrition

Parameter	Frequency
Blood sugar	2–3 times a day while increasing glucose infusing rate;
	Once a day while on stable glucose infusion rate
Urine sugar	Once per nursing shift
Serum electrolytes	Twice a week initially, then weekly
Blood urea	Twice a week initially, then weekly
Calcium, magnesium and phosphorus	Weekly
Serum albumin	Weekly
Packed cell volume	Weekly
Liver function tests	Weekly
Serum triglycerides	Weekly
Anthropometry	
weight	Daily
Head circumference	Weekly

PREVENTION OF INFECTION

Hospital-acquired infection (HAI) is a major complication of PN. All efforts should be made to avoid HAI.

- Aseptic precautions during preparation of PN
- Use of laminar flow
- No compromise on disposables
- Trained staff
- No reuse of the PN solutions
- No interruption of the venous line carrying PN

QUALITY IMPROVEMENT

The following process and outcome indicators should be audited in neonatal units which use parenteral nutrition:

1. Incidence density of central line associated bloodstream infection (per 1000 catheter days)
2. Incidence rate of central catheter occlusion necessitating catheter removal
3. Incidence rate of parenteral nutrition associated cholestasis
4. Proportion of eligible neonates who receive parenteral nutrition.

PN WORKSHEET

Steps of charting parenteral nutrition include:

1. Determine birth weight, present weight and weight change since 24 hrs previous to start of parenteral nutrition therapy. Birth weight is used to plan nutrient and fluid intake till baby starts gaining weight and weight on the day of calculation exceeds birth weight. Thereafter weight on the day of therapy is used for all calculations.

2. Depending on day of birth and fluid status of the neonate, determine total fluid to be administered over the 24 hrs period. The amount of parenteral nutrition is determined by subtracting enteral feed and intravenous drugs volume from total fluid amount.

3. Plan amino acids, lipids, glucose and electrolytes (sodium and potassium) to be given over 24 hrs.

4. Calculate amount of each PN component used.

5. Take lipid suspension in one syringe and add MVI into it. To account for some volume loss in dead space of the syringe and fluid administration set, one can take additional 20% amount in syringe (overfill). Rate of administration can be calculated by dividing total volume (before overfill) by duration of administration (24 hrs).

6. In second syringe, amino acids, dextrose, electrolytes and trace elements are mixed together. In this solution also, to account for some volume loss in dead space of the syringe and fluid administration set, one can take additional 20% amount of each constituent. More than one syringe can be used if volume to be administered exceeds syringe capacity.

7. Lipids, amino acids and electrolytes to be used are calculated based on formula given above. After taking into account fluid allowance consumed for each component, remaining fluid is used for administration of glucose. Total grams of glucose to be administered can be calculated by multiplying glucose infusion rate with birth weight and 1.44. Different glucose strength solution can be used to provide the amount of dextrose in the allocated fluid (left after taking into consideration all other constituents of parenteral nutrition).

Table 28.6 provides sources of PN components.

Table 28.6: Sources of parenteral solutions

Component	Source	Concentration
Proteins	Aminoven, Primene	6% and 10%
Lipids	Intralipid	10%, 10% PLR (phospholipids reduced), 20%
Glucose	Dextrose	5%, 10%, 25%, 50%
NaCl	NaCl	0.9%, 3%
KCl	KCl	15%, 20%
Calcium	Calcium gluconate	10%
Multivitamin	Adult MVI	–
Trace elements	Celcel, TMA	–
Magnesium sulfate	Magnesium sulfate	50%

REFERENCES

1. Vlaardingerbroek H, van Goudoever JB, Van den Akker CH. Initial nutritional management of the preterm infant. Early Hum Dev 2009;85:691–5.

2. Te Braake FW, Van den Akker CH, Riedijk MA, Van Goudoever JB. Parenteral amino acid and energy administration to premature infants in early life. Semin Fetal Neonatal Med 2007;12:11–8.

3. Hulzebos CV, Sauer PJ. Energy requirements. Semin Fetal Neonatal Med 2007;12:2–10.

4. Koletzko B, Goulet O, Hunt J, Krohn K, Shamir R. 1. Guidelines on Paediatric Parenteral Nutrition of the European Society of Paediatric Gastroenterology, Hepatology and Nutrition (ESPGHAN) and the European Society for Clinical Nutrition and Metabolism (ESPEN), Supported by the European Society of Paediatric Research (ESPR). J Pediatr Gastroenterol Nutr 2005;41 Suppl 2:S1–87.

5. Ziegler EE, Thureen PJ, Carlson SJ. Aggressive nutrition of the very low birth weight infant. Clin Perinatol 2002;29:225–44.

6. Van den Akker CH, Vlaardingerbroek H, van Goudoever JB. Nutritional support for extremely low-birth weight infants: abandoning catabolism in the neonatal intensive care unit. Curr Opin Clin Nutr Metab Care 2010;13:327–35.

7. Heird WC, Discoll J. Total parenteral nutrition. NeoReviews 2003;4:e137–9.

8. Kanarek K, Santeiro M, Malone J. Continuous infusion of insulin in hyperglycemic low-birth weight infants receiving parenteral nutrition with and without lipid emulsion. J Parenter Enteral Nutr 1991;15:417–20.

9. Henry B. Pediatric Parenteral Nutrition Support. In: Nevin-Folino N, ed. Pediatric Manual of Clinical Dietetics: Faulhabes, 2003;495–514.

10. Shulman RJ. New developments in total parenteral nutrition for children. Curr Gastroenterol Rep 2000;2:253–8.

11. Poindexter BB, Karn CA, Denne SC. Exogenous insulin reduces proteolysis and protein synthesis in extremely low birth weight infants. J Pediatr 1998;132:948–53.

12. Aba-Sinden A, Bollinger R. Challenges and controversies in the nutrition support of the preterm infant. Support Line 2002;2: 2–15.

13. Haumont D, Deckelbaum RJ, Richelle M, et al. Plasma lipid and plasma lipoprotein concentrations in low birth weight infants given parenteral nutrition with twenty or ten percent lipid emulsion. J Pediatr 1989;115:787–93.

14. Gutcher GR, Farrell PM. Intravenous infusion of lipid for the prevention of essential fatty acid deficiency in premature infants. Am J Clin Nutr 1991;54:1024–8.

15. Ziegler EE, O'Donnell A, Nelson S. Body composition of the reference fetus. Growth 1976;40:320–41.

16. Puangco MA, Nguyen HL, Sheridan MJ. Computerized PN ordering optimizes timely nutrition therapy in a neonatal intensive care unit. J Am Diet Assoc 1997;97:258–61.

17. O'Grady NP, Alexander M, Dellinger EP, et al. Guidelines for the prevention of intravascular catheter-related infections. The Hospital Infection Control Practices Advisory Committee, Center for Disease Control and Prevention, U.S. Pediatrics 2002;110:e51.

18. Butler-O'Hara M, Buzzard CJ, Reubens L, McDermott MP, DiGrazio W, D'Angio CT. A randomized trial comparing long-term and short-term use of umbilical venous catheters in premature infants with birth weights of less than 1251 grams. Pediatrics 2006;118:e25–35.

29

Cranial Ultrasonogram

Newborn babies born preterm and sick term infants are at risk of brain injury. Cranial ultrasonogram (CUS) is the choice for routine neuroimaging in NICU as it can be readily performed at the bedside. CUS is relatively safe and serial repetitive examinations are possible even in critical sick neonates.[1]

Systematically done CUS helps in diagnosis of brain injury in at risk infants as well as aids in predicting long-term neuro-developmental outcome.[1]

INDICATIONS FOR CUS[2,3]

- Screening neurosonogram in preterm infants to rule out hemorrhage or parenchymal brain injury
  - All infants <32 weeks or <1500 g.
  - Infants of 32 to 34 weeks gestation or 1500 to <1800 g birth weight who had significant sickness during neonatal period like need for extensive resuscitation, ventilation or exchange transfusion or had illnesses such as sepsis, necrotizing enterocolitis, etc.
- To evaluate for hydrocephalus.
- To evaluate patients with signs and/or symptoms of central nervous system disorder, e.g. seizures, encephalopathy, CNS infections, facial malformations.
- For follow-up or surveillance of previously documented abnormalities including prenatal abnormalities.

Timing of Screening CUS[1,3]

The following are the broad guidelines for timing of CUS screening in NICU (Table 29.1).

Table 29.1: Timing of CUS screening in preterm neonates in NICU

Timing	Group I		Group II
	<32 weeks or <1500 g, 32–34 weeks or 1500 to <1800 g with risk factors[&]		Bigger infants with neurological symptoms
1st Scan	Day 1–3*		As clinically indicated
	Normal	Abnormal	
2nd Scan	7–14 days	As decided clinically— may require scanning more often	Consider at 1–2 weeks after the first scan
3rd Scan	3–4 weeks	3–4 weeks	Term[#]
4th Scan	Term	6–8 weeks or term, whichever earlier	
5th Scan	–	Term	Term

[&]Need for extensive resuscitation, no antenatal steroids, ventilation, surfactant therapy, NEC, pneumothorax, shock requiring therapy (fluids or inotropes), unstable blood pressures, exchange transfusions, sepsis, etc.
*Timing of first scan can be decided by clinical condition and sickness level.
[#]Consider other modality of imaging like CT/MRI based on clinical need.

1. Routine screening of well preterm babies
   - First scan at 3 days to 1 week
   - Second scan at 3–4 weeks
   - Third scan at 40 weeks post menstrual age or at discharge whichever is earlier
2. Follow up scans in infants with CUS abnormalities
   - Follow-up scans at 1–2 weeks interval as per clinical decision
3. Sick symptomatic term/preterm infants
   - Immediately after birth or when indicated clinically.

Note: *The frequency of CUS examinations may be intensified in the following circumstances: sudden deterioration in clinical state, sepsis, necrotizing enterocolitis, episodes of apneas and/or bradycardias, sudden decrease in hemoglobin level, neurological symptoms, ventricular dilatation, and before and after major surgery.*

Table 29.2 provides classification of various abnormalities detected on CUS.

Table 29.2: Classification of abnormalities in CUS

Pathology		Description
Intraventricular hemorrhage (IVH)	Volpe's grading[4]	**Grade I**: Germinal matrix hemorrhage with minimal or no ventricular dilatation (<10% of ventricular area in parasagittal view)
		Grade II: Ventricular bleed occupying 10–50% of ventricular area with bleed in parasagittal view
		Grade III: Ventricular bleed occupying >50% of ventricle
		Separate notation parenchymal echo density representing periventricular hemorrhagic infarction
Periventricular leukomalacia (PVL)	De Vries grading[5] evolution	**Transient flare:** IPL (usually bilateral) persisting for at least 48 hours without cysts
		Grade I: Mild PVL or persistent flare/IPL (usually bilateral) persisting for at least 7 days without cystic evolution
		Grade II: Cystic PVL, IPL persisting for 7 days and evolving into localized small fronto-parietal cysts; lesions not involving occipital cortex
		Grade III: Multiple cysts in parieto-occipital white matter
		Grade IV: IPL with evolving cysts in deep white matter and sub-cortical region
Ventricular dilatation	Levene Index[6]	Normative size of lateral ventricles from 26–40 weeks infants measured in coronal section at the level of 3rd ventricles. Smoothened centile curves permit early detection of ventricular dilatation secondary to cerebral atrophy. Hydrocephalus is defined as ventricular size exceeding the 97th centile by 4 mm.
White matter echo density and echo lucency		Indicator of white matter injury and predicts poor neurodevelopmental outcome
Cerebral malformations		Cystic lesions, vein of Galen malformation, corpus callosal agenesis, etc. may be picked up by CUS

IPL: Intra Parenchymal Lesion

SPECIFICATIONS OF CUS IN NICU[1,2]

Standard Views

Two standard views are used—the coronal and sagittal views with anterior fontanels as the acoustic windows.

Coronal Views

- The coronal view conventionally has the patient's right side on the left side of the image.
- The right or left side of the patient should be clearly marked on the images.
- Representative coronal views angling from anterior to posterior should include sequentially the following:
  - The frontal lobe and frontal horns of the lateral ventricles,
  - The septum pellucidum corpus callosum and portions of the frontal, parietal and temporal lobes,
  - The caudothalamic groove and basal ganglia,
  - The bodies of the lateral ventricles, and
  - The posterior portions of the temporal lobes, occipital lobes, fourth ventricle.

Sagittal Views

- The sagittal view, by convention, should place the anterior aspect of the brain on the left side of the image.
- The right side, midline or left side should be clearly annotated.
- Sequential representative sagittal views are obtained with appropriate degrees of left and right transducer angulation. On each side, these views should include:
  - Caudothalamic groove
  - Lateral ventricle with demonstration of the occipital horn and its choroid plexus
  - Periventricular white matter
  - Sylvian fissure and the middle cerebral artery branches (angiographic sylvian triangle equivalent).
- A midline sagittal view should include the corpus callosum, the cavum septum pellucidum, the third ventricle, the area of the aqueduct of Sylvius, the fourth ventricle, the vermis of the cerebellum and the cisterna magna.

Supplementary Views

The following are the supplemental acoustic windows used in CUS:

- Temporal windows: Visualization of the brainstem, upper part of the cerebellum and circle of Willis, and for Doppler flow measurements.
- The posterior fontanel: Visualization of the occipital horns of the lateral ventricles (enabling early detection of intraventricular hemorrhage, IVH), the occipital parenchyma and the cerebellum.
- The mastoid fontanels: Optimal and detailed visualization of the cerebellum (vermis and hemispheres), fourth ventricle, aqueduct and cisterna magna. Early detection of posterior fossa bleeds is possible in this view.

Note: *Consider performing supplementary views especially in preterm <30 weeks, suspected malformations and cases with ventricular dilatation or IVH.*

Transducer

- CUS is conducted with sector or curved linear transducers that can fit within and image through the anterior fontanels.
- Standard frequency of 5–8 MHz is recommended ideally as multi-frequency probe.
- In term infants, lower transducer frequency of 5 MHz may be used for better visualization of deeper structures (i.e. the basal ganglia/thalami/posterior fossa).
- Preterm infants where less penetration is needed or for detailed visualization of superficial areas, such as the cortex, sub-cortical white matter and brain's convexity, the transducer frequency may be increased (up to 10 MHz), allowing a very high resolution but limited penetration.

Note: *With higher transducer frequencies, the resolution improves at the expense of penetration and vice versa.*

Focus Points

For standard CUS procedures, it is best to have the focus point aimed at the ventricular or periventricular areas.

All scans are to be performed by trained radiologist or neonatologist with digital archiving of all abnormal scans. The finding should duly be recorded in patient medical records.

DOPPLER IMAGING IN CUS

There is a limited role of Doppler (pulse waved Doppler of anterior or middle cerebral artery) in assessing cerebral perfusion especially in the following settings. The flow related indices like resistive index (RI) of Pourcelot or the pulsatility index (PI) may be used as surrogates of cerebral perfusion and intracranial pressure and may predict outcome (Fig. 29.1).[7, 8]

- Cerebral blood flow (CBF) estimation in infants with HIE, shock
- Monitoring infants with hydrocephalus and decide timing of treatment
- In preterm infants with significant PDA to assess severity of ductus (diastolic steal)
- The flow related indices may be predictive of white matter injury.

Resistive Index (RI)

$$= \frac{\text{Systolic flow (S)} - \text{Diastolic flow (D)}}{\text{Systolic flow (S)}}$$

Normal: 0.60–0.85; low: <0.60 (low resistance, increased CBF)

High: >0.85 (high resistance, reduced CBF)

In hydrocephalus—indication for treatment:
- RI > 0.71 without pressure provocation
- RI > 0.90 with pressure provocation*

Pulsatility Index (PI)

$$= \frac{\text{Systolic flow (S)} - \text{Diastolic flow (D)}}{\text{Mean blood flow velocity (M)}}$$

Normal: 0.5–1.05; less widely used than RI

*Applying inward pressure at anterior fontanel for 5 seconds and measuring blood flow velocities.[8]

Fig. 29.1: Resistive and pulsatility indices

EVIDENCE SUPPORTING NEUROIMAGING IN NICU[3]

American Academy of Neurology: Practice Parameter Neuroimaging of the Neonate

Imaging for the Preterm Neonate[*]

- Routine screening cranial ultrasonography (CUS) should be performed on all infants of 30 weeks gestation once between 7 and 14 days of age and should be optimally repeated between 36 and 40 weeks postmenstrual age.
- There is insufficient evidence for routine MRI of all very low birth weight preterm infants with abnormal results of cranial US.

Imaging for the Term Infant

Non-contrast CT should be performed to detect hemorrhagic lesions in the encephalopathic term infant with a history of birth trauma, low hematocrit or coagulopathy. If CT findings are inconclusive, MRI should be performed between days 2 and 8 to assess the location and extent of injury. The pattern of injury identified with conventional/diffusion weighted MRI may provide diagnostic and prognostic information for term infants with evidence of encephalopathy.

Recommendations

- CUS plays an established role in the management of preterm neonates of 30 weeks gestation.
- CUS also provides valuable prognostic information when the infant reaches 40 weeks postmenstrual age.
- For encephalopathic term infants, early CT should be used to exclude hemorrhage; MRI should be performed later in the first postnatal week to establish the pattern of injury and predict neurologic outcome.

PREDICTION OF NEURODEVELOPMENTAL OUTCOME WITH CUS

Evidence for prognostic values of CUS and MRI in predicting neurodevelopmental outcome is limited by few good quality

---

*This frequency of scans as per these guidelines seems inadequate and we recommend more frequent scans as detailed in Table 29.1.

studies. Even though superiority of MRI as imaging modality is well established, it is not yet clear whether it adds significantly to prediction of outcomes. Carefully performed serial CUS seems to provide as much information as MRI.[9] In a recent study, Horsche et al[10] in 72 infants <27 weeks gestation, contemporaneously done CUS and MRI at 40 weeks corrected age, showed acceptable agreement with none of the infants with normal CUS findings (n = 28; 40%) having moderate or severe MRI abnormalities. Moreover, all infants with severe MRI abnormalities (n = 3; 4%) were picked up by CUS as well (Table 29.3).

Table 29.3: Pooled estimates for prediction of abnormal neurodevelopmental outcome at 2 years by CUS[11]

CUS abnormality	Cerebral palsy*	
	Likelihood ratio positive (95% CI)	Positive predictive value (95% CI)
Normal	0.5 (0.4–0.7)	5 (4–6)
Grade I/II IVH	1 (0.4–3)	9 (4–22)
Grade III	4 (2–8)	26 (13–45)
Grade IV	11 (4–31)	53 (29–78)
Cystic PVL	29 (7–116)	74 (42–92)
Ventricular dilatation	3 (2–4)	22 (17–28)
Hydrocephalus	4 (1–13)	27 (10–56)

(Adapted with permission)

*Note that these are based on Western data.

*Normal scan refers to absence of hemorrhage within the brain parenchyma or ventricles, cysts or ventricular dilation. The grade of IVH (intraventricular hemorrhage) is given according to the Papile classification. PVL indicates periventricular leukomalacia. Ventricular dilation indicates moderate to severe ventricular dilation not meeting the criterion for hydrocephalus. Hydrocephalus indicates massive ventricular dilation >4 mm above the 97th centile.

*Likelihood ratio denotes how many times the test is likely to be positive (abnormal ultrasound result) in patients with cerebral palsy as compared to patients without cerebral palsy.

*Positive predictive value is the probability that a patient with a specific abnormality on cranial ultrasound will have abnormal neuromotor function.

*Heterogeneity among studies have been high (80–90%) and baseline prevalence of CP was taken as 9% for estimation based on EPIPAGE study (Pediatrics 2006;117:828–35).

REFERENCES

1. Van Wezel-Meijler G, Steggerda SJ, Leijser LM. Cranial ultrasonography in neonates: role and limitations. Semin Perinatol 2010; 34:28–38.

2. ACR-AIUM-SPR-SRU practice guidelines for performance of neurosonography in neonates and infants [ubterbet]. 2012 (Cited 2013. June 27):www.acr.org or/media/E9BAF 42FDBD44II AA159F7743.pdf.

3. Ment LR, Bada HS, Barnes P, Grant PE, Hirtz D, Papile LA, J Pinto–Martin, Rivkin M, Slovis TL. Practice Parameter: Neuroimaging of the Neonate. Neurology 2002;58:1726–1738.

4. Volpe JJ. Neurology of the Newborn. 4th edn. Philadelphia, PA: WB Saunders 2001;428–493.

5. De Vries LS, Eken P, Dubowitz LMS. The spectrum of leucomalacia using cranial ultrasound. Behav Brain Res 1992;49:1–6.

6. Levene MI. Measurement of the growth of the lateral ventricles in preterm infants with real time ultrasound. Arch Dis in Childhood 1981;56:900–4.

7. Evan DH. Doppler ultrasound and the neonatal cerebral circulation: methodology and pitfalls. Bio Neonate 1992;62:271–9.

8. Taylor GA, Madsen JR: Neonatal hydrocephalus: hemodynamic response to fontanelle compression—correlation with intracranial pressure and need for shunt placement. Radiology 1996;201:685.

9. De Vries LS, Van Haastert IL, Rademaker KJ, et al. Ultrasound abnormalities preceding cerebral palsy in high-risk preterm infants. J Pediatr 2004;144:815–20.

10. Horsch S, Skiöld B, Hallberg B, et al. Cranial ultrasound and MRI at term age in extremely preterm infants. Arch Dis Child Fetal Neonatal 2010;95:F310–14.

11. Nongena P, Ederies A, Azzopardi DV, Edwards AD. Confidence in the prediction neurodevelopmental outcome by cranial ultrasound and MRI in preterm infants. Arch Dis Child Fetal Neonatal 2010;95:F388–90.

30

Blood Components Transfusion

Sick neonates often receive transfusion of blood products. Preterm neonates comprise the most heavily transfused group of patients and about 85% of extremely low birth weight newborns receive a transfusion by the end of their hospital stay.[1,2]

Blood components used in modern day practice include red blood cell components, platelet concentrates and plasma rather than whole blood. Transfusion of blood products in the vulnerable neonates need to be strictly regulated to avoid the inherent risks of transfusion such as transmission of infections.[3]

DONOR SELECTION

Donor selection is done according to predefined criteria. Usually voluntary (not replacement) donors who do not require any remuneration are preferred over paid donors. Donors should be provided with educational materials on blood donation, blood components and the important benefits to patients.

The donors should be given a questionnaire to identify any health risk factors which can be of concern to themselves and the recipients. They should be provided information on the protection of personal data including confirmation that there will be no disclosure of the information concerning the donor. The results of the tests performed should also be provided to the donors.[4]

Collection of Blood

About 450 to 500 mL blood is collected by puncturing vein in the antecubital area after appropriate antiseptic precautions. Blood is collected into bags prefilled with an anticoagulant which is comprised usually of citrate, phosphate and dextrose or other preservatives. The shelf life of the stored blood depends upon the nature of the preservative used.

Apheresis is a technique by which blood components are produced from whole blood donation by selectively collecting one or more components directly from donors and returning the rest to the circulation. Apheresis can be used to collect platelets, plasma, red cells or granulocytes from the donor. The main advantage of apheresis collections are that more than one dose of platelets or red cells can be collected from one donor per donation, thus reducing multiple donors' exposure to the patient.[5]

Testing of Donated Blood

All donations are tested for mandatory microbiological markers (hepatitis B and C, HIV and syphilis). A proportion of donations also undergo testing for other viruses (e.g. CMV) and additional typing, such as extended blood grouping and human leukocyte antigen (HLA) typing, for patients with specific requirements.[4–6]

PRESERVATION AND STORAGE

As there are very few clinical indications for transfusion of whole blood, vast majority of the blood is processed into its basic components: red cells, platelets and plasma (Fig. 30.1). This is achieved by centrifugation of whole blood in the primary

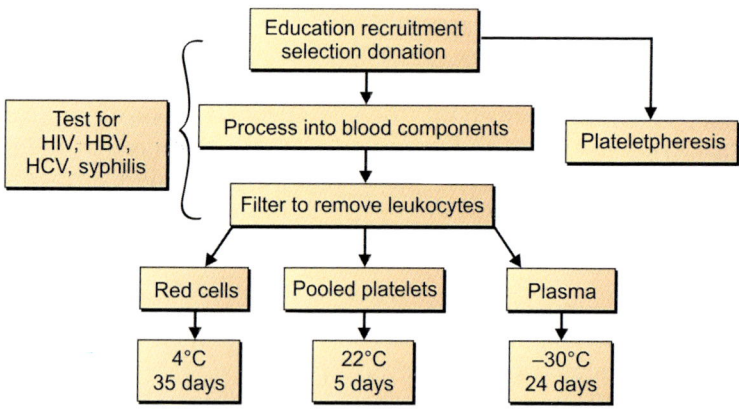

Fig. 30.1 Collection, processing and storage of blood

collection pack followed by manual or automated extraction of the components into satellite packs.

The initial storage temperature of whole blood determines the nature of the components that can be produced from it. For platelet production, whole blood must be processed on the day of blood collection or stored overnight at 22°C. However, for the production of red cells, whole blood can be stored at 4°C for 48–72 hours prior to separation. Plasma is separated from whole blood on the day of collection or from blood that has been stored at 22°C for up to 24 hours.[4, 5]

Preservation of Whole Blood

In the past, whole blood was stored with acid citrate dextrose (ACD) as the preservative initially. Later less acidic citrate phosphate dextrose (CPD) was used. Both ACD and CPD conferred a shelf life of 21 days. Subsequently adenine was added to the preservative thus forming CPD-A which improved the ATP content of the stored blood and increased the shelf life to 35 days.

PRESERVATION OF RED CELLS

Additive Solutions

With the advent of component therapy and preferential use of red cells for transfusion, preparation of red cell concentrates resulted in inadvertent removal of the preservatives, thus resulting in decreased red cell shelf life. To circumvent this problem, red cell additive solution was developed which allowed maximum recovery of plasma and preparation of red cell concentrate with a final hematocrit of 60%. Three types of additive solutions are available: AS-1, AS-3 and AS-5.

This new blood collection system has a primary bag containing CPD anticoagulant and a satellite bag containing an additive solution. Blood is collected in the CPD bag. Once the plasma is removed from the whole blood, the additive solution is added to the red cells. The red cells can be stored for six weeks at 2–6°C. The additive solution should be added to red cells within 72 hours since phlebotomy. Additive solution having mannitol is not routinely used for exchange or neonatal transfusion.[4]

Frozen Red Cells

Frozen red cells are primarily used for autologous transfusion and the storage of rare blood group. Red cells which are less than 6 days old are frozen rapidly after addition of cryopreservative agent containing glycerol. Glycerol prevents damage to red cells when frozen by maintaining a liquid phase and also by preventing hypertonicity. Frozen red cells can be stored for 10 years. Frozen red cells have to be thawed and deglycerolized before use. Frozen red cells once thawed can be stored at 2–6°C for only 24 hours.

SPECIAL RBC PREPARATIONS

Leukocyte Depletion

Leukocyte depletion or reduction is done to reduce the concentration of leukocytes to less than $5 \cdot 10^6$ leukocytes per unit of RBCs by using special filters.

Leukocyte reduction helps in preventing non-hemolytic febrile transfusion reactions (NHFTR1), HLA alloimmunization, transmission of leukotropic viruses (CMV, EBV and HTLV-1), transfusion related graft *versus* host disease (GVHD) and transfusion related acute lung injury (TRALI).[4]

Mukagatare and associates reported that leukocyte reduction significantly decreased the rate of all transfusion reactions from 0.49–0.31% (P <0.001), the rates of febrile non-hemolytic transfusion reactions from 0.35 to 0.24% (P <0.002) and the rate of allergic reactions from 0.05 to 0.01% (P <0.001).[7]

Implementation of universal WBC reduction has been found to decrease the incidence of bronchopulmonary dysplasia (OR 0.42; 0.25 to 0.70), retinopathy of prematurity (OR 0.56; 0.33 to 0.93) and necrotizing enterocolitis (OR 0.39; 0.17 to 0.93).[8]

Gamma Irradiation

Gamma irradiation of blood components is done to inactivate donor T cells and the associated risk of transfusion associated GVHD, which may occur in immunosuppressed patients, very small babies, in large volume transfusions and during intrauterine transfusions[9] or when the donor is related.

Irradiation reduces the shelf life of RBCs to 28 days and also causes leakage of potassium out of RBCs.[10] Irradiated RBCs should be used within 4 hours in neonates to avert the risk of hyperkalemia.

Irradiated RBCs are recommended for babies with birth weight below 1.2 kg. It may be preferable for any transfusions till 4 months of age.

Washed RBCs

Washing RBCs with saline is done to remove plasma and to reduce potassium in the RBCs. Washed RBCs are recommended for intrauterine transfusions, exchange transfusions and large volume transfusions (more than 20 mL/kg). For patients with immunoglobulin A deficiency or severe allergic or anaphylactoid reactions to red cells, it may be necessary to remove >90% of plasma by washing and re-suspending red cells in saline.[3]

CMV Reduced RBCs

CMV reduced RBCs reduce the risk of transmission of CMV infection, which may be a cause of considerable concern in newborns especially preterm infants. CMV reduction can be achieved by either leukoreduction of blood components or by pre-selecting donors who are CMV negative.

A meta-analysis of the available controlled studies indicates that CMV–seronegative blood components are more efficacious than WBC–reduced blood components in preventing transfusion–acquired CMV infection.[11]

Red Cells for Intrauterine Transfusion (IUT)

Red cells are transfused *in utero* to treat severe fetal anemia. In order to keep the volume transfused to a minimum, they are prepared by removing some of the plasma from whole blood to achieve a high hematocrit of 70–90%. Because of concerns over the potential toxicity of adenine and mannitol in red cell additive solutions, red cells for IUT and exchange transfusion are prepared and stored in plasma.

PLATELETS

Random Donor Platelets (RDP)

Platelets can be isolated from the whole blood donations or by apheresis. From whole blood, platelets can be produced either by platelet rich plasma (PRP) method or buffy-coat method. In the PRP method, whole blood is subjected to 'soft spin' initially which separates the whole blood into PRP and red cells. The PRP is then subjected to a 'hard spin' to remove plasma and concentrate the platelets. In the buffy-coat method, whole blood is subjected to a 'hard spin' and buffy-coat separated. The buffy-coats from four to six donations are then pooled with a unit of plasma or platelet additive solution and then subjected to a 'soft spin' and the PRP removed.[4,5]

Single Donor Platelets (SDP)

SDP units are obtained by a process called plateletpheresis wherein multiple units of platelets are collected from single donor and the RBCs and platelet poor plasma are returned to the donor. The procedure is repeated 4 to 6 times, yielding 4 to 6 units of platelets from one individual. It is especially useful to prevent alloimmunization in multiple transfused patients.

Both SDPs and RDPs are irradiated. The concentration of platelets is more in SDP than in RDP, with SDP having a platelet concentration of 3×10^{11}/unit and RDP having a concentration of 0.5×10^{10} per unit. In neonatal transfusion practice, RDP is generally adequate to treat thrombocytopenia. SDP is required only if prolonged and severe thrombocytopenia is anticipated, requiring multiple platelet transfusions. Platelets should be stored at 22–24°C with continuous gentle agitation in platelet incubator and agitator. Maintenance of pH above 6.0 is essential and the function of platelets depends on the permeability of the storage bag to oxygen and carbon dioxide.

Platelets stored in bags made of polyolefin have longer half life up to about 7 days. However, it is recommended to store platelets in new bags for 5 days only from the date of collection of blood. Platelets are stored with agitation at 22 ± 2°C for up to 5 days. 'Washed platelets' can be used in patients with anaphylactic reactions to the plasma component. Washed platelets have a shelf life of only 24 hours.

GRANULOCYTES

Granulocytes are normally collected by apheresis and contain mainly neutrophils, and some lymphocytes, red cells and platelets. Granulocytes can also be prepared from buffy-coats. Granulocyte transfusion should provide a dose of at least 1×10^{10} neutrophils.

Granulocytes should be transfused as soon as possible after collection or preparation but can be stored at 22°C for up to 24 hours without agitation and are irradiated prior to transfusion to prevent transfusion associated GVHD. Post transfusion recovery of granulocytes in circulation and migration into inflammatory loci is better if transfused within 8 hours of storage than granulocytes stored for 24 hours.[12]

FRESH FROZEN PLASMA (FFP)

FFP is produced by rapidly freezing the plasma within 8 hours of collection in order to preserve the activity of coagulation factors V and VIII which are relatively labile.

Frozen plasma components can be stored for up to 24 to 36 months depending on the storage temperature, which is usually below −30°C. Once thawed, FFP should be used immediately but can be stored for up to 24 hours at 4°C.[13]

CRYOPRECIPITATE

It is prepared from FFP by thawing at 2 to 4°C. Undissolved cryoprecipitate is collected by centrifugation and supernatant plasma is aseptically expressed into a satellite bag.

Cryoprecipitate can be stored for 12 months at −18°C or lower. Thawed cryoprecipitate can be stored for 6 hours at 2–6°C and pooled cryoprecipitate kept at 2–6°C should be used within 4 hours.[13]

Indications for PRBC Transfusion in Neonatal Practice

PRBCs are the most commonly used blood product in neonatal transfusions.[2,3] Preterm infants requiring intensive care are in need of repeated PRBC transfusion because of their immaturity, ongoing illness and the need for repeated sampling. Transfusion of PRBCs results in resolution of symptomatic anemia and improvement in tissue oxygenation. PRBC transfusion in preterm neonates should be restricted to minimum to prevent complications which are unique to them such as increased incidence of retinopathy of prematurity (ROP), CMV infection and even necrotizing enterocolitis (NEC). To achieve this, transfusion guidelines in neonates should ensure reduction in the number of transfusions and donor exposures.

Restrictive versus Liberal Transfusion

In order to limit the number of transfusions and the number of donors as well, restrictive transfusion policy is recommended. In general for young, mechanically ventilated preterm infants, the capillary hemoglobin should not be less than 11.5 g/dL; for older, stable infants, the hemoglobin should not be allowed to fall below 7.5 g/dL.

What is Evidence?

Cochrane review by Whyte et al on low *versus* high hemoglobin threshold for blood transfusion in very low birth weight infants did not find any significant difference in the combined outcome of death or serious morbidity at first hospital discharge (RR 1.19; 0.95 to 1.49).[14]

The guidelines for transfusion of PRBC vary according to gestation, postnatal age, level of sickness and hematocrit provided in Tables 30.1 and 30.2.

Table 30.1: Guidelines for packed red blood cells (PRBCs) transfusion thresholds for preterm neonates[3,15]

S.No.	Levels of respiratory support	Oxygen requirement	<28 days (PCV)	>28 days (PCV)
1.	Assisted ventilation	$FiO_2 > 0.3$	<40	<30
		$FiO_2 < 0.3$	<35	
2.	CPAP	Any FiO_2	<30	<25
3.	Spontaneously breathing		*Any age*	
	a. Symptomatic anemia*	$FiO_2 \geq 0.35$	<35	
		$FiO_2 > 0.21 - 0.34$	<30	
	b. Oxygen therapy	$FiO_2 > 0.21$	<25	
	c. Room air		<20	

*Symptomatic anemia is defined as presence of one of the following: (i) more than 9 apneic episodes in 12 hours; (ii) two or more such episodes requiring bag and mask ventilation in 24 hrs while on adequate methylxanthine therapy; (iii) HR >180/min or RR >80/min sustained for 24 hrs or more; (iv) weight gain less than 10 g/day for 4 days on 100 kcal/kg/day; (v) requiring surgery.

Table 30.2: Guidelines for packed red blood cells (PRBCs) transfusion thresholds for term neonates[16]

Condition	Hb (g/dL)
Severe cardiac or pulmonary disease	<13
Moderate pulmonary disease	<10
Major surgery	<10
Symptomatic anemia	<8

Practical Issues

1. *Amount of transfusion to be given*

   It has been seen that transfusion with PRBC at a dose of 20 mL/kg is well tolerated and results in an overall decrease in number of transfusions as compared to transfusions done at 10 mL/kg. There is also a higher rise in hemoglobin with a higher dose of PRBCs.[17]

2. *Properties of RBC products used in neonatal transfusion*

   a. Fresh RBCs (less than 7 days old) with high 2, 3-DPG levels ensure higher tissue oxygen delivery. They also reduce the risk of hyperkalemia.

   b. Multiple donor exposures in small and sick neonates can be prevented by reserving a bag of fresh PRBC for up to 7 days for a newborn and withdrawing small aliquots as and when required.

3. *Choosing the blood group for neonatal transfusions*[18]

   a. It is preferable to take samples from both mother and the newborn, for initial testing prior to transfusion. Mother's sample should be tested for blood group and for any atypical red cell antibodies.

   b. ABO compatibility is essential while transfusing PRBCs. Though ABO antigens may be expressed only weakly on neonatal erythrocytes, neonate's serum may contain transplacentally acquired maternal IgG anti-A and/or anti-B.

   c. Blood should be of newborn's ABO and Rh group. It should be compatible with any ABO or atypical red cell antibody present in the maternal serum.

   d. In exchange transfusions for Rh hemolytic disease of newborn, blood transfused should be compatible with mother's serum. Ideally Rh negative blood of the baby's ABO group has to be used after cross matching with maternal serum. If compatible ABO group is not available then group O and Rh negative blood can be used.

4. *Volume and rate of transfusion*
   a. Volume of packed RBC = Blood volume (mL/kg) × (desired minus actual hematocrit)/hematocrit of transfused RBC.
   b. Rate of infusion should be less than 10 mL/kg/hour in the absence of cardiac failure.
   c. Rate should not be more than 2 mL/kg/hour in the presence of cardiac failure.
   d. If more volume is to be transfused, *it* should be done in smaller aliquots.
   e. Meticulous monitoring of input, output and vital signs are mandatory during blood transfusion.

5. *Expected response*

   Each transfusion of 9 mL/kg of body weight should increase hemoglobin level by 3 g/dL.

PLATELET TRANSFUSION

Thrombocytopenia is defined as platelet count less than 1.5 lakh/cubic mm.[19] Presence of thrombocytopenia leads to an increase in risk of bleeding. Dysfunctional platelets in the presence of normal platelet counts may also cause bleeding tendency. Thrombocytopenia has been observed in 1–5% of newborns at birth.[20–22] Severe thrombocytopenia defined as platelet count of less than 50,000/cubic mm may occur in 0.1–0.5% of newborns.[22,23] In NICU, there is a higher incidence; with thrombocytopenia being observed in up to 22–35% of all admitted babies. Significant proportions (20%) of these episodes of thrombocytopenia are severe.[24,25] Thus, a large number of neonates are at risk of bleeding due to thrombocytopenia in NICU (Table 30.3).

Practical Issues

1. Platelets should never be filtered through a micropore blood filter before transfusion as it will considerably decrease the number of platelets.

Table 30.3: Indications for platelet transfusion in non-immune thrombocytopenia in newborn[19]

1. Platelet count less than 30,000/cubic mm: transfuse all neonates, even if asymptomatic
2. Platelet count 30,000 to 50,000/cubic mm: consider transfusion in
   a. Sick or bleeding
   b. Newborns less than 1000 gm or less than 1 week of age
   c. Previous major bleeding tendency (IVH grade 3–4)
   d. Concurrent coagulopathy
   e. Requiring surgery or exchange transfusion
3. Platelet count more than 50,000 to 99,000/cubic mm: transfuse only if actively bleeding

2. Female Rh-negative infants should receive platelets from Rh-negative donors to prevent Rh sensitization from the contaminating red blood cells.
3. The usual recommended dose of platelets for neonates is 1 unit of platelets per 10 kg body weight, which amounts to 5 mL/kg. The predicted rise in platelet count from a 5 mL/kg dose would be 20 to 60,000/cubic mm.[24,25] Doses of up to 10–20 ml/kg may be used in case of severe thrombocytopenia.

GRANULOCYTE TRANSFUSION

Granulocyte concentrates have limited therapeutic effectiveness in general except for bacterial sepsis or disseminated fungal infection unresponsive to antibiotics in infants. The concentrate should be CMV seronegative and be irradiated as it contains large number of lymphocytes but leukofilters should not be used for granulocyte transfusions. Cochrane review on the effect of granulocyte transfusion on suspected or confirmed sepsis with neutropenia did not find any reduction in mortality when compared to placebo (RR 0.89, 95% CI 0.43 to 1.86).[26]

INDICATIONS FOR TRANSFUSING FRESH FROZEN PLASMA

FFP has traditionally been used for a variety of reasons, including volume replacement, treatment of disseminated intravascular coagulopathy (DIC), during the treatment of a bleeding neonate, for prevention of intraventricular hemorrhage and in sepsis.[3] It has not been shown to have any survival benefits in most of these conditions and currently, the only valid indications for transfusing FFP in a newborn include:

1. Disseminated intravascular coagulopathy
2. Vitamin K deficiency bleeding
3. Inherited deficiencies of coagulation factors

Other rare indications include patients with afibrinogenemia, von Willebrand factor deficiency, congenital antithrombin III deficiency, protein C or S deficiency—when specific factor replacement is not available. It is also used for reconstitution of blood for exchange transfusion.

Indications for Use of Cryoprecipitate

Cryoprecipitate contains about 80 to 100 U of factor VIII in 10–25 mL of plasma, 300 mg of fibrinogen and varying amounts of factor XIII.[13]

1. Congenital factor VIII deficiency
2. Congenital factor XIII deficiency
3. Afibrinogenemia and dysfibrinogenemia
4. von Willebrand disease

Practical Issues

1. FFP should be compatible with recipient's ABO red cell antigens.
2. Volume of FFP to be transfused is usually 10–20 mL/kg.
3. Volume of cryoprecipitate to be transfused is usually 5 mL/kg.

TRANSFUSION ASSOCIATED RISKS

Blood transfusion reactions may be broadly classified as
1. Infectious
   a. Viruses
   b. Bacteria
   c. Parasites
   d. Prions
2. Non-infectious
   a. Acute
      i. Immune mediated reactions
      ii. Non-immune mediated reactions
   b. Delayed

INFECTIOUS COMPLICATIONS

In India, it is mandatory to test every unit of blood collected for hepatitis B, hepatitis C, HIV/AIDS, syphilis and malaria.[27] However, transfusion transmitted infections are still a considerable risk because of the relative insensitivity of screening tests and several other organisms besides those tested for, which may be transmitted through blood.

Viral Infections

Transmissible diseases can be caused by viruses like human immunodeficiency virus (HIV), hepatitis B and C viruses (HBV and HCV) and cytomegalovirus (CMV). Other uncommon viruses like hepatitis G virus and human herpesvirus-8 have also been detected. Viral infections contaminate platelet products more commonly than RBC products due to a higher temperature used for storage of platelet products.[28] Though screening for HIV, HBV and HCV is mandatory in blood banks, other viruses still present an unaddressed problem. Insensitivity of pathogen testing is also an issue and risk of viral infections with blood transfusions remains real. Risk of post transfusion hepatitis B or C in India is about 10% in adults despite routine testing because of low viremia and mutant strain undetectable by routine ELISA.[29] HIV prevalence among blood donors is different in various parts of the country.

CMV: Transfusion related CMV infections in newborns were initially identified in the year 1969 and since then transfusion associated CMV transmission is a well known entity. It has been reported that there is a seroconversion rate of 10–30% in preterm newborns transfused with CMV positive blood. Leuko-depletion and selection of CMV negative donors decreases the risk of transfusion transmitted CMV.[30]

Bacterial Infections

Bacteria in donor blood are derived from either asymptomatic bacteremia in the donor or from inadequate skin sterilization leading to bacterial contamination of the blood. Platelets are at a higher risk of causing bacterial infection than other blood components as they are stored at room temperature, leading to rapid multiplication of infectious organisms. The highest fatality is seen when the contaminating organism is a gram-negative bacteria. In case of a febrile non-hemolytic reaction post transfusion, bacterial contamination always remains a possibility. It generally causes a higher rise in temperature than other febrile transfusion reactions.

Parasites

Plasmodium, trypanosome and several other parasites may be transmitted through blood, depending on the endemicity of the area. Transfusion transmitted malaria is not uncommon in India and may occur in spite of blood bag testing as the screening tests for malaria are insensitive.[29]

Prions

Variant Creutzfeldt-Jakob disease (CJD) is an established complication of blood transfusion and has been reported since 2004. It is thought to have an incubation period of approximately 6.5 years. There is no easy test as yet to detect the presence of prions. It is not very clear whether leukoreduction prevents transmission of CJD.[28] Restricted transfusions and avoidance of transfusions unless essential, are the only ways currently to prevent transmission.

NON-INFECTIOUS COMPLICATIONS

These can be further sub-classified as acute and delayed complications. Of them, acute complications are again divided into two, say, immune mediated and non-immune mediated reactions.

Acute Immune Mediated Reactions

Immune Mediated Hemolysis

Acute hemolytic transfusion reactions are a common cause of transfusion related fatality in adult patients, but these are rare in neonates. Newborns do not form red blood cell (RBC) antibodies; all antibodies present are maternal in origin.

a. Newborns must be screened for maternal RBC antibodies including ABO antibodies if non-O RBCs are to be given as the first transfusion.

b. If the initial results are negative, no further testing is needed for the initial 4 postnatal months.

Infants are at a higher risk of passive immune hemolysis from infusion of ABO-incompatible plasma present in PRBC or platelet concentrates. Smaller quantities of ABO-incompatible plasma (less than 5 mL/kg) are generally well tolerated. Newborns do not manifest the usual symptoms of hemolysis that are observed in older patients, such as fever, hypotension and flank pain. An acute hemolytic event may be present as increased pallor, presence of plasma free hemoglobin, hemoglobinuria, increased serum potassium levels and acidosis. Results of the direct antiglobulin (Coombs') test may confirm the presence of an antibody on the RBC surface. Treatment is mainly supportive and involves maintenance of blood pressure and kidney perfusion with intravenous saline bolus of 10 to 20 mL/kg along with forced diuresis with furosemide. Enforcing strict guidelines for patient identification and issue of blood, and minimizing human error is essential in preventing immune mediated hemolysis.

Transfusion Related Acute Lung Injury (TRALI)

It refers to non-cardiogenic pulmonary edema complicating transfusion therapy. It is a common and under-reported complication occurring after therapy with blood components. It has been associated with all plasma-containing blood products, most commonly whole blood, packed RBCs, fresh frozen plasma and platelets. It has also been reported after the transfusion of cryoprecipitate and IVIG. The most common symptoms associated with TRALI are dyspnea, cough and fever associated with hypo- or hypertension. It occurs most commonly within the initial 6 hours after transfusion. The presence of anti-HLA and/or anti-granulocyte antibodies in the plasma of donors is implicated in the pathogenesis of TRALI. Diagnosis requires a high index of suspicion and confirmation of donor serum cross-reacting antibodies against the recipient. Treatment is mainly supportive in this self-limiting condition.[31,32]

Febrile Non-hemolytic Transfusion Reactions (FNHTRs)

These reactions are suspected in the absence of hemolysis with an increase in body temperature of less than 2°C. For reactions associated with a temperature rise of greater than 2°C or with hypotension, bacterial contamination should also be suspected and a Gram stain and microbial culture performed on the remaining blood product.

Allergic Reactions

Allergic reactions are caused by presence of preformed immunoglobulin E antibody against an allergen in the transfused plasma and are a rare occurrence in newborns. In some cases, release of residual cytokines or chemokines (e.g. RANTES) from stored platelets may also cause allergic reactions. These reactions are generally mild and respond to anti-histaminics. Severe anaphylactic reactions are rare.

Acute Non-immune Mediated Reactions

Fluid Overload

Neonates are at increased risk of fluid overload from transfusion because the volume of the blood component issued may exceed the volume that may be transfused safely into neonates. Care should be taken to ensure that, in the absence of blood loss, volumes infused do not exceed 10 to 20 mL/kg. There is no role for routine use of furosemide while transfusing newborns.

Metabolic Complications[33]

These complications occur with large volume of transfusions like exchange transfusions.

a. *Hyperkalemia*: In stored blood, potassium levels tend to be high. It has been seen that after storage for around 42 days, potassium levels may reach 50 mEq/L in a RBC unit.[34] Though small volume transfusions do not have much risk of metabolic disturbances, large volume transfusions may lead to hyperkalemia. Washing PRBCs before reconstituting with FFP before exchange transfusion helps in preventing this complication.

b. *Hypoglycemia:* Blood stored in CPD blood has a high content of glucose leading to a rebound rise in insulin release 1–2 hours after transfusion. This may lead to hypoglycemia and routine monitoring is necessary, particularly after exchange transfusion (after 2 and 6 hours), to ensure that this complication does not occur.

c. *Acid–base derangements*: Metabolism of citrate in CPD leads to late metabolic alkalosis. Metabolic acidosis is an immediate complication occurring in sick babies who cannot metabolize citrate.

d. *Hypocalcemia and hypomagnesemia* are caused by binding of these ions by citrate present in CPD blood.

Delayed Complications

Alloimmunization

Alloimmunization is an uncommon occurrence before the age of 4 months and is caused by transfusion of blood products which are mismatched for highly immunogenic antigens like Rh.[35]

Transfusion Associated Graft versus Host Disease (TAGVHD)

Newborns are at risk for TAGVHD, if they have received intrauterine transfusions, exchange transfusions or are very small or immunocompromised. Unchecked donor T cell proliferation is the cause of TAGVHD and it can be effectively prevented by leucoreduction of the transfused blood products in at risk patients.

REFERENCES

1. Bell EF, Strauss RG, Widness JA, Mahoney LT, Mock DM, et al. Randomized trial of liberal *versus* restrictive guidelines for red blood cell Transfusion in preterm infants. Pediatrics 2005; 115:1685–1691.
2. Ohls RJ. Transfusions in the preterm neonates. NeoReviews 2007;8:377–386.
3. Murray NA, Roberts IAG. Neonatal transfusion practice. Arch Dis Child FN 2004;89:101–107.
4. McClelland Ed. In: Handbook of transfusion medicine. United Kingdom blood services. 4th edn. TSO Publishers. London 2007; p. 5–22.
5. James V (Ed). In: Guidelines for blood transfusion services in the United Kingdom. 7th edn. TSO Publishers. London 2005; p. 21–32.
6. Dhingra N (Ed). In: Screening donated blood for transfusion transmissible infections. WHO Recommendations 2010.
7. Mukagatare I, Monfort M, deMarchin J, Gerard C. The effect of leukocyte-reduction on the transfusion reactions to red blood cells concentrates [French]. Transfus Clin Biol 2010;17:14–19.

8. Fergusson D, Hebert PC, Lee SK, et al. Clinical outcomes following institution of universal leukoreduction of blood transfusions for premature infants. JAMA. 2003;289:1950–1956.

9. Schroeder ML. Transfusion-associated graft-*versus*-host disease. Br J Haematol 2002;117:275–287.

10. Pelszynsky MM, Moroff G, Luban NLC, Taylor BJ, Quinones RR. Effect of γ irradiation of red blood cell units on T-cell inactivation as assessed by limiting dilution analysis: implications for preventing transfusion-associated graft *versus* host disease. Blood 1994; 83:1683–1689.

11. Vamvakas EC. Is white blood cell reduction equivalent to antibody screening in preventing transmission of cytomegalovirus by transfusion? A review of the literature and meta-analysis. Transfus Med Rev 2005;19:181–199.

12. Strauss RG. Transfusion therapy for neonates. Am J Dis Child 1991;145:904–911.

13. Brandon S. Poterjoy, Cassandra D. Josephson. Platelets, frozen plasma and cryoprecipitate: what is the clinical evidence for their use in the neonatal intensive care unit? Semin Perinatol 2009; 33(1):66–74.

14. Whyte R, Kirpalani H. Low *versus* high haemoglobin concentration threshold for blood transfusion for preventing morbidity and mortality in very low birth weight infants. Cochrane Database of Systematic Reviews 2011, Issue 11. Art. No.: CD000512. DOI: 10.1002/14651858.CD000512.pub2.

15. Cloherty JP, Eichenwald EC, Stark AR Eds. In: Manual of neonatal care. 7th edn. Lippincott William and Wilkins USA 2011; p. 441.

16. Behrman ER (Ed). Red blood cell transfusions and erythropoietin therapy. In Nelson Textbook of Pediatrics 19th edn, Elseviers, 2010; p.1647.

17. Paul DA, Leef KH, Locke RG, Stefano JL. Transfusion volume in infants with very low birth weight: a randomized trial of 10 *versus* 20 ml/kg. J Pediatr Hematol Oncol 2002;24:43–6.

18. Chatterjee K, Sen A. Step by step blood transfusion services. 1st edn. New Delhi. Jaypee; 2006; p. 238–300.

19. Roberts I, Murray NA. Neonatal thrombocytopenia: causes and management. Arch Dis Child FN 2003;88:F359–64.

20. Hohlfeld P, Forestier F, Kaplan C, Tissot JD, Daffos F. Fetal thrombocytopenia: a retrospective survey of 5,194 fetal blood samplings. Blood 1994;84:1851–6.

21. Burrows RF, Kelton JG. Incidentally detected thrombocytopenia in healthy mothers and their infants. N Engl J Med 1988;319:142–5.

22. Sainio S, Jarvenpaa A-S, Renlund M, Riikonen S, Teramo K, et al. Thrombocytopenia in term infants: a population-based study. Obstet Gynecol 2000;95:441–6.

23. Uhrynowska M, Niznikowska-Marks M, Zupanska B. Neonatal and maternal thrombocytopenia: incidence and immune background. Eur J Haematol 2000;64:42–46.

24. Castle V, Andrew M, Kelton J, Girm D, Johston M, et al. Frequency and mechanism of neonatal thrombocytopenia. J Pediatr 1986;108: 749–55.

25. Murray NA, Howarth LJ, McCloy MP, Letsky EA, Roberts IAG. Platelet transfusion in the management of severe thrombocytopenia in neonatal intensive care unit (NICU) patients. Transfus Med 2002;12:35–41.

26. Pammi M, Brocklehurst P. Granulocyte transfusions for neonates with confirmed or suspected sepsis and neutropenia. Cochrane Database Syst Rev. 2011 Oct 5;(10):CD003956.

27. Choudhury LP, Tetali S. Ethical challenges in voluntary blood donation in Kerala, India. J Med Ethics. 2007;33:140–2.

28. Madjdpour C, Heindl V, Spahn DR. Risks, benefits, alternatives and indications of allogenic blood transfusion. Minerva Anestesiol 2006;72:283–98.

29. Choudhury N, Phadke S. Transfusion transmitted diseases. Indian J Pediatr 2001;68:951–8.

30. Bowden RA, Slichter SJ, Sayers M, Weisdorf D, Cays M, et al. A comparison of filtered leukocyte—reduced and cytomegalovirus (CMV) seronegative blood products for the prevention of transfusion—associated CMV infection after marrow transplant blood 1995;86:3598–3603.

31. Yang X, Ahmed S, Chandrasekaran V. Transfusion-related acute lung injury resulting from designated blood transfusion between mother and child: a report of two cases. Am J Clin Pathol 2004;121:590–2.

32. Looney MR, Gropper MA, Manhay MA. Transfusion—related acute lung injury—a review. Chest 2004;126:249–258.

33. Martin CR, Cloherty JP. Neonatal hyperbilirubinemia. In: Cloherty JP, Eichenwald ER, Stark AR (Eds). Manual of neonatal care. 5th edn. Philadelphia: Lippincott Williams and Wilkins. 2004;p.185–221.

34. Strauss RG. Transfusion approach to neonatal anemia. Neo-Reviews 2000;1:e74–80.

35. Galel SA, Fontaine MJ. Hazards of neonatal blood transfusion. Neo Reviews 2006;7:e69–75.0.

31

Pain and Developmental Supportive Care

Developmental care refers to set of actions like reduction in noise and light, minimal handling, effective pain prevention and treatment aimed at reducing the stresses in the NICU and optimizing neurobehavioral outcome.[1] Developmental care interventions are potentially beneficial to sick neonates especially those born prematurely to cope with the adverse external environment in NICU and organize all sensory inputs. Structured developmental supportive programs like Newborn Individualized Development Care and Assessment Program (NIDCAP) combines various measures to provide individualized care based on each baby's need.

Developmentally Supportive Care: What is Evidence?

A Cochrane meta-analysis (2006) included 36 RCTs and examined the effects of developmental care interventions like positioning, clustering of nursery care activities, modification of external stimuli and individualized developmental care interventions (e.g. NIDCAP).
- Modest beneficial effects in the form of decreased moderate-severe chronic lung disease, decreased incidence of necrotizing enterocolitis and improved family outcomes.
- Limited long-term positive effect on behavior and motor outcome at 5 years corrected age.

INTEGRATION OF CORE MEASURES

For operationalizing of evidence-based developmental care program,[1] the following core measures are proposed:
1. Protected sleep
2. Pain and stress management
3. Developmentally supportive activities of daily living
4. Family centered care
5. Creating a healing environment

These five-point patient centered measures need to be integrated into the routine clinical practice and its performance needs systematic audit, so as to reap best results (Table 31.1).

Table 31.1: Evidence-based core developmental care strategies in NICU

Core measures	Practice parameters
Protected sleep	• All non-emergent care-giving is provided while infant is awake (no disturbance while baby is sleeping). · Promote sleep by facilitative tuck, swaddling and skin-to-skin care. • Light and sound levels are minimized. Day-night pattern is simulated by reducing lights in night to facilitate nocturnal sleep. • Family education on care-giving activities that promote safe sleep.
Prevent and treat pain	• Assess if baby suffers from pain once during each nursing shift and during all procedures using a validated score (refer to pain section). • Provide non-pharmacologic and/or pharmacologic measures to reduce pain for all stressful and/or painful procedures. • Care-giving activities are adapted to minimize pain and stress. • Parents are educated regarding infant pain and involved in its management.
Provide containment	• Provide containment by keeping the infant in flexed posture by support of hand during procedures and transport.
Provide developmentally supportive care	• Use boundaries around the infants to maintain them in flexed posture (similar to in utero posture) (Fig. 31.1). Provide non-nutritive sucking while the infant is being fed by gavage or paladai by allowing the baby to suck on mother's finger or breast. • Provide lactation counseling and support to initiate and maintain lactation in the mother. • Protect the integrity of skin during application and removal of adhesive products (minimize use or do not strap to achieve hemostasis after sampling, instead just put a dry cotton swab and hold it for some time. Adhesive should be removed only after 72 hrs of application once it has loosened from skin surface. Wet the plaster before removal).
Provide family centered care *(do not consider infant as a solo entity)*	• Disease has serious impact on social fabric of the family. Consider individuals beyond infant and issues beyond disease such as those related to financial condition and relationship within family. Consider cost-benefit ratio of treatment/investigation modality that you plan to employ.

Contd...

Table 31.1: Evidence-based core developmental care strategies in NICU (Contd...)

Core measures	Practice parameters
	• Allow the parents to visit the infant in NICU and to have conversation with the treating team. Involve parents in decision making regarding treatment of the infant. Family observations and input regarding their infants are sought by the clinical care providers.
	• Family is supported in parenting activities such as skin-to-skin care, holding the baby, feeding, dressing, diapering, singing and all infant care interactions.
	• Babies in NICU should be divided to available nurses on the shift so that all care-giving activities of a baby should be carried out by the allotted nurse of that baby. The practice of 'task-specific' allotment of nurses (such as one nurse responsible for feeding, another for injections to all babies) must be avoided.
	• Practice 'primary nursing'. That means one nurse becomes 'primary nurse' of a baby and that baby always gets allotted to the primary nurse in whatever shift duty she comes. Her name should be recorded on bedside identification tag and communicated to the family. 'Primary nurse' of the baby is responsible for keeping a close liaison with family and physicians for holistic care of the baby.
Healing environment	• Minimize sound, lights and strong smells (e.g. spirit). Do not place anything on incubator. Close the incubator doors gently. Cover incubator with a cloth sheet to minimize light. Do not use procedure light unnecessarily. Do not speak too loudly. Do not drag chairs in NICU.
	• Make sure that health professionals follow caring behaviors such as adherence to hand hygiene protocols, cultural sensitivity, open listening skills and an empathic relationship with families.
	• Do not perform investigation for a routine. Consider utility of an investigation before you do it. If it is unlikely to change your management, it is unnecessary and potentially harmful by causing pain and increasing the infection risk.
	• Promote free and healthy communication between physicians, nurses and other professionals working in NICU. A cohesive team is more likely to avoid errors and provide healing touch.

Modified as per feasibility in developing country settings

PAIN ASSESSMENT AND MANAGEMENT

Preterm infants have well developed pain preception mechanisms, but do not have those required for pain modulation as in term infants or an adult. Repeated stimuli in latter result in

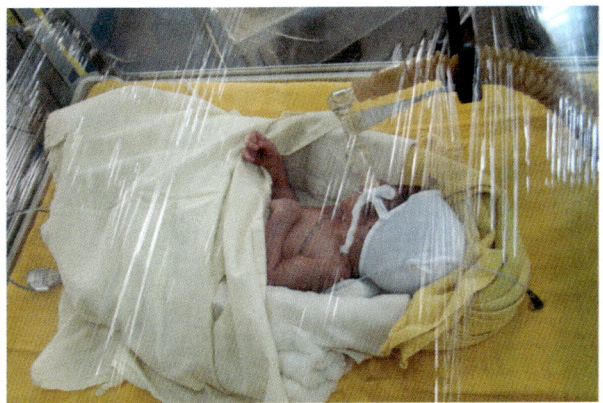

Fig. 31.1: Boundaries to promote in utero posture of the infant

Note that boundary is tall enough to contain the baby and the cloth sheet should be tied at ends so as to maintain the round shape of it. Warmer bassinet has been covered using a thin plastic sheet to minimize insensible water losses in very preterm infants.

progressive attenuation of pain while it result in increasing severity of pain in the former. Therefore, preterm infants not only perceive pain but do it at much more intensity as well as for much longer time.

Pain has lasting adverse effects on infant's brain development which manifests later as abnormal pain perception, behavioral abnormalities, cognitive defects and learning disabilities.[4] Hence, routine assessment and management of pain forms an important part of the developmental supportive care.[2]

Assessment of pain, an integral part of any pain prevention program is challenging in neonates. Use Premature Infant Pain Profile (PIPP; Table 31.2) for assessment of acute pain.[3]

GENERAL MEASURES FOR PREVENTING OR REDUCING PAIN

Pain is managed most effectively by preventing, limiting or avoiding noxious stimuli. The following measures in combination are followed to minimize pain:
- Avoid bright light, loud noise
- Limit the number of painful procedures and handling
- Avoiding unnecessary investigations

Table 31.2: Premature infant pain profile (PIPP)[3]

S. No.	Parameters	Score			
		0	1	2	3
1.	What is gestation weeks of infant?	≥36	32–35[6/7]	28–31[6/7]	≤28
2.	Score behavioral state before the procedure (15 sec).	Active awake *Eyes-open Facial movements +*	Quite awake *Eyes-open No facial movements*	Active sleep *Eyes-closed Facial movements +*	Quite/sleep *Eyes-closed No facial movements*
3.	Record baseline HR and find out maximum HR during the procedure.	0–4/min increase	5–14/min	15–24/min	≥25/min
4.	Record baseline SO_2 and find out minimum SO_2 during the procedure.	0–2.4% fall	2.5–4.9% fall	5–7.4% fall	≥7.5% fall
5.	Observe the infant for 30 sec immediately after the procedure (for brow bulge, eye squeeze and naso-labial furrow).	None (0–9% of time)	Minimum (10–39% of time)	Moderate (40–69% of time)	Maximum (≥70% of time)

Health professionals should record PIPP score of all babies once/nursing shift and before the procedures. The issue of pain should be discussed on the rounds. The minimum score is 0 and maximum score is 21. Higher is the score, greater the pain. Score <5: no pain; 6–10: moderate pain; and >10: severe pain.

- Bundling of investigations and nursing interventions
- Swaddling, facilitated tucking, distraction measures like talking, music, etc.
- Hold the baby with firm grip during procedures. Avoid feathery touch or stroking.

NON-PHARMACOLOGICAL MEASURES

The environmental and behavioral interventions that do not use pharmacological agents are collectively called non-pharmacological measures. These include:

1. Sucrose/glucose solution induced analgesia
2. Breastfeeding/breast milk supplementation
3. Skin-to-skin care
4. Non-nutritive sucking using pacifiers

The non-pharmacological measures are thought to alleviate pain by activating gate control mechanism, secretion of endogenous endorphins, diversion of attention and by pre-emptying hypersensitivity.[4]

Sucrose Analgesia

Sucrose administration is particularly useful for short procedures like venipuncture, heel prick, etc. Oral administration of concentrated sucrose solution (24–50%) acts by release of endogenous opioids like beta-endorphin. Analgesic effect lasts for 5–8 min and should be combined with other non-pharmacological measures for maximum benefit. Alternative to sucrose is dextrose which is less widely used (Table 31.3).

Table 31.3: Dose of sucrose/dextrose for analgesia[6,9]

Concentration	For babies who are NPO	Preterm (<32 weeks)	Late PT/term
24% Sucrose/ 25% dextrose	0.1–0.2 mL	0.1–0.5 mL	0.2–1.0 mL

The sucrose solution is given orally by a syringe 2–3 min before procedure and may be repeated 1–2 min after the procedure. Intragastric administration has no analgesic effect.

Breastfeeding and Breast Milk Supplementation

Breastfeeding and breast milk supplementation is almost as effective as sucrose analgesia in reducing pain in newborns undergoing single painful procedure (Table 31.4).

PHARMACOLOGICAL MEASURES

The pharmacological measures can be broadly divided into the following:
- Local anesthetic agents
- Systemic agents: Opioids, acetaminophen

   Non-steroidal anti-inflammatory Drugs (NSAIDs) are generally not used in newborns as analgesics.

Local Anesthetics

Local anesthesia is particularly useful for management of acute procedure related pain with the exception of heel lances.[7] It can be either topically applied on intact skin or injected subcutaneously.

Table 31.4: Evidence supporting non-pharmacological analgesic measures in neonates

Agent	Evidence	Findings
Sucrose (24%)	Cochrane meta-analysis[1] 44 studies, 3496 infants	• Reduction in pain scores (PIPP) • Decreases physiological indicators of pain (heart rate increase) • Less behavioral indicators of pain (duration of cry, facial action).
Breast milk and breastfeeding	Cochrane meta-analysis[1] 11 studies	• Less duration of cry, lesser increase in heart rate • Lesser PIPP score • Lesser increase in neonatal facial coding score • Breastfeeding was better than breast milk supplementation.
Non-nutritive sucking, skin-to-skin care, swaddling, facilitated tucking, music	Systematic Reviews[4] 13 RCT 2 Meta-analyses	• Favorable effect on heart rate, respiration and oxygen saturation, on the reduction of motor activity, and on the excitation states after invasive measures • Non-nutritive sucking, swaddling and facilitated tucking are particularly useful • Combination of measures always provides better analgesia.

The common topical preparations marketed are:

1. Eutectic mixture of local anesthetics (EMLA): It is a mixture of two local anesthetics, namely, lidocaine and prilocaine that comes as 5% cream.
2. Tetracaine (4%)
3. Liposomal lidocaine 4% cream

The dose of EMLA is 1–2 g with contact period of 30 min to 1 hour. Apply the cream over 2–3 cm^2 area with 1–2 mm thickness and cover with transparent (tegaderm) dressing. For maximal analgesic effect, the topical anesthetics should be combined with other non-pharmacological measures like sucrose analgesia or breast milk supplementation.

The major drawback is the delayed onset of action and a contact period of at least 1 hour prior to the procedure, which makes it unsuitable for emergent procedures. The risk of methemoglobinemia associated with repeated use of EMLA cream, is not seen with newer preparations like tetracaine gel.

For emergent procedures, subcutaneous local anesthetic injection (lidocaine hydrochloride 2%) is preferred over the topical creams.

Systemic Agents

Opioids: The opioid drugs are the mainstay in the management of severe pain related to mechanical ventilation, endotracheal intubation and post surgical pain in neonates. The two most commonly used agents are morphine and fentanyl.

a. **Morphine:** Morphine has slower onset of action with mean onset at 5 min and peak effect at 15 min. It is metabolized in the liver to morphine-3-glucuronide, an opioid antagonist and morphine-6-glucuronide, a potent analgesic. Newborn babies especially preterm infants mainly produce morphine-3-glucuronide leading to emergence of tolerance after 2–3 days of therapy.

   The observed side effects include hypotension, need for prolonged ventilation, delay in reaching full feeds and rarely bronchospasm secondary to histamine release.[12]

b. **Fentanyl:** Fentanyl is a synthetic opioid analgesic. It is 50 to 100 times more potent and more rapid in onset of action as compared to morphine. Fentanyl is preferred over morphine in infants with hypotension as cardiovascular side effects are lesser.[2,8] The unique side effect of fentanyl is chest wall rigidity especially if given as rapid intravenous bolus.

   The other opioids used are methadone, sulfentanil, remifentanil, etc. which are used for short procedures like endotracheal intubation and short neonatal surgeries.

ANALGESIA FOR SPECIFIC PROCEDURES

Elective and Semi-elective Intubation

Intubation of neonates in awake state is associated with increase in heart rate, greater fall in oxygen saturations/heart rate, increased intracranial pressure, increased risk of IVH, airway trauma and failure of procedure especially in inexperienced hands[10] (Table 31.5).

The AAP committee on fetus and newborn recommends avoiding awake intubation of newborn babies except in

Table 31.5: Sedation for elective intubation

The preferred regimen includes:

1. Inj. Fentanyl 1–4 mcg/kg, given slow IV over 3–5 min
2. Inj. Atropine 0.02 mg/kg (minimum dose should be 0.1 mg)
3. Inj. Vecuronium 0.1 mg/kg administered IV, 2–3 minutes prior to the procedure

Avoid using paralytic agents in case experienced person is unavailable for intubations.

emergent situations like delivery room intubation and in cases where intravenous access is unavailable.[4]

The AAP recommends:

• Analgesic agents or anesthetic dose of a hypnotic drug should be given.

• Vagolytic agents and rapid-onset muscle relaxants should be considered.

• Use of sedatives alone such as benzodiazepines without analgesic agents should be avoided.

• A muscle relaxant without an analgesic agent should not be used.

Tables 31.6 and 31.7 provide details on how to provide analgesia in different procedures.

Table 31.8 provides details of different analgesic agents.

Table 31.6: Analgesic measures for routine bedside procedures

Procedures	Analgesic measures recommended			
	General measures	Sucrose analgesia*	Breast milk*	Facilitated tucking/ caressing
Venipuncture Sampling#	+	+	±	+
Heel prick#	+	+	+	+
Subcutaneous/IM injection	+	+	+	+
Adhesive tape removal	+	+	+	+
IV cannulation	+	+	±	+

* Either sucrose analgesia or breastfeeding can be adopted depending on the availability and feasibility; for slightly longer procedure, sucrose analgesia is preferred over breast milk/breastfeeding.
# Venipuncture should be the preferred mode of blood sampling as heel lance is more painful.

Table 31.7: Analgesic measures for specific procedures[6]

Procedures	Intubated	Non-intubated
Arterial puncture/ cannulation Lumbar puncture PICC line placement	• Inj. Morphine 0.1–0.2 mg/kg IV • EMLA cream locally • Sucrose analgesia	• EMLA cream locally • Sucrose analgesia • General measures
Chest tube placement	• Inj. Morphine 0.1–0.2 mg/kg IV • Local infiltration with Lignocaine 2% • Sucrose analgesia	• Inj. Morphine 0.1 mg/kg IV* • Local infiltration with Lignocaine 2% • Sucrose analgesia
Chest drain removal	• Inj. Morphine 0.1–0.2 mg/kg • Sucrose analgesia • General measures	• EMLA cream locally • Sucrose analgesia • General measures
ROP screening	• Inj. Morphine 0.1–0.2 mg/kg IV • Local anesthetic eye drops • Sucrose analgesia • Postscreen—paracetamol	• Local anesthetic eye drops • Sucrose analgesia • Postscreen—paracetamol
ROP laser surgery	• Inj. Morphine 0.1–0.2 mg/kg IV • Local anesthetic eye drops • Sucrose analgesia • Postoperative—paracetamol 15 mg/kg q 6 hourly for 1–2 day	• Inj. Morphine 0.1–0.2 mg/kg IV* • Local anesthetic eye drops • Sucrose analgesia • General measures • Postoperative—paracetamol 15 mg/kg q 6 hourly for 1–2 day
CT/MRI-for sedation	• Inj. Morphine 0.1–0.2 mg/kg IV • Inj. Midazolam 0.1–0.3 mg/kg IV • IV Midazolam 0.1–0.2 mg/kg IV single dose	• Oral chloral hydrate 50–100 mg/kg • Oral Trichlophos 20 mg/kg

*In non-ventilated babies, while using opioids—watch for apnea/respiratory depression; IV Naloxone should be kept ready and used in case of respiratory depression or apnea (0.1 mg/kg or 0.25 ml/kg IV); Inj. Fentanyl may be substituted for Inj. Morphine; dose 1–4 mcg/kg, slow IV over 3–5 min.

NB: *Even ventilated patients on opioid infusion during procedures need additional analgesic measures.*

Table 31.8: Drugs and dosages of analgesic/sedative medications commonly used in NICU

Drug	Dose	Preparation/Administration	Pharmacology	Adverse effect
Morphine	Bolus: 100–200 mcg/kg slow IV over 5 min Infusion: 10–20 mcg/kg/hr IV	1 mL=15 mg Dilute in: NS/10D/5D to make a maximum concentration of 5 mg/mL Incompatible with phenytoin, phenobarbitone	Narcotic analgesic Onset: 5 min Peak: 15 min T$\frac{1}{2}$: 9 hrs	Respiratory depression Bradycardia Hypotension Ileus, urinary retention Tolerance
Fentanyl	Bolus: 1–5 mcg/kg IV slow IV over 5–10 min Infusion: 1–5 mcg/kg/hour IV	1 mL = 50 mcg Dilute in: NS/5D/10D Incompatible with phenytoin, phenobarbitone	50–100 times more potent than morphine; Rapid onset; less hypotension than morphine T$\frac{1}{2}$: 1–15 hrs; short acting benzodiazepine	Respiratory depression Chest wall rigidity with rapid push Urinary retention Tolerance
Midazolam	Bolus: 0.1–0.2 mg/kg slow IV Infusion: 0.01–0.06 mg/kg/hour Intranasal/sublingual route (dose 0.2–0.3 mg/kg) may also be used	1 mL = 1 mg Dilute in: NS/5D/10D Incompatible with NaHCO$_3$, fat emulsion	Sedation only, no analgesic effect T$\frac{1}{2}$: 4–6 hrs in term infants; preterm variable up to 22 hrs; not recommended in neonates esp. preterm	Respiratory depression Myoclonic jerk Hypotension (esp. with rapid push)

Contd...

Table 31.8: Drugs and dosages of analgesic/sedative medications commonly used in NICU (Contd.)

Drug	Dose	Preparation/Administration	Pharmacology	Adverse effect
Vecuronium	0.1 mg/kg	Available as powder (1 vial = 10 mg/20 mg) Dilute in 5D/NS to make 1 mg/mL)	Non-depolarizing muscle relaxant; Onset 1–2 min duration of action 1–2 hours emergent intubation as premedication Consider using during non-intubation as premedication	Respiratory depression Hypotension Avoid routine use in ventilated neonates
Paracetamol	10–15 mg/kg/dose PO 6–8 hrly 30 mg/kg/dose per rectal	Syp 5 mL = 125 mg Drops 1 ml = 100 mg Suppositories 80 mg	Rectal route erratic absorption	
Chloral hydrate	25–75 mg/kg PO/rectally	1 ml = 100 mg	No analgesia, only sedation Administer with feeds (high osmolality, may cause GI intolerance)	Bradycardia Gastric irritation Contraindicated in hepatic/renal dysfunction
EMLA cream	1–2 g for 1 hr	Lidocaine-priiocaine 5% (e.g. Oint Prilox available in India) 5 g/30 g with tegaderm dressing	Delayed onset: ½–1 hr Not effective for heel lance	Methemoglobinemia

MECHANICAL VENTILATION

Mechanical ventilation is a painful and uncomfortable experience which might adversely affect the course of acute illness as well as long-term neurodevelopment.[5] However, there is insufficient evidence for routine use of pharmacological measures in all ventilated infants.[11]

Indications for continuous infusion of opioids in ventilated neonates are:

- Postoperative patients especially in the first 48–72 hours.
- Illnesses like meconium aspiration syndrome or congenital diaphragmatic hernia with PPHN.
- Asynchrony or fighting with ventilator. Rule out causes like ventilator malfunction, tube block or inappropriate settings before infant is sedated for this indication.

Avoid use of midazolam especially in preterm babies. Do not use paralytic agents routinely in ventilated babies.

Analgesia/Sedation in Ventilated Neonates: What is Evidence?

A Cochrane meta-analysis (2005) including 13 studies and 1505 infants concluded that there is insufficient evidence to recommend routine use of opioids. However, when used, morphine is safer than midazolam showing reduction in pain severity as noted by lower PIPP scores and there is no long-term/short-term reduction in morbidity/mortality.

REFERENCES

1. Coughlin M, Gibbins S, Hoath S. Core measures for developmentally supportive care in neonatal intensive care units: theory, precedence and practice. Journal of Advanced Nursing 2009; 65(10):2239–48.

2. American Academy of Pediatrics, Committee on Fetus and Newborn and Section on Surgery; Canadian Paediatric Society, Fetus and Newborn Committee. Prevention and Management of Pain in the Neonate: An Update. Pediatrics 2006;118:2231–41.

3. Stevens B, Johnston C, Petryshen P, Taddio A. Premature infant pain profile: development and initial validation. Clin J Pain 1996;12:13–22.

4. Cignacco E, Hamers JP, Stoffel L, van Lingen RA, Gessler P, McDougall J, Nelle M. The efficacy of non-pharmacological

interventions in the management of procedural pain in preterm and term neonates. A systematic literature review. Eur J Pain 2007;11:139–52.

5. Stevens B, Yamada J, Ohlsson A. Sucrose for analgesia in newborn infants undergoing painful procedures. Cochrane Database of Systematic Reviews 2004, Issue 3. Art. No.: CD001069.

6. Shah PS, Aliwalas LL, Shah VS. Breastfeeding or breast milk for procedural pain in neonates. Cochrane Database of Systematic Reviews 2006, Issue 3. Art. No.: CD004950.

7. Lehr VT, Taddio A. Topical anesthesia: clinical practice and practical considerations. Semi Perinatology 2007;31:323–29.

8. Saarenmaa E, Huttunen P, Leppaluoto J, et al. Advantages of fentanyl over morphine in analgesia for ventilated newborn infants after birth: a randomized trial. J Pediatr 1999;134:144–50.

9. Carbajal R, Eble B, Anand KJS. Premedication for tracheal intubation in neonates: confusion or controversy. Seminars in Perinatology 2007;31:309–17.

10. Kumar P, Denson SE, Mancuso TJ. Premedication for non-emergency endotracheal intubation in the neonate. Pediatrics 2010; 125;608–15.

11. Hall RW, Boyle E, Young T. Do ventilated neonates require pain management? Seminars in Perinatology 2007;31:289–97.

12. Hall RW, Shbarou RM. Drug of choice for sedation and analgesia in newborn: ICU. Clin Perinatol 2009;36:15–26.

32

Chest X-ray—Use and Interpretation

INDICATIONS

The indications for a chest X-ray include:
1. For evaluating the initial cause of respiratory distress
2. For suspected cardiac or pericardial disease
3. To check position of endotracheal tube, umbilical venous or arterial lines, peripherally inserted central catheters or chest tubes
4. For evaluating cause of worsening respiratory distress in a ventilated neonate after ruling out mechanical problems (tube block/secretions/dislodgement) or ventilator dysfunction.

Some conditions where X-rays are *not* indicated include:
1. Routine/daily X-rays in ventilated neonates
2. Routine pre/post extubation X-rays
3. After re-intubation in a neonate where the optimal "tip-to-lip" distance is known based on initial X-ray
4. Evaluation of an isolated episode of desaturation/apnea.

INTERPRETATION

While describing an X-ray, the following vital observations need to be made:[1,2]
• Projection (AP versus PA film)
• Exposure (hard versus soft films)
• Rotation
• Soft tissue/bone
• Lungs:
  – Expansion
  – Parenchymal appearance—lucency, nature of opacities, fissure
  – Cardiac and diaphragmatic margins

- Cardiac:
  - Cardiothoracic ratio/cardiac size
  - Pulmonary vascular markings
  - Specific chamber enlargement

Projection

The following features distinguish AP from a PA film:

- In PA films, the scapulae lie posterolaterally and are away from the lung fields, whereas they tend to overlap the lungs in AP films.
- Due to its anterior placement, the heart appears larger in AP rather than PA film.
- The cervico-thoracic vertebral end plates are tangential to the AP projection beam, making them prominently seen in AP view, while the lamina appears more prominent in PA view.
- The ribs appear to be more horizontally placed in AP than PA view.

Practical Tip

Most neonatal chest X-rays are AP films, unless the baby is made to lie prone.

Exposure

- Lucency of soft tissue shadow—darker the soft tissue, more is the exposure.
- Ease of visibility of retrocardiac vertebrae—if the retrocardiac vertebrae are easily seen, the film is over exposed.
- Relative lucency of lung fields.

Rotation

The chest X-ray is said to be rotated if:

- The distance of the posterior ends of ribs from the midline of spine are unequal on either side. The film is rotated to that side on which the distance appears greater.
- Medial end of clavicles are not equidistant from the midline.

The first criterion is usually more helpful as the lower chest tends to be rotated more commonly than the upper chest, as the latter is usually stabilised at the time of taking X-rays.

Soft Tissue/Bone

The importance of carefully looking at the bones cannot be over-emphasised especially for picking up changes of osteopenia and fractures. This is not discussed in detail here.

Thymus—Normal and Abnormal

The thymus may create some challenge in the interpretation of neonatal chest X-rays. One needs to differentiate its normal from abnormal appearance.

Normally, thymus appears as a bilateral smoothly outlined superior mediastinal fullness blending with the cardiac silhouette. Some normal variants of thymus:

- "Notch sign"—uniform enlargement of thymus on both sides with prominent notch on inferior left border
- "Sail sign"—characteristic sail like border of normal thymus, more commonly seen on right side
- Undulating waviness of the lateral border of thymus due to indentation of ribs

INTERPRETATION OF LUNG FIELDS

Lung Expansion

Normal lung expansion: Up to 6 ribs anteriorly and 8 ribs posteriorly. This follows the normal position of the diaphragm between 5th and 7th anterior ribs.

The radiological features of hyper-expansion are:

1. Presence of more than 6 ribs anteriorly and 8 ribs posteriorly
2. Flattening of diaphragm
3. Increased lucency of lung fields (blackness)
4. Air under the heart/herniation of lung to opposite side
5. Ribs more horizontal

However, the evaluation of lung expansion by counting the number of ribs (or intercostal spaces) above the diaphragm can be tricky in newborns due to two reasons:

1. This technique represents the expansion in two dimensions only. But newborns, unlike older infants and children, have highly compliant thoracic cage, which can easily expand in the antero-posterior dimension as well.

2. Lesser diaphragmatic excursions occur during inspiration in neonates as compared to older children.

CHARACTERISTIC APPEARANCE OF COMMON DISEASE CONDITIONS

Respiratory Distress Syndrome (RDS)

The condition is caused by the deficiency of surfactant production by type II alveolar cells, which results in alveolar collapsibility with over inflation of larger alveoli and resultant transudation of proteinaceous fluid into alveoli, creating the classical hyaline membranes. The radiological features of the condition are:

- Under-aerated lungs
- Reticulo-granularity (presence of air in the terminal bronchioles and alveolar ducts against a background of alveolar atelectasis)
- Air bronchograms (with progress of disease, more and more distal airways collapse, leaving the proximal bronchi which stand out as air bronchograms. Note that air bronchograms may be absent in an expiratory film)
- Diffuse granularity
- In severe cases or in expiratory films, these findings may be replaced by white-out lungs due to diffuse alveolar atelectasis

The severity of RDS has been classified based on radiological findings as follows:

Mild: Normal/decreased aeration, reticulo-granularity

Moderate: Decreased aeration, air bronchograms and indistinct diaphragm and heart borders.

Severe: Confluent opacification of lungs with loss of mediastinal and diaphragmatic borders.

Transient Tachypnea of Newborn (Retained Fluid Syndrome)

This is a condition resulting from the delayed clearance of fetal lung fluid, overloading the interstitium, lymphatics and cardiovascular system. X-ray picture is characterised by:

- Prominent hilum with perivascular streaky shadows
- Prominent interlobar fissure

- Small pleural effusion
- There may be mild cardiomegaly
- Normal to increased lung volume

Pulmonary Interstitial Emphysema (PIE)

It is caused by the dissection of air from alveoli into the parenchyma and interstitium of lungs and perivascular sheaths of vessels, tracking towards the hilum. X-ray appearance is characterised by

- Radiolucent streaks—linear or irregular, branching/cystic spaces (honeycomb like) or pneumatoceles.
- PIE may present with linear or cystic changes. Linear lucencies of PIE may be differentiated from air bronchograms in that the latter are generally smooth and branching, in contrast to interstitial air which is coarser and non-branching.

Pneumothorax

This results from the dissection of extra-alveolar air to the hilum, followed by rupture into pleural space. Increased radio-lucency of the ipsilateral lung and sharpness of mediastinal border are the earliest signs of pneumothorax. The characteristic X-ray findings are:

- Clear border of collapsed lung
- Absent lung markings beyond the collapsed lung border [This differentiates pneumothorax from vertical skin folds]
- May or may not be accompanied by mediastinal shift
- Herniation of the pneumothorax bounded by parietal pleura into the contralateral side
- The thymus is compressed by pneumothorax whereas it is elevated by pneumomediastinum.

Pneumomediastinum

It is the presence of air adjacent to the heart outlining the thymus and *elevating it.*

Meconium Aspiration Syndrome (MAS)

The radiological appearance may range from hyper-expansion to collapse:

- Gross hyper-expansion of lungs

- Bilateral nodular opacities (this represents areas of focal alveolar atelectasis with focal alveolar over distension in between).
- Sometimes, a large piece of meconium can obstruct the bronchus leading to emphysema of one lung/lobe and compression of the other lung.

Pneumonia

- The radiological picture is variable and may range from reticulo-granularity to lobar or segmental consolidation.
- Asymmetry of reticulo-granular pattern with air bronchograms may be seen.
- Coarse granular patchy infiltrates with irregular areas of hyper inflation.

Pleural Effusion

- Detected by the blunting of posterior and later, the lateral costophrenic angle (only in erect film).
- In supine radiographs, there is decreased translucency of the lung with preserved pulmonary vascular markings.
- If enough fluid is present, it is seen as a peripheral band separating the lung and lateral chest wall.

Bronchopulmonary Displane

The radiological appearance is variable and depends on the postnatal age (Northway et al)

Stage I (2–3 days)—air bronchograms, reticulo-granularity (similar to RDS)

Stage II (4–10 days)—opacification; coarse irregular densities

Stage III (10–20 days)—small generalised radiolucent cysts

Stage IV (1 month)—dense fibrotic strands, generalised cystic areas, hyper-inflated lungs

Types of Bubbles in Chest X-ray

There are three types of bubbles in chest X-ray which are as follows:

Type I   : Seen in RDS
          Small and uniform, rounded
          1–2 mm in diameter

More prominent in lung bases
Due to over distension of the terminal airways
Become less pronounced on expiration

Type II : Seen in pulmonary interstitial emphysema (PIE)
Nodular and tortuous in shape
Peribronchial and perivascular in location
Do not empty on expiration

Type III : Larger than the first two types of bubbles
Irregular shaped
Seen in focal hyper-aeration syndrome, e.g.
bronchopulmonary dysplasia
Also become less pronounced on expiration, like
type I bubbles.

CONGENITAL DIAPHRAGMATIC HERNIA

Bochdalek defects present with a well defined dome shaped soft tissue opacity usually on the left chest. Importantly, intestinal loops may be gasless in the first few hours of life and the classical appearance of gas filled loops in the chest may appear only few hours after birth.

Morgagni hernias are seen as opacities adjacent to the right costophrenic angle.

Tracheoesophageal Fistula

A soft rubber tube is better than an infant feeding tube for the radiological diagnosis of TEF. The X-ray shows coiling of the tube in the upper esophagus. If one desires to delineate the extent of gap between the upper and lower pouch, a lateral X-ray is preferable. Absent stomach gas suggests associated esophageal atresia.

INTERPRETATION OF THE CARDIAC SHADOW IN X-RAY[3]

The most important features to be noted are:

1. Cardiac size
2. Pulmonary vasculature
3. Shape and size of different chambers/cardiac situs

Cardiac Size

This may be assessed simply by measuring the cardiothoracic ratio (CT ratio). CT ratio is the largest transverse diameter of the heart divided by the smallest internal diameter of the chest.

A CT ratio of more than 0.6 suggests cardiomegaly in newborns.

Pulmonary Vasculature

Normally, it is difficult to appreciate pulmonary vascular markings in the lateral third of the lung fields as well as in the lung apices.

Increased pulmonary vascularity is said to be present when the pulmonary vessels are seen in the lateral third of the film or in the lung apices or if the right pulmonary artery which is visible in the right hilus appears wider than the trachea.

Decreased pulmonary blood flow/PBF (oligemia) is diagnosed by the relative blackness of lung fields with small lung hilum (Table 32.1).

Table 32.1: Causes of decreased and increased PBF

Causes of decreased PBF	Causes of increased PBF
Tricuspid valve: Tricuspid atresia Ebstein's anomaly	Acyanotic: Ostium primum/secundum ASD
Right ventricle:	Ventricular septal defect
Tetralogy of Fallot	Patent ductus arteriosus
Pulmonary stenosis (PS)	Cyanotic: Admixture lesions without PS–
Arterial:	Transposition of great arteries
Peripheral pulmonary artery stenosis	Total anomalous pulmonary venous drainage
Pulmonary atresia	Persistent truncus arteriosus
Persistent truncus (type IV)	Single ventricle

Specific Chamber Enlargement

In an AP view, the right heart border is formed above downwards by superior vena cava (SVC), ascending aorta (AA), right atrial appendage (RAA) and the right atrium (RA). The left heart border is formed by the aortic arch (AoA), main pulmonary artery (PA), left atrial appendage (LAA) and the left ventricle (LV). This forms the basis for diagnosing various chamber enlargements. Note that the right ventricle (RV) does not contribute to either of the borders and usually presents with an up-turned apex, when enlarged. Left atrial enlargement results in splaying of the carina and double left heart border appearance. Specific X-ray picture in congenital heart disease is provided (Table 32.2).

Table 32.2 Specific X-ray picture in congenital heart lesions

Heart lesion	X-ray picture
Ventricular septal defect	Prominent pulmonary vascular markings, left atrial and ventricular enlargement
Patent ductus arteriosus	Prominent main pulmonary artery, left atrial and ventricular enlargement
Coarctation of aorta	"Reverse 3 sign" along the upper left heart border-hypoplastic aortic knob along with left ventricular prominence; inferior rib border notching
Tetralogy of Fallot	"Coeur en sabot" (boot shaped) heart—caused by a small pedicle (atretic PA) with an up-turned apex due to RV hypertrophy; pulmonary oligemia
Truncus arteriosus	Narrow pedicle, frequently accompanied by absent thymus
Total anomalous pulmonary venous connection (supracardiac)	"Snowman" appearance caused by the dilated vertical vein, innominate vein and SVC, pulmonary plethora
Transposition of great arteries	"Egg on side" appearance due to the narrow pedicle created by the parallel orientation of aorta and pulmonary artery

LINE POSITIONS

Umbilical Arterial Line

- High: Between T6 and T9 vertebrae
- Low: Between L3 and L4 vertebrae

Umbilical Venous Line

0.5 to 1 cm above the diaphragm

Endotracheal Tube Tip

At least 2 cm above carina OR between the lower border of T2 to upper border of T3 thoracic vertebrae.

Percutaneous Central Line (PICC)

When inserted from upper limb, the line must have crossed the first rib and passed medially with the tip lying between T3 and T6 vertebrae.

Practical Tips

While doing an X-ray

- Follow aseptic precautions.
- Adequate hand hygiene is a must for all including radiographer.
- Always make note and discuss the exposure settings with the radiographer in order to optimise image quality. A rough guide is to use 30–50 kV (kilo Volts) and 4–10 mA (milliAmps).
- Avoid direct contact of the X-ray plate with the baby to prevent hypothermia. Always place the X-ray plate in the separate tray meant for that purpose.
- In small babies, beware of hypothermia as the radiant warmer is tilted away during the X-ray and provide extra heat source if necessary. X-ray can be done through an incubator safely.
- Instruct health care providers to wear lead apron and use gonad shield for the baby. Maintain safe distance for health care professionals when an X-ray is being filmed in order to prevent radiation hazard.
- Expose only the area of interest and remove chest leads, tubings, etc. from the field.
- Make sure that the baby is not rotated.
- As far as possible, quieten the baby to avoid swings in respiratory depth.

While reading an X-ray

- Read schematically, jumping to the diagnosis may entail the risk of missing additional details.
- Correlate findings with clinical details.
- Make note of age in hours/days, serial sequence number and interventions done before (such as surfactant administration) and after the X-ray (pulling out a deeply placed endotracheal tube).
- Use of a view box and magnifying glass for reading X-ray is the ideal

REFERENCES

1. Deorari A, Kumar P, Murki S. Workbook on CPAP: science, evidence and practice. 2nd edn. Neonatal chest X-ray interpretation, New Delhi, 2011;p. 59–64.

2. Swischuk LE. Imaging of the newborn, infant and young child. 5th edn. Philadelphia: Lippincott Williams and Wilkins: Respiratory system, 2004;p. 1–108.

3. Abdulla R. Heart Diseases in Children: A Pediatrician's Guide. Chicago: Springer: Chapter 2, Cardiac Interpretation of Pediatric Chest X-ray, 2011;p. 17–34.

33

Dressing for Open Neural Tube Defects (NTD)

DRESSING OF OPEN NEURAL TUBE DEFECT

- Handle the infant with sterile, non-latex gloves and with sterile clothing and sheets.
- Cover the lesion with non-adhesive dressing like paraffin gauze followed by wet saline gauze.
- Place one end of a small orogastric tube (size 6 Fr) between the two layers of saline gauze and connect the other end to a syringe containing sterile saline solution.
- Place a ring of curlex around the lesion to prevent pressure on the sac.
- Cover the entire lesion with cling wrap and make a single wrap around the infant's chest or abdomen to keep it in place.
- Inject 0.5 cc saline every 2 hours to keep the dressing moist.
- Change the dressing once per day or when soiled/displaced.

Step 1

Make a ring with cotton gauze of size, slightly larger than the lesion. Cover the ring with cling wrap to make it water resistant.

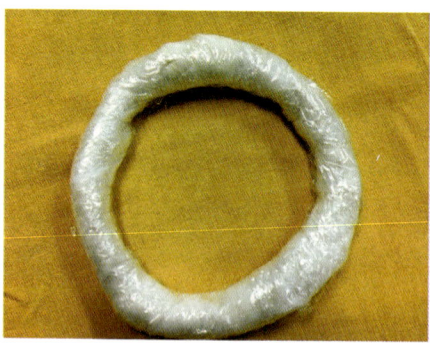

Step 2

Place tegaderm on the skin surrounding the lesion.

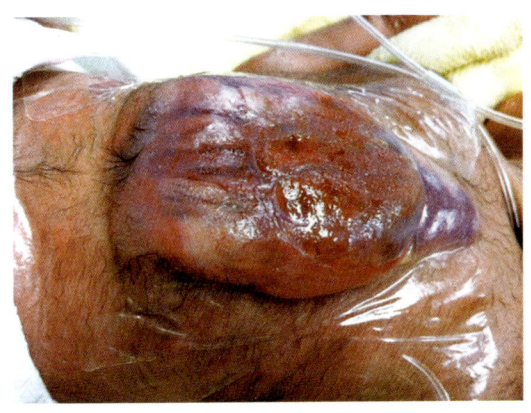

Step 3

Cover paraffin gauze over the lesion.

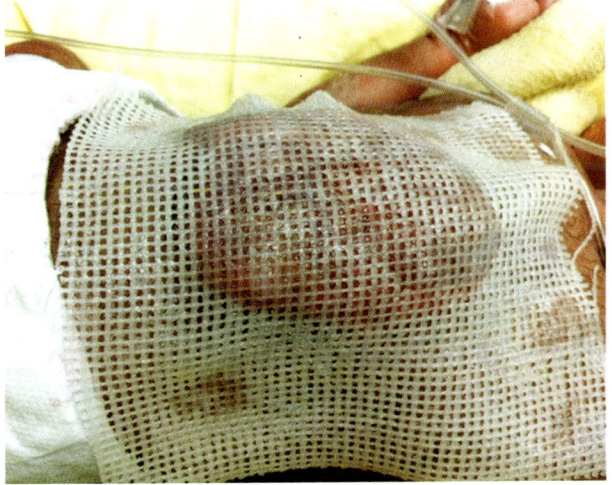

Step 4

Place sterile saline soaked gauze over the paraffin gauze.

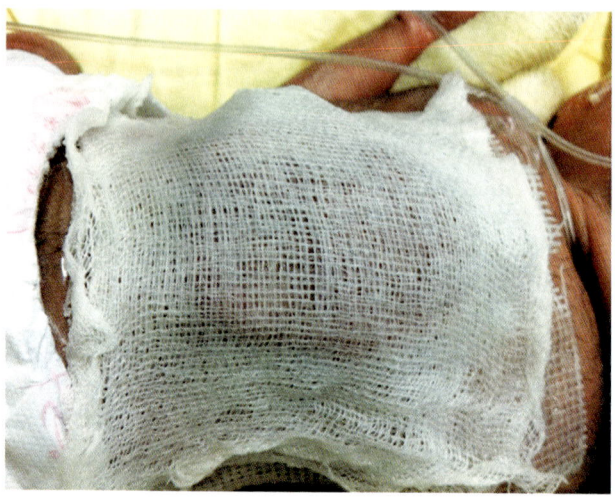

Step 5

Insert the smallest OG tube or a scalp vein tube (with needle cut) between the two layers of gauze. Connect the other end to a syringe containing sterile saline.

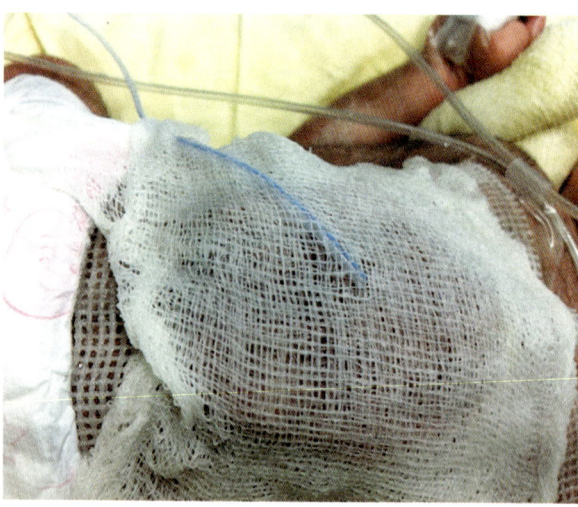

Step 6

Place the ring around the dressing to hold it in place and to support the lesion.

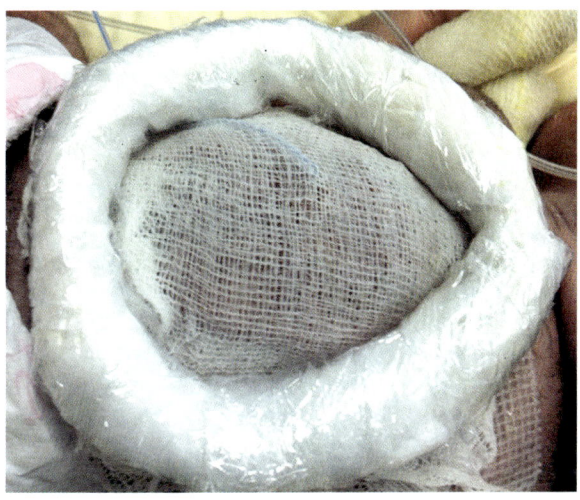

Step 7

Nurse the infant prone or side lying only. Inject 0.5 mL saline via the OG tube every 2 hourly to keep it moist.

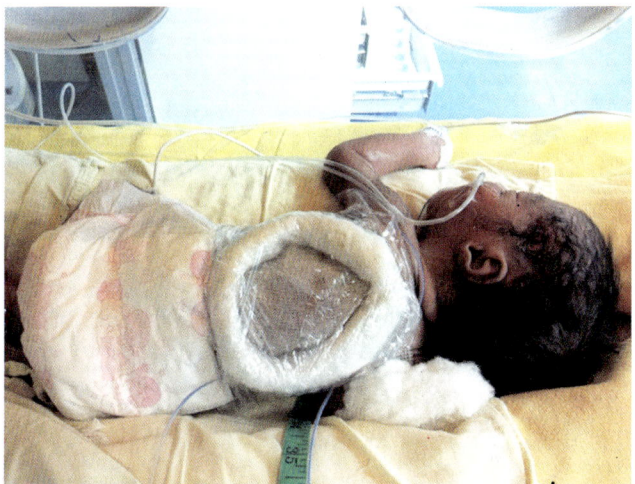

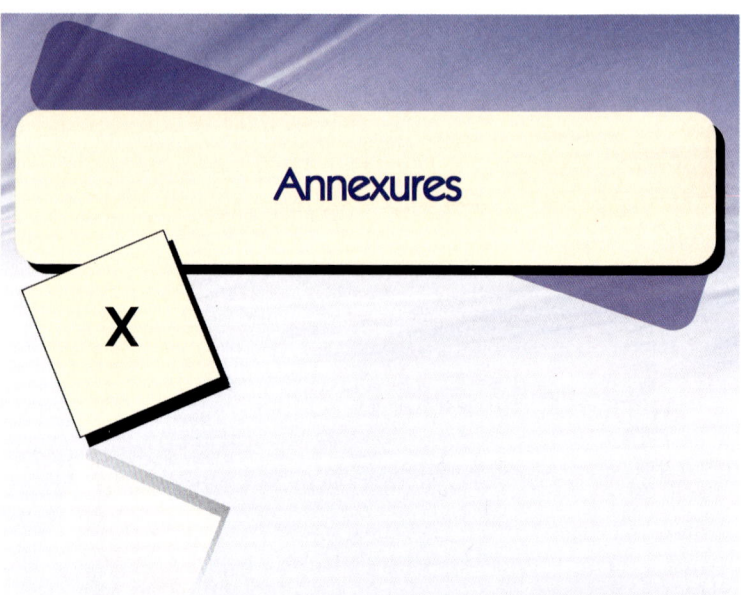

Annexures

X

Annexures

A1—RESEARCH PRIORITIES FOR MD, DNB THESES

Research questions	Subjects	Study designs	Interventions/ Exposure	Outcomes to be measured
NORMAL NEWBORN CARE				
1. What are the benefits and harms of delayed cord clamping?	Term IUGR (In utero growth <10th centile)	RCT	I: Delayed cord clamping (2 to 3 minutes) C: Immediate cord clamping	• Short term: Hematocrit, rates of polycythemia, serum bilirubin levels during neonatal period • Fe status and clinical anemia at 3 and 6 months • Neurodevelopment at 18 to 24 months
2. Is footprint of baby a reliable method to ascertain the identity of a neonate?	Term normal neonates	Descriptive	Nil	• Proportion of footprints reliable enough to determine the identity of neonate, when presented to experts
3. What is the feasibility, reliability and cost effectiveness of use of biometric system for identification of the mother - baby dyad?	Term normal neonates	Descriptive/RCT	I: Use of biometric system C: Conventional system, e.g. footprint	• The feasibility, cost and reliability • Correct identity establishment by an expert

Contd...

A1—RESEARCH PRIORITIES FOR MD, DNB THESES

Research questions	Subjects	Study designs	Interventions/Exposure	Outcomes to be measured
4. What is the safest method for clamping the cord?	Term normal neonates	RCT	Subjects can be randomized to three methods of clamping of cord, e.g. commercial clamp, thread, rubber band	• Rates of cord slippage, oozing of blood • Need for re-clamping in the first 24 hrs • Parental satisfaction and acceptability • Cost
5. What are the rates, reasons (post discharge morbidities), age and outcomes of babies who need readmission after discharge following birth hospitalization in the first month of life?	• Term normal neonates • Late preterm neonates • Very preterm neonates	Cohort study	Nil	• Rate, reasons (post discharge morbidities), age and outcomes of re-admissions
6. What is the optimum hospital stay of healthy term and late preterm neonates?	Healthy term and late preterm neonates (Two sub-groups of babies delivered by vaginal route and cesarean section)	RCT	Different hospital stays such as: For normally delivered neonates: 24 hr *versus* 48 hr *versus* 72 hr For cesarean babies: 48 hr *versus* 72 hr *versus* 96 hr	• Exclusive breastfeeding; Rate (6 wk, 6 mo) and adequacy (% weight loss by day 7) • Re-admissions rates for morbidities-hyperbilirubinemia, excessive weight loss, sepsis • Maternal morbidities (need collaboration with Ob-Gyn).

Contd...

Research questions	Subjects	Study designs	Interventions/Exposure	Outcomes to be measured
				• Family satisfaction • Cost to the hospital and the family
THERMAL PROTECTION				
7. What is the epidemiology of hyperthermia in neonates?	Neonates with hyperthermia	Observational (prospective cohort)	None	• Incidence density, season, relationship with ambient temperature, humidity and clothing, manifestations • Treatment required • Outcomes—short term and at 18 months (neuro-development)
8. What is the efficacy of devices made up of phase changing materials (PCMs) meant for thermal protection?	LBW neonates after initial stabilization	RCT	I: PCM device C: Incubator/radiant warmer	• Average axillary and core temperatures • Incidence of cold stress and hypothermia • Morbidity, mortality rates • Hospital stay • Cost of therapy • Weight gain during hospital stay
POST-RESUSCITATION CARE OF ASPHYXIATED BABIES				
9. Does restricting fluid intake improve the outcomes in asphyxiated babies?	Asphyxiated neonates requiring intensive care	RCT	Normal maintenance fluids *versus* two-thirds of maintenance fluid depending on day of postnatal life	**Efficacy:** Rates and severity of HIE, seizures, SIADH (S.Na), mortality by 28 days, neuro-development at 18 months

Contd...

Research questions	Subjects	Study designs	Interventions/Exposure	Outcomes to be measured
				Safety: Hypotension requiring fluid or inotropic support, acute renal failure
10. Does supplementing IV calcium routinely improve the outcomes in asphyxiated babies?	Asphyxiated neonates requiring intensive care	RCT	IV calcium 4 to 8 mL/kg/day of calcium gluconate *versus* placebo during initial 3 days of life	**Efficacy:** Rates and severity of HIE, seizures, incidence of hypocalcemia, survival, neurodevelopment at 18 months **Safety:** Extravasations, skin damage, cardiac arrest
11. Does aminophylline prevent occurrence of renal failure in asphyxiated neonates?	Asphyxiated neonates requiring intensive care	RCT	IV aminophylline *versus* placebo during initial 3 days of life	Urine output, renal function, survival, neurodevelopment at 18 months
NEONATAL SEIZURES				
12. What is the epidemiology of seizures in term and preterm neonates in resource restricted settings?	Neonates admitted with seizures	Cohort study (for incidence); Case series for others	None	• Incidence, etiology and type of neonatal seizures • Age at onset of seizures • EEG changes during ictal and inter-ictal periods • Need for therapy (which AED, how long) • Short- and long-term (18 months) outcomes of neonates with seizures
13. What is the optimal first-line AED for term	Neonates with seizures	Randomized trial	Phenobarbitone *versus* alternate therapy	• Seizure control rates (clinical as well as EEG)

Contd...

Research questions	Subjects	Study designs	Interventions/Exposure	Outcomes to be measured
neonates with seizures following HIE?				• Time taken to achieve control of seizures • Mortality, hospital stay • Neurodevelopmental outcomes at 18–24 months age
14. What is the optimal second-line AED in term asphyxiated neonates with seizures refractory to phenobarb/phenytoin/other first-line agent?	Neonates with seizures uncontrolled with phenobarbitone and are requiring 2nd line drug	Randomized trial	Comparison of different drugs	Same as above
15. What is the optimal timing and method of discontinuation of AEDs in newborns whose seizures are controlled on current AED treatment (for e.g. stopping AED after 72 hours *versus* after 2–4 weeks; abrupt stoppage of phenobarbitone *versus* gradual tapering followed by stopping)?	Neonates with seizures treated with AED	Randomized trial/cohort study	Comparison of different approaches: • Stopping AED after 72 hrs *versus* after 2–4 weeks • Abrupt stoppage of phenobarbitone *versus* gradual tapering followed by stopping	• Seizure recurrence • Neurodevelopmental outcomes at 18–24 months age

Contd...

Research questions	Subjects	Study designs	Interventions/Exposure	Outcomes to be measured
NEONATAL SEPSIS				
16. Does antimicrobial stewardship (AMS) reduce antibiotics usage in NICU?	All babies admitted to NICU	Before and after study	AMS as formulated by the unit based on prevalent flora, antimicrobial resistance (AMR) and the available best evidence. The practices are guided by a written policy	• Antibiotics usage rate • Use of higher antibiotics • Hospital stay • Cost
17. What is the rate of medication errors with regard to antibiotic prescription in NICU?	All babies admitted to NICU in the last two years	Prospective study	None	Rates of medication errors and associated harms and estimated additional costs due to it
CHRONIC LUNG DISEASE (CLD)				
18. What is the epidemiology of CLD in Indian NICUs?	Preterm infants <34 weeks ap.	Cohort study (for incidence); Descriptive cohort for natural history	None	• Gestation specific incidence of mild, moderate and severe BPD • Natural course of the disease including the need for home oxygen, age at stoppage of oxygen therapy, etc.
19. What is the long-term (12 months of age) pulmonary outcomes of preterm neonates with BPD?	Preterm infants with BPD and gestation matched infants without BPD	Cohort study	None	• Pulmonary function tests at 12 months of age • Need for long-term bronchodilator treatment • Incidence of severe respiratory tract infections

Contd...

Research questions	Subjects	Study designs	Interventions/Exposure	Outcomes to be measured
20. What are the neuro-developmental outcomes at 18–24 months of age of preterm neonates with BPD?	Preterm infants with BPD and gestation matched babies without BPD	Cohort study	None	requiring admission in the first year of life Incidence of moderate or severe disability (defined as presence of any one of the following—cerebral palsy, motor or mental DQ <70, visual or hearing deficit, epilepsy)
21. What is the efficacy and safety of different interventions (permissive hypercapnia, InSuRE approach, diuretics, etc.) on the incidence and severity of BPD in preterm neonates?	Preterm neonates at risk of/having BPD	Randomized trial/cohort study	I: Permissive hypercapnia, InSuRE approach, diuretics, etc. C: Alternative strategy/placebo	• Incidence of BPD • Duration of oxygen therapy, duration of hospital stay, need for home oxygen, etc.
22. What is the efficacy and safety of aggressive nutrition intervention on the incidence and severity of BPD in preterm neonates?	Preterm neonates at risk of BPD (gestation <32 wks)	Randomized trial	I: Higher calories and protein intake C: Standard intake	• Incidence of BPD • Duration of oxygen therapy, duration of hospital stay, need for home oxygen, etc.

Contd...

Research questions	Subjects	Study designs	Interventions/Exposure	Outcomes to be measured
APNEA				
23. Is humidified high flow nasal cannula (HHFNC) at least as effective as CPAP in preterm neonates with apnea of prematurity refractory to methylxanthines?	Preterm neonates with apnea of prematurity already on methylxanthine but still having recurrent apnea	RCT	I: HHHFNC C: CPAP	• **Need of intubation or nasal IPPV** • **Number of apneas per day** • **Number of desaturations per day** • **Need of bag and mask ventilation**
24. What is the epidemiology of apnea in Indian NICUs?	Preterm neonates <37 wks	Cohort study	None	Incidence density, etiology, severity, therapeutic needs. Time to resolve apnea, neurodevelopmental outcome
25. Do preterm neonates (<28 weeks) need higher dose of maintenance caffeine for treating recurrent apneas of prematurity?	Extremely preterm neonates with apnea of prematurity having recurrent apneas	RCT	Caffeine therapy at different doses starting from lowest recommended dose	Pharmacokinetic and pharmacodynamic effects of caffeine
JAUNDICE				
26. Are the parents able to correctly detect significant jaundice?	Neonates with jaundice (all severity level)	Diagnostic test in a cohort	Test: Visual estimation of jaundice by the parents Gold standard: Visual estimation of jaundice by the pediatrician and TSB	Sensitivity; specificity and likelihood ratios

Contd...

	Research questions	Subjects	Study designs	Interventions/Exposure	Outcomes to be measured
27.	Is double surface Ptx more effective than single surface Ptx in neonates with unconjugated hyperbilirubinemia?	Neonates with non-hemolytic jaundice	Randomized trial	I: Double surface phototherapy C: Single surface Ptx	Failure of phototherapy, duration of phototherapy and rate of bilirubin decline
28.	What is the temperature variation under different phototherapy devices?	Neonates with hyperbilirubinemia undergoing phototherapy using different types of phototherapy devices (straight lamps, CFL, LED, halogen lamp)	Cohort study	None	Measurement of ambient and baby's temperature every 2 to 4 hours
29.	What is the efficacy of blue green (turquoise) light phototherapy *versus* blue light phototherapy?	Neonates with non-hemolytic jaundice	Randomized trial	I: Turquoise light phototherapy C: Blue light phototherapy	Failure of phototherapy, duration of phototherapy and rate of bilirubin decline
30.	What are the predictors of jaundice in ABO settings?	Neonates with ABO setting (mother being 'O' and baby either 'A' or 'B')	Cohort study	Monitor the infants for presence and absence of risk factors	**Predictors:** Clinical-weight, gestation, sickness, type of feeding **Biochemical:** Cord TSB, rate of rise, DCT, hemolysis in peripheral smear, reticulocyte count

Contd...

Research questions	Subjects	Study designs	Interventions/Exposure	Outcomes to be measured
31. When should photo-therapy be stopped: one or two TSB values below cut-offs?	Neonates with non-hemolytic jaundice	Randomized trial	I: PTx stopped when one TSB value is below age specific cut-off C: PTx stopped when two consecutive TSB values are below age specific cut-off	• Need for re-initiation of phototherapy • Duration of phototherapy • Rate of bilirubin decline
32. What is the population attributable risk of feeding inadequacy for hyperbilirubinemia in jaundice?	Late preterm and term neonates	Cohort study	Measure birth weight and weight at 72 hrs precisely to calculate % weight loss. Collect info on other risk factors such as oxytocin use, cephalhematoma, blood group incompatibility, G6PD deficiency, mutations, ethnicity and others.	• Follow the infants for development of hyper-bilirubinemia • Calculate adjusted odds ratio, attributable risk and population attributable risk for feeding inadequacy

FEEDING OF LBW BABIES

Research questions	Subjects	Study designs	Interventions/Exposure	Outcomes to be measured
33. What is the efficacy and safety of two existing preparations of HMFs in Indian market on the short- and long-term neuro-developmental and growth outcomes (O) in preterm VLBW infants (P)?	Very preterm infants	RCT	I: HMF-1 C: HMF-2	• Weight-for-age, height-for-age and weight-for-height at 40 wks, 12 months of corrected age • Short-term effects as feed intolerance, NEC, sepsis and hospital stay • Incidence of moderate or severe disability (defined as presence of any one of the

Contd...

Research questions	Subjects	Study designs	Interventions/Exposure	Outcomes to be measured
				following—cerebral palsy, motor or mental DQ <70, visual or hearing deficit, epilepsy) at 18 months
34. What is the comparative efficacy and safety of routine abdominal circumference and conditional gastric residual volume measurement (I) with routine pre-feed gastric residual volume measurement alone (C) for feed intolerance in stable preterm infants on gavage feeding (P)?	Very preterm infants	RCT	I: Monitoring for feed intolerance by routine abdominal circumference and conditional gastric residual volume measurement C: Routine pre-feed gastric residual volume measurement alone (C)	• Time taken to reach full feeds • Time to regain birth weight • Duration of hospital stay • Incidence of NEC stage II or more
35. What is the safety and efficacy (O) of early discharge from the hospital of VLBW infants?		RCT	*Two trials* 1. Weight of 1400–1500 g (I) *versus* 1600–1800 g (C) 2. Discharging once the baby is on cup/direct breast feeding (C) *versus* when baby is stable but still on tube feeding (I)	**Safety**: Major morbidities such as apnea, sepsis, aspiration, hypothermia **Efficacy**: Weight-for-age, height-for-age, and weight-for-height at 40 wks, 12 months of corrected age. Parental satisfaction
36. What is the efficacy of massage (I) as com-		RCT	I: Massage C: No massage	• Weight-for-age, height-for-age and weight-for-height

Contd...

Research questions	Subjects	Study designs	Interventions/Exposure	Outcomes to be measured
pared to no massage (C) on growth, morbidities, workload of nurses and parental satisfaction (O) in preterm VLBW infants (P)?				at 40 wks, 12 months of corrected age • Short-term effects as feed intolerance, apnea, NEC, sepsis, CLD and hospital stay • Incidence of moderate or severe disability (defined as presence of any one of the following—cerebral palsy, motor or mental DQ <70, visual or hearing deficit, epilepsy) at 18 months
37. What is the impact of different doses of vitamin D supplementation on the vitamin D levels and morbidities among preterm, term SGA and term AGA infants?	Preterm, term SGA and term AGA infants	RCT or prospective, cohort	Different doses of vitamin D, e.g. 400 *versus* 800 IU/day	Vitamin D and PTH levels, bone mineral density, incidence/prevalence of different morbidities
38. How does the amount and composition of breast milk change over time in mothers of exclusively breastfed preterm infants?	Preterm mother-infant dyad	Prospective cohort	None	Breast milk output using manual or isotopic methods and breast milk constitution including various micronutrients

Contd...

Research questions	Subjects	Study designs	Interventions/Exposure	Outcomes to be measured
39. What is the impact of in-hospital lactation counseling support on duration of exclusive breastfeeding among mothers of very preterm infants?	Very preterm infants (<32 weeks gestation)	RCT or prospective cohort	In-hospital lactational counseling by trained nurses	Duration of exclusive breastfeeding
HYPOCALCEMIA				
40. What is the incidence of neonatal hypocalcemia, age at onset, clinical manifestations and short term outcomes? (Epidemiology of hypocalcemia)	At-risk neonates	Cohort study	None	Incidence, age at onset in hours, clinical manifestation, neurological findings, outcomes, etc.
41. What are the long-term outcomes of neonatal hypocalcemia?	At-risk infants	Cohort study	None	Neurodevelopment outcomes at 18 months
42. Does routine prophylactic calcium supplementation in at-risk babies improve the clinical outcomes?	At-risk neonates	Randomized control trial	I: Prophylactic calcium supplementation at 40 mg/kg/dL to at-risk babies C: No calcium	• Incidence of asymptomatic and symptomatic hypocalcemia • Complications of therapy such as thrombophlebitis, arrhythmias, gastrointestinal

Contd...

Research questions	Subjects	Study designs	Interventions/Exposure	Outcomes to be measured
POLYCYTHEMIA				
43. What is the incidence, age at onset, clinical manifestations and short-term outcomes of polycythemia in neonates?	At-risk neonates	Cohort	None	Incidence, age at onset in hours, clinical manifestation, neurological findings, outcomes • side effects and nephrocalcinosis • Other morbidities, long-term outcomes
44. Does partial exchange transfusion helps in improving short-term and long-term outcomes in asymptomatic polycythemia?	Asymptomatic neonates with polycythemia	Randomized control trial	I: Treat with PET C: No PET	• Alleviation of symptoms or reducing the incidence of symptoms related to polycythemia • Neurodevelopmental outcomes at 18–24 months of age
45. Does partial exchange transfusion improve the functional parameters of different organ systems such as myocardial performance, middle cerebral and mesenteric	Neonates with polycythemia	Before and after study	Measurement of the parameters before and after PET	• Estimation of different parameters by ultrasound before and after PET

Contd...

Research questions	Subjects	Study designs	Interventions/Exposure	Outcomes to be measured
flow and pulmonary artery pressure?				
46. How does hematocrit values vary in at-risk neonates during initial 48 to 72 hrs and does cord/2 hrs hematocrit value predict subsequent polycythemia?	At-risk neonates	Cohort study by enrolling at-risk infants	Nil	• Variation in hematocrit during initial 48–72 hrs • Diagnostic utility (sensitivity, specificity, PPV, NPV and likelihood ratios) of cord/2 hrs hematocrit for subsequent development of polycythemia
HYPOGLYCEMIA				
47. What is the incidence of neonatal hypoglycemia, age at onset, clinical manifestations and short-term outcomes? (Epidemiology of hypoglycemia)	At-risk neonates	Cohort study by enrolling at-risk infants	Nil	• Incidence • Age at which it is detected in hours • Rate of occurrence of different clinical manifestation • Neurological examination at discharge and MRI findings • Neurodevelopmental outcome at 18–24 months of age
48. Does asymptomatic hypoglycemia need treatment with intravenous glucose?	Neonates with asymptomatic hypoglycemia	Randomized control trial	I: Treat with IV fluids C: Oral feeds only, no IV fluids (unless symptoms appear)	Neurodevelopmental outcome at 18–24 months of age

Contd...

Research questions	Subjects	Study designs	Interventions/Exposure	Outcomes to be measured
49. What is the accuracy of point of care reagent strips when compared to lab values (gold standard) for detecting hypoglycemia?	At-risk neonates requiring blood glucose monitoring	Diagnostic evaluation study	Nil	• Estimation of correlation and agreement between two methods • Sensitivity, specificity, PPV, NPV

FOLLOW-UP OF HIGH RISK NEONATES

Research questions	Subjects	Study designs	Interventions/Exposure	Outcomes to be measured
50. What is the spectrum of various post discharge morbidities in high risk infants?	All high risk infants discharged from level 2–3 neonatal units	Prospective cohort or cross sectional	None	Incidence/prevalence of various post discharge morbidities
51. What is the growth trajectory of exclusively breastfed preterm and term SGA infants in infancy?	Preterm and term SGA infants	Prospective cohort	None	Serial growth parameters from birth preferably including skin fold thickness
52. What is the difference in growth trajectory among preterm and term SGA infants on exclusive breastfeeding as compared to those on other types of feeding, e.g. formula feeding in early infancy?	Preterm and term SGA infants	Prospective cohort	None	Serial growth parameters from birth preferably including skin fold thickness

Contd...

Research questions	Subjects	Study designs	Interventions/Exposure	Outcomes to be measured
53. What is the role of parent administered post discharge early stimulation and intervention program in promoting neuro-developmental outcome among high-risk infants?	High-risk infants discharged from NICU	RCT or prospective cohort	Parent administered early stimulation/intervention *versus* standard care	Neurodevelopmental outcome at 12 months CA
54. What is the impact of post discharge breast-feeding support and counseling (through telephonic conversation or personal contact) on duration of exclusive breastfeeding among mothers of very preterm infants?	Very preterm infants (<32 weeks gestation)	RCT or prospective cohort	Post discharge breastfeeding support and counseling (through telephonic conversation or personal contact)	Duration of exclusive breast-feeding
55. What is the psycho-social and financial impact of a high-risk birth on the parents/family?	Parents/family of all high risk infants	Prospective cohort or cross sectional	None	Various psychosocial components using standardized scales and cost of care borne by the family and hospital
56. How does the neuro-logical examination of	Preterm and term healthy infants	Cross sectional	None	Neurological examination of preterm and term infants using

Contd...

Research questions	Subjects	Study designs	Interventions/Exposure	Outcomes to be measured
healthy preterm infants at term corrected age differ from healthy term born infants?				standardized neurological examination
57. Does early intervention in form of physical exercises during initial hospital stay in preterm infants affect later motor development?	Preterm infants	RCT	Early physical exercises during initial hospital stay *versus* no such exercises	Motor development using standardized scales at 9–12 months of age
58. What is the difference in growth and neuro-developmental outcome of preterm infants initiated on complementary feeding at different postnatal/corrected ages?	Preterm infants	Prospective or retrospective cohort study	None	Growth and neurodevelopment in relation to time of initiation of complementary feeding
59. What is the spectrum of various ophthalmo-logical abnormalities in high-risk infants (both with and without ROP) at 6–9 months of age?	All high-risk infants	Prospective cohort or cross sectional study	None	Comprehensive ophthalmo-logical evaluation of all high-risk infants by a trained ophthalmologist at 6–9 months of age
60. Which is the best hear-ing screening strategy	All high-risk infants failing initial hearing	Diagnostic test evaluation	OAE *versus* screening BERA *versus* OAE followed	Positive predictive value of different strategies, with

Contd...

Research questions	Subjects	Study designs	Interventions/Exposure	Outcomes to be measured
for high risk infants— OAE *versus* screening BERA *versus* OAE followed by screening BERA for those who fail initial OAE?	screening		of screening BERA for those who fail OAE	diagnostic BERA as gold standard
61. What is the sensitivity and specificity of screening tools like TDSC or DDST-II for detecting abnormal neurodevelopment in high risk infants till 6 months of age?	All high-risk infants till 6 months of age	Prospective cohort or cross sectional	None	Screening test and formal developmental evaluation using DASII at monthly intervals
62. What is the spectrum of auditory neuropathy spectrum abnormalities in otherwise healthy late preterm and term neonates with severe jaundice?	Otherwise healthy late preterm and term neonates with hyper-bilirubinemia requiring exchange transfusion as per American Academy of Pediatrics	Prospective cohort	None	Comprehensive auditory evaluations (tympanometry, oto-acoustic emission tests and auditory brainstem evoked responses) performed by an audiologist unaware of the severity of jaundice
63. What is the neuro-developmental out-come of term small for gestational age infants?	Term small for gesta-tional age infants	Prospective cohort	None	Standardized neurodevelop-ment assessment at 18–24 months of age

Contd...

Research questions	Subjects	Study designs	Interventions/Exposure	Outcomes to be measured
RETINOPATHY OF PREMATURITY				
64. What is the visual outcome of neonates with ROP?	Neonates eligible for screening of ROP a) Spontaneous regression of ROP b) ROP needing laser ablation c) No ROP	Cohort study	Nil	Visual acuity, visual field, refractive errors and anatomical abnormalities in retina (foveal thickness, retinal folds, etc.), color vision
65. What are the factors determining spontaneous regression of ROP?	Neonates eligible for screening of ROP a) Spontaneous regression of ROP b) ROP needing laser ablation	Cohort study with enrolment at initiation of screening OR Case control study with regressed OR treated ROP	Nil	Risk ratios for possible factors like intrauterine growth status, antenatal steroid exposure, postnatal nutrition (macro/micro nutrient intake, weight gain), sepsis, respiratory support
66. What is the role of genetic factors in epidemiology of ROP?	Neonates eligible for screening of ROP a) Spontaneous regression of ROP b) ROP needing laser ablation c) No ROP	Cohort study with enrolment at initiation of screening OR Case control study with regressed OR treated ROP OR No ROP	Nil	Association between ROP outcome and putative genetic factors like VEGF polymorphism

Contd...

Research questions	Subjects	Study designs	Interventions/Exposure	Outcomes to be measured
67. Which measures can reduce incidence of ROP in a particular unit?	All neonates eligible for screening of ROP	Before and after intervention study	Quality improvement measures delivered individually or combined, e.g. education of health care providers, oxygen saturation monitoring, ROP screening protocols	Incidence of ROP and its subtypes
68. How to reduce pain experienced by neonates during screening for ROP?	All neonates eligible for screening of ROP	Randomized cortrolled trial	Possible interventions include topical anesthetic drops in combination with oral sucrose, swaddling or other pharmacological/non-pharmacological measures	Pain measured by validated pain scores, e.g. premature infant pain profile
69. What are the long-term outcomes in neonates who receive bevacizumab for treatment of ROP?	Neonates with ROP a) Laser ablation OR b) Bevacizumab	Randomized controlled trial OR national/regional registry	Laser ablation *versus* intravitreal bevacizumab Nil	Visual acuity, visual field, refractive errors and anatomical abnormalities in retina (foveal thickness, retinal folds, etc.), color vision
CPAP				
70. What is the comparative efficacy of different pressure sources used for delivery of CPAP—bubble CPAP, IFD, ventilator-derived CPAP—in (a) preterm	Neonates requiring CPAP therapy	RCT	Different pressure sources	**For objective (a):** • Need for mechanical ventilation in the first 7 days of life • Incidence of CLD • Duration of CPAP and hospital stay

Contd...

Research questions	Subjects	Study designs	Interventions/Exposure	Outcomes to be measured
neonates with RDS and (b) in post-extubation settings?				**For objective (b):** • Need for re-intubation in the next 3 to 7 days after extubation • Incidence of CLD • Duration of CPAP and hospital stay
71. What is the comparative efficacy of CPAP delivered by nose mask with that by short binasal prongs in preterm neonates with RDS?	Neonates requiring CPAP therapy	RCT	Nasal mask *versus* short prong	• Need for mechanical ventilation in the first 7 days of life • Incidence of CLD • Duration of CPAP and hospital stay • Incidence of nasal trauma
72. What is the comparative efficacy of two different initial CPAP pressure levels—5 cm H_2O *versus* 7–8 cm H_2O—in preterm neonates with RDS?	Neonates requiring CPAP therapy	RCT	5 cm H_2O *versus* 7–8 cm H_2O	Same as above plus incidence of air-leaks
73. What is the comparative efficacy of different strategies used for withdrawal of CPAP namely, stopping CPAP completely, decreasing	Neonates requiring CPAP therapy	RCT	Accordingly	• Time to successfully coming off NCPAP altogether • Need for endotracheal intubation and mechanical ventilation in the next 7 days after enrolment

Contd...

Research questions	Subjects	Study designs	Interventions/Exposure	Outcomes to be measured
the CPAP to predefined level of airway pressure and then stopping it completely, removing NCPAP for a pre-determined number of hours each day until NCPAP is able to be stopped completely (graded time off)[19] in stable preterm neonates?				• Total duration of CPAP support (from birth) • Incidence of CLD

KMC

Research questions	Subjects	Study designs	Interventions/Exposure	Outcomes to be measured
74. What is the feasibility and safety of KMC in small or sick infants?	Small (<1200 g) or infants with sickness (with respiratory distress, infection, asphyxia, oxygen requirement, intravenous fluids)	RCT	I: KMC C: No KMC (conventional care)	• Safety • Feasibility • Mortality • Hospital stay • Confidence of health providers and mothers
75. What is the safety and efficacy of KMC in home setting/community setting?	Low birth weight neonates after discharge	Cluster RCT	I: KMC C: No KMC (conventional care)	• Safety • Confidence of mothers • Mortality • Feedback
76. What are the barriers (from health facility as well as family and	Mothers/KMC caregivers (other family members)	Qualitative research (feedback	Nil	• Questionnaire (incorporating barriers in KMC care-giving)

Contd...

Research questions	Subjects	Study designs	Interventions/Exposure	Outcomes to be measured
community perspectives) in successful implementation of KMC?		questionnaire/ focus group discussions)		
77. What are the requirements for successful KMC (such as that of privacy, special attire, chair/cot)?	Mothers/KMC caregivers (other family members)	Qualitative research (feedback questionnaire)	Nil	Feedback questionnaire
TPN				
78. Can parenteral nutrition be delivered through peripheral venous catheter?	Preterm neonates needing parenteral nutrition	Randomized controlled trial	Peripherally inserted central catheter *versus* peripheral venous catheter	• Energy, amino acids, lipids delivered • Weight gain • Rate of hospital-acquired bloodstream infections
79. For what duration can umbilical venous catheter be used without increasing risk of infection?	Preterm neonates needing parenteral nutrition	Randomized controlled trial	Different durations, e.g. 7 *versus* 14 days	Rate of hospital-acquired bloodstream infections
80. What are the complications of parenteral nutrition in SGA neonates?	Preterm SGA and AGA neonates	Prospective cohort study	Exposure: SGA Control: AGA	**Rate of complications:** • Neonatal cholestasis • Age at full feeds • Weight gain • Rate of hospital-acquired blood stream infections

Contd...

Research questions	Subjects	Study designs	Interventions/Exposure	Outcomes to be measured
81. What are the benefits and harms of providing aggressive parenteral nutrition?	Preterm neonates needing parenteral nutrition	Randomized controlled trial	Starting full dose parenteral nutrition immediately after birth *versus* gradually building up the dose administered	• Energy, amino acids, lipids delivered • Weight gain • Rate of hospital-acquired bloodstream infections • Metabolic profile: Serum ammonia, blood pH, triglycerides
82. Should dose of lipids be restricted in neonates under phototherapy?	Preterm neonates needing parenteral nutrition and with significant hyper-bilirubinemia	Randomized controlled trial	Lipid restricted to 1–1.5 g/kg/d *versus* full dose 3 g/kg/d	• Free bilirubin • Concentration of free radicals/oxidative metabolites • Brainstem auditory evoked response
83. What is the quality of delivery of parenteral nutrition?	Neonates needing parenteral nutrition as per unit protocol	Prospective cohort study	None	• Proportion of neonates who get parenteral nutrition as per evidence-based unit protocol • Rate of catheter related complications • Rate of parenteral nutrition related complications • Energy and metabolite actually administered
BLOOD COMPONENTS				
84. What is the effect of implementation of strict transfusion guide-	All neonates admitted in NICU receiving transfusion	Before and after study	Implementation of strict transfusion criteria	Number of transfusions, donor exposure, transfusion associated complications

Contd...

Research question	Subjects	Study design	Interventions/Exposure	Outcomes to be measured
lines in the transfusion practices in NICU?				
85. What is the effect of lower cut-off for PRBC transfusion on the growth parameters of VLBW infants at discharge?	All VLBW neonates admitted in NICU receiving transfusion	Randomized trial	PRBC transfusions at two different cut-off levels	Growth parameters such as weight, length and OFC at birth and discharge; time taken to discharge
PAIN				
86. What are the effects of developmental supportive care like NIDCAP and pain management protocols on long-term neurodevelopmental outcomes in preterm and term neonates?		RCT/Prospective cohort	I: Supportive development program and pain management program, e.g. NIDCAP C: Standard care	Psychomotor and mental developmental index as measured by Bayley scale of infant development or other suitable objective scales like DASII-2 at 18–24 months. Objective neurological assessment at 18–24 months.
87. What is the efficacy and safety of dextrose 25% *versus* sucrose 24% in procedural analgesia in NICU?		RCT	Dextrose 25% *versus* sucrose 24%. For procedures like venipuncture, ROP examination, IV cannulation, arterial puncture, lumbar puncture	Pain assessment by standardized pain scales like PIPP; Comparison changes of physiological parameters like heart rate, saturations, respiratory rate, etc. during procedure
88. What is the comparative efficacy of pain assessment tools in NICU?		Cohort study	Compare pain scales with PIPP scale as standard	Validity of different scales as compared to PIPP. Time required for assessment and accuracy by staff nurses and resident doctors.

A2—COMMONLY USED DRUGS

1. Adrenaline

- ❏ Dose: Resuscitation and bradycardia: 0.1 to 0.3 mL/kg of 1:10000 solution IV. IV infusion: 0.1 to 1 mcg/kg/min
- ❏ Adverse effects: Hyperglycemia, tachycardia, elevated lactate, cardiac arrhythmia and renal vascular ischemia
- ❏ Solution compatibility: 5% dextrose, 10% dextrose and normal saline
- ❏ Incompatibility: Ampicillin, aminophylline and sodium bicarbonate.

2. Amikacin

- ❏ Dose: IV

  PMA: 29 weeks lesser:
  - 0–7 days: 18 mg/kg/dose every 48 hrs
  - 8–28 days: 15 mg/kg/dose every 36 hrs
  - 29 days or older: 15 mg/kg/dose every 24 hrs

  PMA: 30–34 weeks
  - 18 mg/kg/dose every 36 hrs for 0–7 postnatal days
  - 15 mg/kg/dose every 24 hrs for ≥8 postnatal days

  PMA: ≥35 weeks
  - 15 mg/kg/dose every 24 hrs for all postnatal days
- ❏ Adverse effects: Neurotoxicity, ototoxicity and nephrotoxicity. Increased neuromuscular blockade when used with neuromuscular blocking agents. Discontinue therapy or adjust dose if there is ototoxicity or nephrotoxicity. Serum half life is prolonged in premature and asphyxiated newborns.
- ❏ Solution compatibility: 5% dextrose, 10% dextrose and normal saline
- ❏ Incompatibility: Ampicillin, amphotericin B, heparin (>1 unit/L) and phenytoin, fat emulsion, phenobarbital, sodabicarb, vancomycin
- ❏ Renal modification

GFR mL/min/1.73 m^2	Dose modification
>50	90%, single dose
10–50	70%, single dose
<10	30%, single dose

3. Aminophylline

- ❏ Dose:
  - Loading: 8 mg/kg over 30 min IV or can be given orally
  - Maintenance: 1.5 to 3 mg/kg/dose orally or IV slow push every 8–12 hours (start maintenance dose 8–12 hrs after the loading dose)

❏ Adverse effects: GI irritation, hyperglycemia, CNS irritability, sleeplessness, associated with renal calcification when concurrently used with furosemide and dexamethasone
❏ Toxicity: Sinus tachycardia, withhold next dose if HR > 180, failure to gain weight, jitteriness, hyperreflexia and seizures
❏ Solution compatibility: 5% dextrose, 10% dextrose and normal saline
❏ Incompatibility: Ciprofloxacin, dobutamine, adrenaline, insulin, cefepime, ceftriaxone and penicillin G.

4. Ampicillin

❏ Dose: Slow IV push or IM
  Group B streptococcal infection: 150–200 mg/kg/day for bacteremia; 300–400 mg/kg/day for meningitis
  PMA ≤ 29 weeks
  • 0–28 days: 25–50 mg/kg/dose every 12 hrs
  • 29 days or more: 25–50 mg/kg/dose every 8 hrs
  PMA: 30–36 weeks
  • 0–14 days: 25–50 mg/kg/dose every 12 hrs
  • 15 days or older: 25–50 mg/kg/dose every 8 hrs
  PMA: 37–44 weeks
  • 0–7 days: 25–50 mg/kg/dose every 12 hrs
  • 8 days or more: 25–50 mg/kg/dose every 8 hrs
  PMA: ≥ 45 weeks
  • 25–50 mg/kg/dose every 6 hrs

❏ Adverse effects: CNS excitation or seizure activity, prolongation of bleeding time, hypersensitivity reactions (maculopapular rash, fever is rare)
❏ Solution compatibility: 5% dextrose and normal saline
❏ Incompatibility: Amikacin, dopamine, adrenaline, gentamicin, midazolam, sodium carbonate and tobramycin.

5. Amphotericin B

❏ Dose: 1–1.5 mg/kg every 24 hours/IV infusion over 2–6 hours
❏ Adverse effects: Hypokalemia, transient increase in serum creatinine, decreased renal blood flow and GFR, injury to tubular epithelium, anemia, thrombocytopenia and fever
❏ Solution compatibility: 5% dextrose and 10% dextrose
❏ Incompatibility: Normal saline fat, amikacin, calcium gluconate, ciprofloxacin, dopamine, fluconazole, gentamicin, meropenem, penicillin G, piperacillin-tazobactam and tobramycin
❏ Renal modification: Dose modification for renal dysfunction is only necessary if serum creatinine increases greater than 0.4 mg/dL from

baseline during therapy, hold for 2–5 days. Alternate day dosing is recommended over decreasing daily dose in patients experiencing renal toxicity.

GFR mL/min/1.73 m^2	Dose modification
>50	q 24 hrs
10–50	q 24 hrs
<10	q 24–36 hrs

6. Caffeine Citrate

- ❏ Dose: 20–25 mg/kg of caffeine citrate IV (over 30 min) or oral
- ❏ Maintenance: 5–10 mg/kg of caffeine (slow IV or oral), to be started 24 hrs after loading dose
- ❏ Adverse effects: Restlessness, vomiting and functional cardiac symptoms. Suggested association with NEC (causality is not proven). Withholding dose if heart rate greater than 180/min
- ❏ Solution compatibility: 5% dextrose
- ❏ Solution incompatibility: Furosemide and ibuprofen.

7. Cefoperazone and Sulbactam

- ❏ Dose: 30–40 mg/kg/dose of cefoperazone (not combined cefoperazone and sulbactam). Infuse over 30 min to 1 hr every 8 hours
- ❏ Adverse effects: Used with caution in hepatic failure. No CSF penetration
- ❏ Solution compatibility: Normal saline, 5% dextrose and 10% dextrose
- ❏ Renal modification:

Cefoperazone

Dose for impaired renal function GFR mL/min/1.73 m^2	Dose modification
>50	100%
10–50	100%
<10	100%

Sulbactam

Dose for impaired renal function GFR mL/min/1.73 m^2	Dose modification
30–50	100%
10–29	50%
<10	25%

8. Cefotaxime

- ❑ Dose: IV infusion over 30 min.
  PMA: 29 weeks or lesser
  - 0–28 days: 50 mg/kg/dose every 12 hrs
  - 29 days or more: 50 mg/kg/dose every 8 hrs
  PMA: 30–36 weeks
  - 0–14 days: 50 mg/kg/dose every 12 hrs
  - 15 days and older: 50 mg/kg/dose
  PMA: 37–44 weeks
  - 0–7 days: 50 mg/kg/dose every 12 hrs
  - 8 days or older: 50 mg/kg/dose every 8 hrs
  PMA: 45 weeks and higher
  - 50 mg/kg/dose every 6 hrs
- ❑ Adverse effects: Rash, phlebitis, diarrhea, leukopenia, granulo-cytopenia and eosinophilia
- ❑ Solution compatibility: 5% dextrose, 10% dextrose and normal saline.
- ❑ Incompatibility: Sodium bicarbonate, vancomycin and azithromycin.
- ❑ Renal modification:

Dose for impaired renal function GFR mL/min/1.73 m^2	Dose modification and duration
>50	q 6 hrly
10–50	q 8–12 hrly
<10	q 24 hrly

9. Ceftazidime

- ❑ Dose: IV infusion over 30 min.
  PMA: 29 weeks or lesser
  - 0–28 days: 30 mg/kg/dose every 12 hrs
  - 29 days or older: 30 mg/kg/dose every 8 hrs
  PMA: 30–36 weeks
  - 0–14 days: 30 mg/kg/dose every 12 hrs
  - 15 days or older: 30 mg/kg/dose
  PMA: 37–44 weeks
  - 0–7 days: 30 mg/kg/dose every 12 hrs
  - 8 days or older: 30 mg/kg/dose every 8 hrs
  PMA: 45 weeks or greater
  - 30 mg/kg/dose every 8 hrs
- ❑ Adverse effects: Rash, diarrhea, elevated hepatic transaminase, eosinophilia and Coombs' test positive
- ❑ Solution compatibility: 5% dextrose, 10% dextrose and normal saline

❑ Incompatibility: Erythromycin, phenytoin, midazolam and vancomycin
❑ Renal modification:

GFR mL/min/1.73 m^2	Dose modification
>50	q 8–12 hrly
10–50	q 24–48 hrly
<10	q 48 hrly

10. Ceftriaxone

❑ Dose:
  • Sepsis: 50 mg/kg every 24 hrs; meningitis: 100 mg/kg loading dose followed by 80 mg/kg every 24 hrs
  • Gonoccocal infection prophylaxis: 25–50 mg/kg/dose as a single dose
  • Gonoccocal infection disseminated: 25–50 mg/kg/dose IV/IM single dose for 7 days, for meningitis 10–14 days
❑ Adverse effects: Eosinophilia, thrombocytosis, leukopenia and gall bladder precipitates. Increase in BUN, creatinine, AST and ALT. Not recommended for use in neonates with hyperbilirubinemia. Calcium containing solutions usage along with ceftriaxone is contraindicated
❑ Solution compatibility: 5% dextrose, 10% dextrose and normal saline
❑ Incompatibility: Aminophylline, calcium chloride, calcium gluconate and vancomycin
❑ Renal modification:

GFR mL/min/1.73 m^2	Dose modification and duration
>50	100%
10–50	100% q 24 hrly
<10	50% q 24 hrly

11. Ciprofloxacin

❑ Dose: 10 mg/kg/dose every 12 hrs over 30–60 min IV
❑ Adverse effects: GI upset, renal failure, rash and seizures. Tendon rupture can occur during or after therapy. Prolongs half life of aminophylline, theophylline and caffeine, hence to be used with caution with these drugs.
❑ Solution compatibility: 5% dextrose
❑ Incompatibility: Antacids and divalent salts

❑ Renal modification:

GFR mL/min/1.73 m²	Dose modification
>50	100%
10–50	50–75%
<10	50%

12. Calcium Gluconate

❑ Dose: Acute symptomatic hypocalcemia: 80–100 mg/kg/dose to be diluted and infused IV over 10–30 min (1 to 2 mL/kg/dose ≈ 10 to 20 mg/kg of elemental calcium. Maintenance dose: 200–800 mg/kg/day for 3–5 days. Oral and IV to be given in the same dose
❑ Adverse effects: Extravasation causes cutaneous necrosis or calcium deposition, bradycardia when given as bolus and gastrointestinal intolerance if given orally
❑ Solution compatibility: Normal saline, 5% dextrose and 10% dextrose
❑ Solution incompatibility: Amphotericin B, ceftriaxone, fluconazole, indomethacin, meropenem, metoclopramide, sodium bicarbonate, lipid emulsions, phosphate and magnesium salts.

13. Cloxacillin

❑ Dose: 25–30 mg/kg/dose IV or orally every 6–8 hrs
❑ Adverse effects: Skin rash, thrombophlebitis and drug fever
❑ Solution compatibility: 5% dextrose and normal saline
❑ Incompatibility: Aminoglycosides, tetracycline and erythromycin.

14. Dexamethasone

❑ Dose:
  • For extubation and airway edema: 0.25–0.5 mg/kg/dose may repeat 8 hrly, max of 4 doses IV
  • BPD:

Length of course	Day	Dose
Short course	1	0.1 mg/kg q 12 h
	2	0.075 mg/kg q 12 h
	3	0.05 mg/kg q 12 h
May repeat if necessary		
Long course	1 and 2	0.1 mg/kg q 12 h
If no response after 48–72 hrs of this dosing, stop		
If responding	3 and 4	0.075 mg/kg q 12h
	5, 6, 7	0.05 mg/kg q 12h
	8	Off
	9	0.05 mg/k q 12 h
	10	END

- Adverse effects: Gastrointestinal hemorrhage, perforation, hyperglycemia, glycosuria, hypertension, sodium and water retention, hypokalemia, increased risk of sepsis, renal stones, osteopenia, inhibition of growth and adrenal insufficiency.
- Solution compatibility: 5% dextrose, 10% dextrose and normal saline.
- Incompatibility: Midazolam and vancomycin.

15. Digoxin

- Dose: Loading dose given for treating arrhythmias and acute congestive heart failure IV slowly over 5–10 min, given as 3 divided doses 8 hourly
- Loading dose
  - PMA $\leq$29 weeks: IV 15 mcg/kg; oral–20 mcg/kg
  - PMA 30–36 weeks: IV 20 mcg/kg; oral– 25 mcg/kg
  - PMA 37–44 weeks: IV 30 mcg/kg; oral– 40 mcg/kg
  - PMA $\geq$45 weeks: IV 40 mcg/kg; oral dose 50 mcg/kg
- Maintenance dose
  - PMA $\leq$29 weeks: IV 4 mcg/kg; oral–5 mcg/kg every 24 hrs
  - PMA 30–36 weeks: IV 5 mcg/kg; oral–6 mcg/kg every 24 hrs
  - PMA 37–44 weeks: IV 4 mcg/kg; oral–5 mcg/kg every 12 hrs
  - PMA $\geq$45 weeks: IV 5 mcg/kg; oral–6 mcg/kg every 12 hrs
- Adverse effects: Cardiac effects, feeding intolerance, vomiting, diarrhea and lethargy
- Solution compatibility: 5% dextrose, 10% dextrose, normal saline and sterile water
- Incompatibility: Dobutamine and propanolol.

16. Dopamine

- Dose: 2–20 mcg/kg/min as continuous infusion
- Adverse effects: Tachycardia, arrhythmia, increase pulmonary artery pressure, extravasation of dopamine can cause sloughing and necrosis
- Solution compatibility: 5% dextrose, 10% dextrose, normal saline and Ringer lactate
- Incompatibility: Ampicillin, furosemide, indomethacin, penicillin G, insulin and sodium bicarbonate.

17. Dobutamine

- Dose: 2–25 mcg/kg/min as continuous infusion
- Adverse effects: Hypotension if hypovolemic, tachycardia at higher doses, arrhythmias, hypertension and cutaneous vasodilation,

increases myocardial oxygen consumption, tissue ischemia with infiltration
- Solution compatibility: 5% dextrose, 10% dextrose, normal saline and Ringer lactate
- Incompatibility: Aminophylline, cefepime, digoxin, ibuprofen, indomethacin, phenytoin, piperacillin–tazobactam and sodium bicarbonate.

18. Domperidone

- Dose: 0.2–0.4 mg/kg per dose, 8th hourly orally
- Adverse effects: Diarrhea, extrapyramidal symptoms, babies with hereditary fructose intolerance should not be given sorbitol based medication. Contraindicated in neonates with gastrointestinal hemorrhage, mechanical obstruction, hepatic impairment, perforation and neonates with long QT or congestive cardiac failure
- Anticholinergic reduces its side effects.

19. Furosemide

- Dose: 1 mg/kg/dose IV or can be given orally. Maximum of 2 mg/kg/dose IV or 6 mg/kg/dose orally
- Preterm infants—24 hourly. Term infants—12 hourly. Consider alternate day therapy for long-term use
- Adverse effects: Nephrolithiasis, osteopenia, cholelithiasis, hypercalciuria, hypokalemia, volume depletion, alkalosis, hyponatremia, ototoxicity
- Solution compatibility: 5% dextrose, 10% dextrose, normal saline and sterile water
- Incompatibility: Ciprofloxacin, dopamine, dobutamine, erythromycin, gentamicin, midazolam and netilmicin.

20. Fosphenytoin

- Dose:
  - Loading dose: 15–20 mg PE/kg IM or IV over at least 10 min
  - Maintenance dose: 4–8 mg PE/kg every 24 hrs
  - (PE: Phenytoin equivalents; 1.5 mg of fosphenytoin is metabolically converted to 1 mg of phenytoin)
- Adverse effects: Drowsiness, venous irritation, Stevens-Johnson syndrome, toxic epidermal necrolysis, increases serum bilirubin level by displacing it from protein binding site
- Solution compatibility: Normal saline, 5% dextrose and 10% dextrose
- Solution incompatibility: Midazolam.

21. Gentamicin

❑ Dosage and route of administration:

PMA: 29 weeks or lesser
- 0–7 days: 5 mg/kg/dose every 48 hrs
- 8–28 days: 4 mg/kg/dose/every 36 hrs
- 29 days or older: 4 mg/kg/dose every 24 hrs

PMA: 30–34 weeks
- 0–7 days: 4.5 mg/kg/dose every 36 hrs
- 8 days or older: 4 mg/kg/dose every 24 hrs

PMA: 35 weeks or older
- 4 mg/kg/dose every 24 hrs

❑ Adverse effects: Renal tubular dysfunction, vestibular toxicity, auditory toxicity and neuromuscular blockade
❑ Solution compatibility: 5% dextrose, 10% dextrose and normal saline
❑ Incompatibility: Ampicillin, furosemide, heparin and indomethacin
❑ Renal modification:

GFR mL/min/1.73 m^2	Dose modification
>50	100%
10–50	2 mg/kg q 12 hrly
<10	1 mg/kg q 24–48 hrly

22. Hydrocortisone

❑ Hypoglycemia: 5 mg/kg/day IV or PO in 2 divided doses 24 to 48 hrs
❑ Shock:

Day	Dose (mg/kg)	Interval (hrs)
Day 1	1	8 hrs × 3 doses
Day 2 follow in 12 hrs with	0.5	12 hrs × 2 doses
Day 3 follow in 12 hrs with	0.25	12 hrs × 2 doses
Day 4 follow in 24 hrs with	0.125	24 hrs × 1 dose

❑ Adverse effects: Hyperglycemia, hypertension, salt retention, water retention, GI perforation, increased risk of disseminated candida infections
❑ Solution compatibility: 5% dextrose, 10% dextrose and normal saline
❑ Incompatibility: Midazolam, phenobarbitone and phenytoin.

23. Ibuprofen

- ❑ Dose: 1st dose 10 mg/kg, 2nd dose and 3rd dose is 5 mg/kg 24 hourly
- ❑ Adverse effects: Infection, active bleeding, thrombocytopenia, coagulation defects, NEC, renal dysfunction, congenital heart disease with duct dependent systemic blood flow
- ❑ Solution compatibility: Normal saline and 5% dextrose
- ❑ Incompatibility: Caffeine citrate and dobutamine.

24. Indomethacin

- ❑ Dose: 3 doses per course/maximum 2 courses at 12–24 hourly intervals
  - Age <48 hrs: 0.2 mg/kg on day 1; 0.1 mg/kg on day 2 and day 3
  - Age 2–7 days: 0.2 mg/kg once a day for three days
  - Age 8 days or more: 0.2 mg/kg on day 1 and 0.25 mg/kg on day 2 and day 3.
- ❑ Adverse effects: Bleeding, thrombocytopenia, coagulation defects, NEC, impaired renal function and hypoglycemia
- ❑ Solution compatibility: 5% dextrose and normal saline
- ❑ Incompatibility: Calcium gluconate, dobutamine, dopamine and gentamicin.

25. Insulin

- ❑ Dose: 0.1–0.2 unit/kg every 6–12 hours.
- ❑ Continuous infusion: 0.01–0.1 unit/kg/hr
- ❑ Adverse effects: Hypoglycemia, insulin resistance, metabolic acidosis
- ❑ Solution compatibility: 5% dextrose, 10% dextrose and normal saline
- ❑ Incompatibility: Aminophylline, dopamine, phenobarbitone and phenytoin.

26. Lorazepam

- ❑ Dose: 0.05–0.1 mg/kg per dose/IV slow push
- ❑ Adverse effects: Respiratory depression, myoclonic jerks in preterm neonates
- ❑ Solution compatibility: Normal saline, 5% dextrose and sterile water
- ❑ Solution incompatibility: Fat emulsion, caffeine and imipenem.

27. Metronidazole

❑ Dose
  • Loading dose: 15 mg/kg/dose orally or IV infusion over 60 min
  • Maintenance dose: Orally or IV infusion over 60 min
  PMA: 29 weeks or lesser
  • 0–28 days: 7.5 mg/kg/dose every 48 hrs
  • 29 days or older: 7.5 mg/kg/dose every 24 hrs
  PMA: 30–36 weeks
  • 0–14 days: 7.5 mg/kg/dose every 24 hrs
  • 15 days or more: 7.5 mg/kg/dose every 12 hrs
  PMA: 37–44 weeks
  • 0–7 days: 7.5 mg/kg/dose every 24 hrs
  • 8 days or more: 7.5 mg/kg/dose every 12 hrs
  PMA ≥45 weeks
  • 7.5 mg/kg/dose every 8 hrs
❑ Adverse effects: Seizures and brownish discoloration of urine
❑ Solution compatibility: 5% dextrose and normal saline
❑ Incompatibility: Aztreonam and meropenem.

28. Midazolam

❑ Dose: 0.05 –0.15 mg/kg over 5 min every 2–4 hrs IV or IM
❑ Continuous infusion: 10–60 mcg/kg/hr
❑ Adverse effects: Respiratory depression, arrest, hypotension and seizures
❑ Solution compatibility: 5% dextrose, sterile water and normal saline
❑ Incompatibility: Ceftazidime, dexamethasone, furosemide, hydrocortisone and sodium bicarbonate.

29. Morphine

❑ Dose: 0.05–0.2 mg/kg per dose over 5 min, repeat every 4 hrs
❑ Continuous infusion: Loading dose 0.1–0.15 mg/kg over 1 hr followed by 0.01–0.02 mg/kg/hr
❑ Adverse effects: Respiratory depression, hypotension, bradycardia, hypertonia, illeus, delayed gastric emptying, seizures and tolerance
❑ Solution compatibility: 5% dextrose, 10% dextrose and normal saline
❑ Incompatibility: Phenytoin, azithromycin and cefepime.

30. Noradrenaline

❑ Dose: 50–100 mcg/kg/min of noradrenaline base as IV.
❑ Adverse effects: Severe vasoconstriction, plasma volume depletion, arrhythmias, bradycardia, peripheral ischemia, larger increase in blood pressure
❑ Solution compatibility: 5% dextrose, 10% dextrose, normal saline and half normal saline
❑ Incompatibility: Aminophylline, phenobarbitone, phenytoin and sodium bicarbonate.

31. Naloxone

❑ Dose: 0.1 mg/kg/IV push, dose needed to reverse narcotic induced depression may be as low as 0.01 mg/kg
❑ Adverse effects: Seizures secondary to acute opioid withdrawal
❑ Solution compatibility: Normal saline and 5% dextrose
❑ Incompatibility: Heparin and alkaline solution.

32. Netilmicin

❑ Dose: IV infusion over 30 min

PMA ≤ 29 weeks
• 0–7 days: 5 mg/kg/dose every 48 hrs
• 8–28 days: 4 mg/kg/dose every 36 hrs
• 29 days or older: 4 mg/kg/dose every 24 hrs

PMA: 30–34 weeks
• 0–7 days: 4.5 mg/kg/dose every 36 hrs
• 8 days or more: 4 mg/kg/dose every 24 hrs

PMA ≥ 35 weeks
• 4 mg/kg/dose every 24 hrs

❑ Adverse effects: Transient and reversible renal tubular dysfunction, ototoxicity and increased neuromuscular blockade when used with other neuromuscular blocking agents
❑ Solution compatibility: 5% dextrose, 10% dextrose and normal saline
❑ Incompatibility: Ampicillin, furosemide, heparin and penicillin G
❑ Renal modification:

GFR mL/min/1.73 m^2	Dose modification
>50	100%
10–50	q 12 hrly
<10	50% q 24 hrly

33. Phenobarbitone

❑ Dose:
  - Loading dose of 20 mg/kg/IV slowly over 10–15 min
  - Refractory seizures: Additional 5 to 10 mg/kg/dose, up to a total of 40 mg/kg
  - Maintenance dose: 3–4 mg/kg/day beginning 12–24 hours after the loading dose q 24 hrly

❑ Adverse effects: Sedation above serum concentration of 40 mcg/ml, respiratory depression at concentration above 60 mcg/ml and thrombophlebitis

❑ Solution compatibility: 5% dextrose, 10% dextrose and normal saline

❑ Incompatibility: Fat emulsion, hydrocortisone, insulin and vancomycin.

34. Phenytoin

❑ Dose:
  - Loading: 15–20 mg/kg IV/infusion over at least 30 min
  - Maintenance: 4–8 mg/kg every 24 hrs/IV slow push or orally

❑ Adverse effects: Avoid using in central lines because of risk of precipitation, extravasation causes inflammation and necrosis. Bradycardia, arrhythmias and hypotension during infusion. High concentrations are associated with seizures.

❑ Solution compatibility: Unstable in any IV solutions

❑ Incompatibility: 5% dextrose, 10% dextrose, amino acid solutions, amikacin, ceftazidime, dobutamine, heparin, insulin, morphine, hydrocortisone and sodium bicarbonate.

35. Piperacillin/Tazobactam

❑ Dose: 50–100 mg/kg/dose of piperacillin IV infusion over 30 minutes

  PMA ≤ 29 weeks PMA
  - 0–28 days: every 12 hrs
  - 29 days or more: every 8 hrs

  PMA: 30–36 weeks
  - 0–14 days: every 12 hrs
  - 15 days or older: every 8 hrs

  PMA: 37–44 weeks
  - 0–7 days: every 12 hrs
  - 8 days or more: every 8 hrs

  PMA ≥ 45 weeks
  - Every 8 hrs

❏ Adverse effects: Eosinophilia, hyperbilirubinemia, elevation in AST, ALT, BUN and serum creatinine
❏ Solution compatibility: 5% dextrose, 10% dextrose, Ringer lactate and normal saline
❏ Incompatibility: Amikacin, dobutamine, gentamicin, netilmicin, tobramycin, azithromycin, amphotericin B and vancomycin
❏ Renal modification of piperacillin:

GFR mL/min/1.73 m^2	Dose modification
>50	100%
10–50	70% q 6 hrly
<10	70% q 8 hrly

36. Prostaglandin E1

❏ Dose:
- Initial: 0.05–0.1 mcg/kg/min by continuous IV infusion, titrate to infants response
- Maintenance: May be as low as 0.01 mcg/kg/min
❏ Adverse effects: Apnea usually occurs during first hour of infusion, hypotension, fever, leukocytosis, cutaneous flushing and brady-cardia are the common symptoms. Uncommon and rare symptoms are seizures, hypoventilation, tachycardia, cardiac arrest, sepsis, diarrhea, DIC, urticaria, bronchospasm, hemorrhage, hypo-glycemia and hypocalcemia
❏ Solution compatibility: 5% dextrose and normal saline
❏ Incompatibility: Aminophylline, ampicillin, caffeine citrate, calcium chloride, cefotaxime, dopamine, dobutamine, furosemide, gentamicin, metronidazole, penicillin G, tobramycin and vancomycin.

37. Vancomycin

❏ Dose: IV infusion over 30 minutes
- Meningitis: 15 mg/kg/dose
- Bacteremia: 10 mg/kg/dose

PMA ≤29 weeks PMA
- 0–14 days: every 18 hrs
- 15 days or older: every 12 hrs

PMA: 30–36 weeks
- 0–14 days: every 12 hrs
- 15 days or older: every 8 hrs

PMA: 37–44 weeks
- 0–7 days: every 12 hrs
- 8 days or more: every 8 hrs

PMA $\geq$ 45 weeks
- Every 6 hrs

- Adverse effects: Nephrotoxicity, ototoxicity, rash and hypotension (Redman syndrome), neutropenia and phlebitis
- Solution compatibility: 5% dextrose, 10% dextrose and normal saline
- Incompatibility: Cefepime, cefotaxime, ceftriaxone, ceftazidime, dexamethasone, heparin, phenobarbitone, piperacillin/tazobactam and ticarcillin
- Renal modification:

GFR mL/min/1.73 m²	Dose modification
>50	100%
10–50	10 mg/kg q 24 hrly
<10	10 mg/kg q 48–72 hrly

38. Vitamin K

❑ Dose:
    <1.5 kg—0.5 mg IM
    >1.5 kg—1 mg IM
    Hemorrhagic disease: 1–10 mg/slow/IV push

❑ Adverse effects: Pain, swelling at IM site, anaphylactoid or hypersensitivity reaction, efficacy decreased in liver disease
❑ Solution compatibility: 5% dextrose, 10% dextrose and normal saline
❑ Incompatibility: Dobutamine and phenytoin.

A3—MEDICATION USE IN G6PD DEFICIENCY

I. Avoid

   i. Anti-malarial, e.g. primaquine, pamaquine

  ii. Sulfonamides, e.g. sulfacetamide, sulfanilamide, sulfame-thoxazole (e.g. septran, bactrim), sulfasalazine

 iii. Anti-bacterials, e.g. nitrofurantoin, nalidixic acid, dapsone, mafenide cream

 iv. Analgesics, e.g. phenacetin, acetanilide, phenazopyridine (pyridium)

  v. Miscellaneous, e.g. quinine, flutamide (eulexin), methylene blue, rasburicase

For more details: *www.g6pddeficiency.org*

A4—DRUGS IN PREGNANCY AND BREASTFEEDING

Drugs during pregnancy—risk to fetus (FDA)		Drugs during breastfeeding—risk to infant (AAP)	
Category	*Risk*	*Category*	*Risk*
A	None	L1	Safest; no risk
B	Possibly none (animal studies but no human studies)	L2	Safer; remote risk
C	Possibly yes. Use if benefits outweigh risks	L3	Moderately safe; Use if benefits outweigh risks
D	Yes. Use if benefits outweigh risks	L4	Possibly hazardous; use in life-threatening or serious conditions not having any safer option
X	Definitive risk. Avoid the drug	L5	Contraindicated
NR	Not reviewed till today		

- Details of drugs use during breastfeeding can be accessed at the following site: http://toxnet.nlm.nih.gov/cgi-bin/sis/htmlgen?LACT
- Details of drugs use during pregnancy can be accessed at the following sites: http://www.tga.gov.au/hp/medicines-pregnancy.htm; http://safefetus.com/index.php
- Drugs in Pregnancy and Lactation: A Reference Guide to Fetal and Neonatal Risk. By Gerald Briggs, Roger K. Freeman, Sumner J. Yaffe. Lippincott Williams & Wilkins, 2011.

Group	Name	Pregnancy	Lactation
Analgesics and NSAID	Acetaminophen	**B**	**L1**
	Ibuprofen	**B** (1, 2 tr) **D** (3 tr)	**L1**
	Indomethacin	**B** (1, 2 tr) **D** (3 tr)	**L3**
	Ketorolac	**B** (1, 2 tr) **D** (3 tr)	**L2**
	Mefenamic acid	—	N
	Naproxen	**B**	**L3** **L4** (chronic use)
	Piroxicam	**B**	**L2**

Contd...

Group	Name	Pregnancy	Lactation
Narcotic analgesics	Codeine	C	L2
	Fentanyl	B	L3
	Methadone	B	L2
	Morphine	B	L3
	Propoxyphene	C	L3
Anesthetics	Halothane	C	L2
	Lidocaine	C	L2
	Methohexital	B	L3
	Thiopental	C	L3
GI	Cisapride	C	L2
	Domperidone	—	L1
Antibiotics	Amoxicillin	B	L1
	Aztreonam	B	L2
	Cephalosporins	B	L1
	Ciprofloxacin	C	L3
	Clindamycin	B	L3
	Erythromycin	B	L1 L3 (early postnatal
	Gentamicin	C	L2
	Nitrofurantoin	B	L2
	Ofloxacin	C	L2
	Penicillin	B	L1
	Streptomycin	D	L3
	Sulbactam	—	NR
	Sulfisoxazole	C	L2
	Tetracycline	D	L2
	Ticarcillin	B	L1
	Trimethoprim/ Sulfamethoxazole	C	L3
Anti-coagulants	Bishydroxycoumarin (dicumarol)	—	NR
	Warfarin	D	L2
Anti-convulsants	Carbamazepine	C	L2
	Ethosuximide	C	L4
	Phenytoin	D	L2
	Valproic acid	D	L2
Anti-fungals	Fluconazole	C	L2
	Ketoconazole	C	L2

Contd...

Group	Name	Pregnancy	Lactation
Anti-histamines	Fexofenadine	C	L2
	Loratadine	B	L1
Anti-virals	Acyclovir	C	L2
	Interferon-alpha	C	L2
Asthma	Terbutaline	B	L2
	Theophylline	C	L3
Contraceptives	Estradiol	X	L3 (may interfere with milk production)
Hormones	Clogestone	—	NR
	Contraceptive pill with estrogen/progesterone	X	L3 (may interfere with milk production)
	Levonorgestrel	X	L2
	Medroxyprogesterone	D	L1 L4 (if used in first 3 days postpartum)
	Norethynodrel	X	L2
	Progesterone	—	L3
Cough	Codeine	C	L3
	Noscapine	—	NR
Decongestants	Pseudoephedrine	C	L3 (acute use) L4 (chronic use)
Anti-diabetic drugs	Insulin	B	L1
	Tolbutamide	D	L3
Diarrhea medications	Loperamide	B	L2
Diuretics	Acetazolamide	C	L2
	Chlorothiazide	D	L3
	Spironolactone	D	L2
Anti-arrhythmics, Anti-hypertensives	Disopyramide	C	L2
	Flecainide	C	L3
	Mexiletine	B	L2
	Procainamide	C	L3
	Quinidine	C	L2
	Captopril	D	L3 (if used after 30 days)

Contd...

Group	Name	Pregnancy	Lactation
	Diltiazem	C	L3
	Enalapril	C (1 tr) D (2, 3 tr)	L2
	Hydralazine	C	L2
	Labetalol	C	L2
	Methyldopa	C	L2
	Metoprolol	B	L3
	Minoxidil	C	L2 (topical) L3 (oral)
	Nifedipine	C	L2
	Propranolol	C	L2
	Verapamil	C	L2
	Digoxin	C	L2
Anti-malarials	Chloroquine	C	L3
	Hydroxychloroquine	C	L2
	Pyrimethamine	C	L4
	Quinine	D	L2
Medications for diagnostic studies	Diatrizoate	—	NR
	Fluorescein	C	L3
	Gadolinium	C	L2
	Iohexol	B	L2
	Iopanoic acid	D	L2
	Metrizamide	B	L2
	Metrizoate	B	L2
Migraine	Sumatriptan	C	L3
Sedatives	Zolpidem	B	L3
Steroids	Methylprednisolone Prednisolone Prednisone	C	L2
Thyroid medications	Carbimazole Methimazole	D	L3
Anti-tubercular agents	Rifampicin	C	L3
	Pyrazinamide	C	L3
	Ethambutol	A	L2
	Isoniazid	A	L3

A5—MANROE CHART

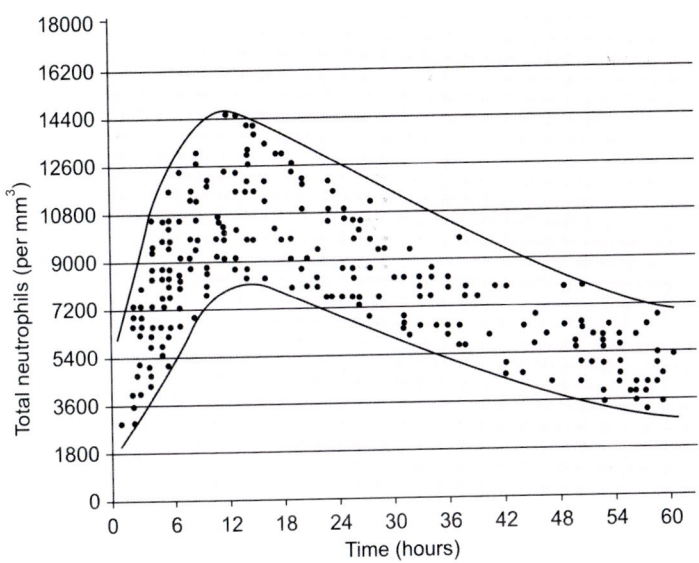

Fig. A5.1: Manroe's chart for absolute neutrophil count for term neonates (reproduced with permission)

(Manroe BL, Weinberg AG, Rosenfeld CR, Browne R. The neonatal blood count in health and disease. I. Reference values for neutrophilic cells. J Pediatr 1979;95:89–98)

A6—MOUZINHO CHART

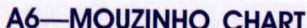

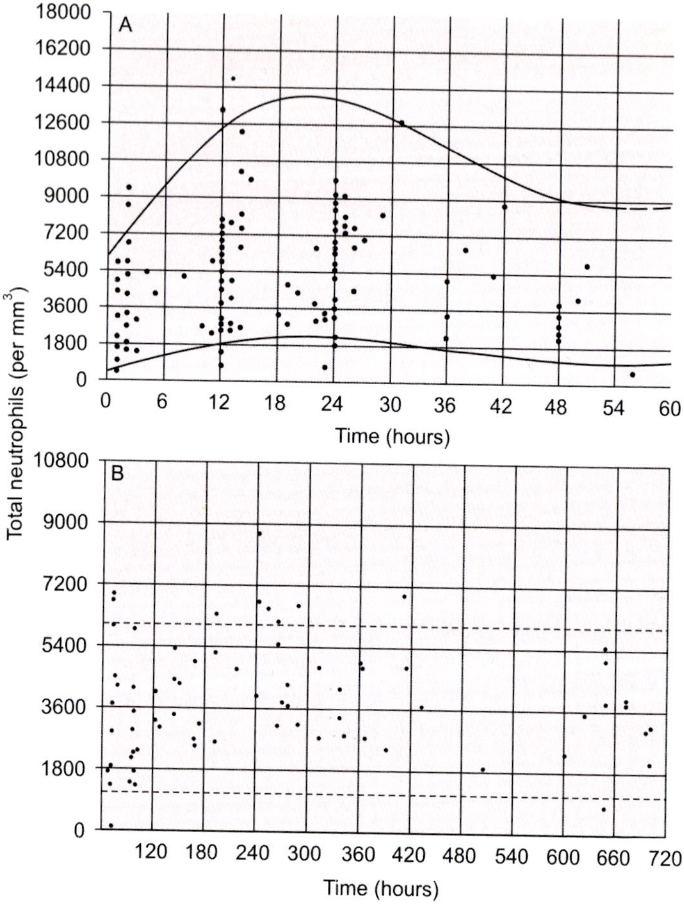

Fig. A6.1: Mouzinho's chart for absolute neutrophil count in very low birth weight neonates (reproduced with permission)

(Mouzinho A, Rosenfeld CR. Revised reference ranges for circulating neutrophils in very-low-birth-weight neonates. Pediatrics 1994;94: 76–82).

A7—UAC/UVC CHARTS

Length of umbilical arterial catheter to be inserted as measured by shoulder–umbilical distance

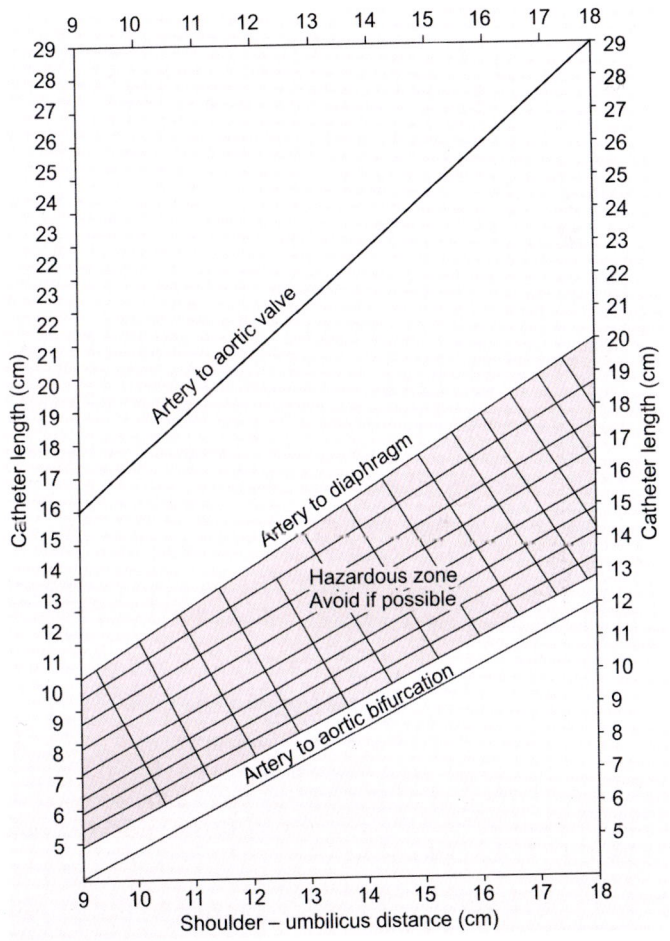

Fig. A7.1: Distance from shoulder to umbilicus measured from above the lateral end of the clavicle to the umbilicus, as compared with the length of **umbilical artery** catheter needed to reach the designated level (reproduced with permission)

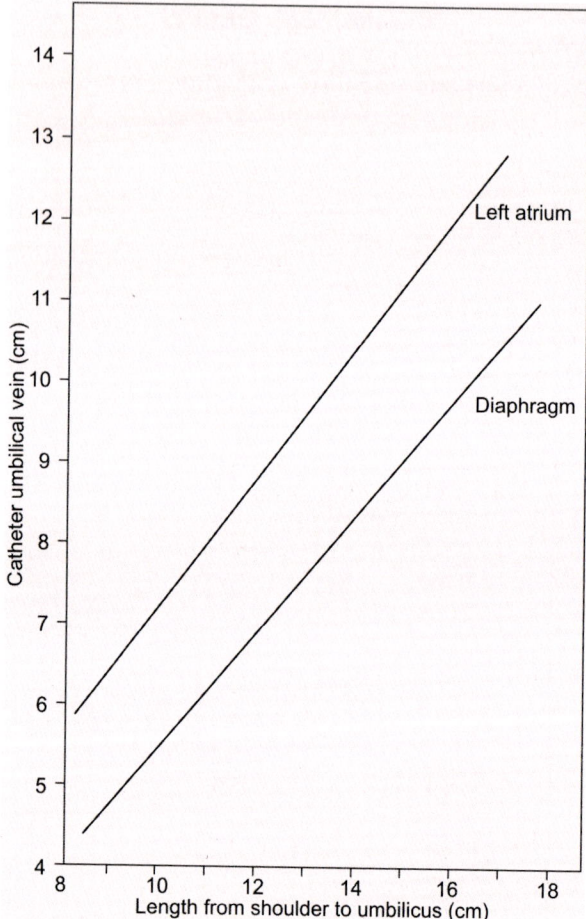

Fig. A7.2: Catheter length for **umbilical vein** catheterization. The catheter tip should be placed between the diaphragm and the left atrium. (Reproduced with permission)

(Ref: Dunn PM. Localization of the umbilical catheter by post-mortem measurement. Arch Dis Child 1966;41:69–75.)

A8—BLOOD PRESSURE CHARTS
(ZUBROW ET AL)

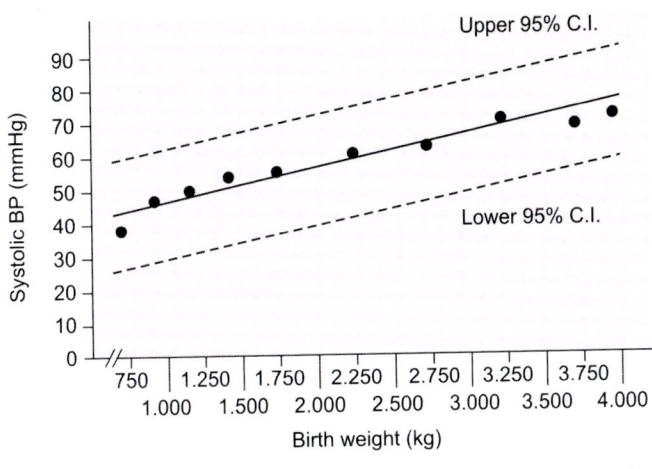

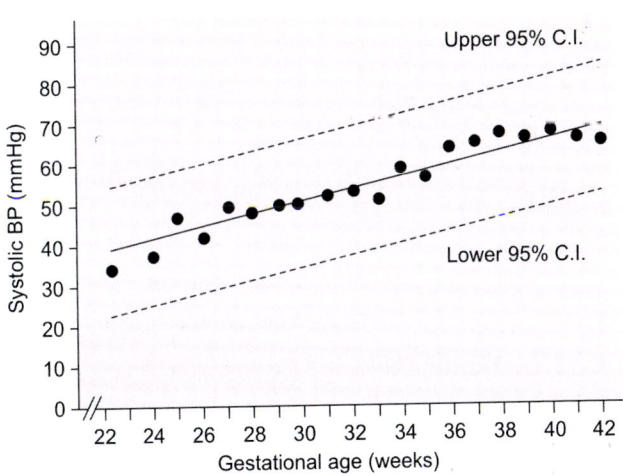

Fig. A8.1(a): Systolic blood pressures (reproduced with permission)

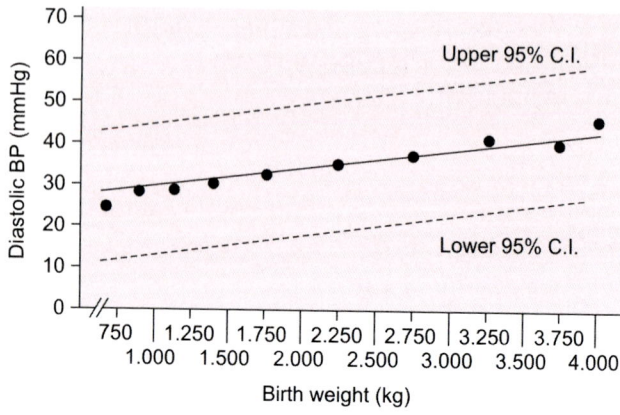

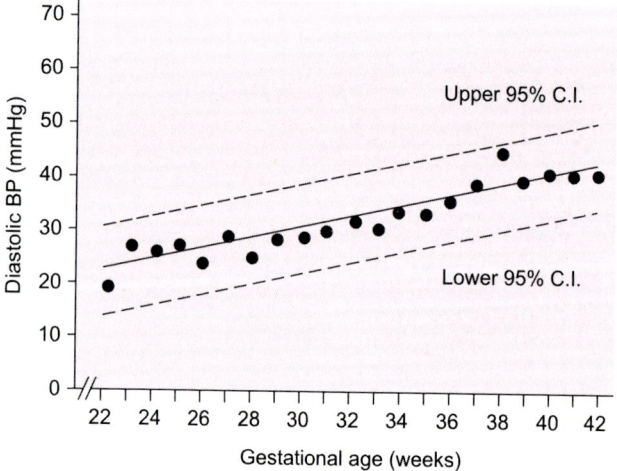

Fig. A8.1(b): Diastolic blood pressures

Fig. A8.1(b): Diastolic blood pressures **by birth weight/gestation on day 1 of life**, with 95% confidence limits (upper and lower dashed lines) (reproduced with permission)

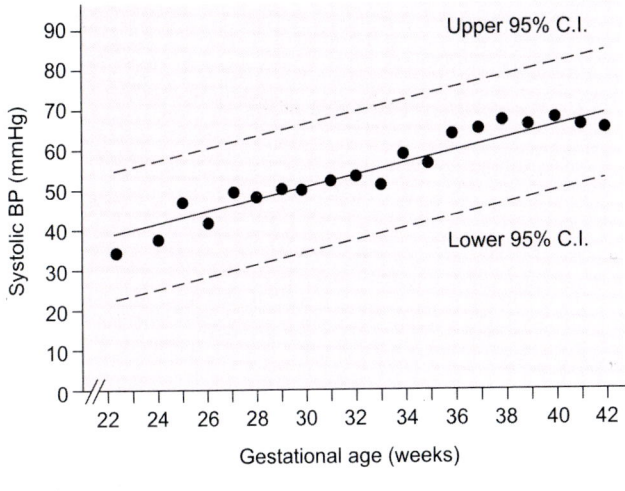

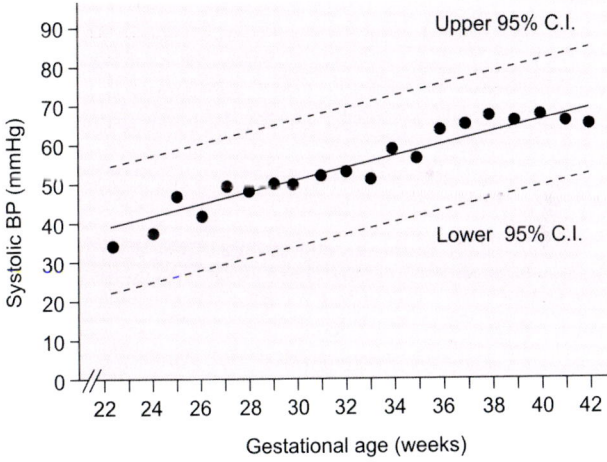

Fig. A8.2: Systolic and diastolic blood pressures by post-conceptional age in weeks, with 95% confidence limits (upper and lower dashed lines) (reproduced with permission)

(Ref: Zubrow AB, Hulman S, Kushner H, Falkner B. Determinants of blood pressure in infants admitted to neonatal intensive care units: a prospective multicenter study. J Perinatol 1995;15:470–79.)

A9—INTERNATIONAL DEATH CERTIFICATE

A death certificate (DC) has two parts–*Part I* deals with direct cause and *Part II* deals with contributory cause of death.

Cause of Death

I.		Approximate interval between onset and death
Disease or condition directly leading to death*	(a) _____ due to or as a consequence of	_____
Antecedent causes	(b) _____	_____
Morbid conditions giving rise to the above cause, stating the under-lying condition last	due to or as a consequence of (c) _____ due to or as a consequence of	_____
II. Other significant conditions contributing to the death, but not related to the disease or condition causing it _____		_____
*This does not mean the mode of dying, e.g. heart failure, respiratory failure. It means the disease, injury or complication that caused death.		

Fig. A9.1: International death certificate

Part I

a. Write the disease or condition that directly caused the death.
b. Write intermediate cause of death, if any.
c. Write the underlying cause of death on the last line.

   If the disease or condition leading directly to death I(a) and the underlying cause of death I(c) happen to be the same—fill in only line I(a).

Part II

Write in this part, some other condition or disease that contributed to the death, but which is not part of the sequence that led to death. If there is none, keep it blank.

Example: A term baby weighing 2200 g born through meconium stained liquor developed meconium aspiration syndrome (MAS) and PPHN and required ventilation for 60 hours. The baby also developed features of HIE stage 2.

On day 5 of life, the baby developed sepsis which progressed to septic shock and acute renal failure. The baby died of hyperkalemia on day 6 of life.

The chain of event: Septic shock → acute renal failure → hyperkalemia

It does not appear that either of MAS, PPHN or HIE contributed to death as the baby had reasonably recovered from all of that.

Therefore, hyperkalemia (a), acute renal failure (b) and septic shock (c) would be filled out in Part 1(a). Part 2 would be left blank. In addition, time interval between its onset and death would be entered for each condition.

A10—ICD-10 CODES

ICD-10 codes	Cause of death	Criteria
Infectious and Parasitic Diseases		
A09	Diarrhea	Frequent/liquid/watery loose or soft stools
		Possibly with fontanelle depressed OR eyes sunken OR urine volume low
A33/A34	Neonatal tetanus	Baby able to suck after birth AND stopped sucking after 3 days AND Baby's body became rigid with or without convulsions; Possibly with umbilical cord inflammation OR fever
Diseases of the Respiratory System		
J22	Acute lower respiratory tract infection	Cough OR fever AND rapid breathing OR difficult breathing with in-drawing of chest (often local term)
Certain Diseases Originating in the Perinatal Period		
P05	Low birth weight (full term pregnancy)	Smaller than average size baby. If weighed, birth weight below 2.5 kilograms AND no other obvious causes of death AND full term pregnancy
		Possibly with poor sucking after birth OR death at 3–7 days
P07	Prematurity (not full term)	Born between 28 and 36 but before 37 weeks of gestation AND no other obvious causes of death
P10	Birth trauma	Bruises at birth OR elongation/swelling/ blood clots over skull OR any limb broken at birth OR convulsions at first 72 hours of birth
		Possibly with instrument delivery or complicated delivery
P21	Asphyxia at birth	Delayed or poor breathing or no breathing at birth OR delayed or no cry at birth AND any sign of life at birth (i.e. exclude stillbirths) OR convulsions in 72 hours
		Possibly with prolonged or difficult labour OR death at 3–7 days OR cold to touch

Contd...

Contd...

ICD-10 codes	Cause of death	Criteria
P36	Bacterial sepsis of newborn	Fever AND no other obvious causes of death (like ARI, diarrhea); possibly with cord infection OR poor sucking OR limp and lethargic, coma
P80	Hypothermia	Central part of the body felt cold AND lethargic AND stopped feeding; possibly with exposure to cold
Other		
Q89	Congenital malformations	Abnormality of head (small, flat, swelling), spine, body, arms or legs reported at birth
		For specific diagnoses refer to codes Q65–88.
P96	Ill defined/unspecified	

[Ref: SRS collaborators: Registrar-General of India/Centre for Global Health Research Prospective Study of 6 Million Indians. Technical document No 5b (available at www.cghr.org), University of Toronto, 2003]

Index